Master the™
NCLEX-RN®

1st Edition

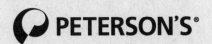

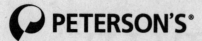

About Peterson's®

Peterson's has been your trusted educational publisher for over 50 years. It's a milestone we're quite proud of, as we continue to offer the most accurate, dependable, high-quality educational content in the field, providing you with everything you need to succeed. No matter where you are on your academic or professional path, you can rely on Peterson's for its books, online information, expert test-prep tools, the most up-to-date education exploration data, and the highest quality career success resources—everything you need to achieve your education goals. For our complete line of products, visit **www.petersons.com**.

For more information, contact Peterson's, 8740 Lucent Blvd., Suite 400, Highlands Ranch, CO 80129, or find us online at **www.petersons.com**.

NCLEX®, NCLEX-RN®, and NCSBN® are registered trademarks of the National Council of State Boards of Nursing, Inc. (NCSBN), which did not collaborate in the development of, and does not endorse, this product.

ISBN: 978-0-7689-4366-5

Printed in the United States of America

10 9 8 7 6 5 4 3 2   21 20 19

First Edition

Contents

Before You Begin ix
    Who Should Use This Book? ix
    How This Book Is Organized ix
    How to Use This Book x
    Special Study Features xi
    Proven Strategies to Raise Your Score xii
    Give Us Your Feedback xiii
    You're Well on Your Way to Success! xiii

PART I: THE REGISTERED NURSING PROFESSION AND THE NCLEX-RN®

1   About the RN Profession and the NCLEX-RN® 3
    Overview 3
    Registered Nurses and Their Career Outlook 3
    Nursing Education 4
    Licensure 4
    NCLEX-RN® Exam Basics 4
    Proven Test-Taking Strategies and Study Techniques 6
    NCLEX-RN® Test Plan 7
    Top 10 Strategies for Choosing the Correct Answer 19
    Summing It Up 21

PART II: DIAGNOSING STRENGTHS AND WEAKNESSES

2   Practice Test 1: Diagnostic Test 25
    Answer Sheet 25
    Answer Key and Explanations 43
    Diagnostic Test Assessment Grid 57

PART III: NCLEX-RN® REVIEW

3   Safe and Effective Care Environment 61
    Overview 61
    Client Needs for Management of Care 61
    Case Management 62
    Client Rights 63
    Concepts of Management 65
    Information Security and Confidentiality 66
    Legal Rights and Responsibilities 66
    Client Needs for Safety and Infection Control 67
    Handling Hazardous and Infectious Materials 70
    Reporting of Incident/Event/Irregular Occurrence/Variance 72

Safe Use of Equipment 72

Home Safety 74

Summing It Up 75

Practice Questions: Safe and Effective Care Environment 77

Answer Key and Explanations 79

4 Health Promotion and Maintenance.. 81

Overview...81

The Aging Process..81

Ante/Intra/Postpartum and Newborn Care 91

Developmental Stages and Transitions 97

Health Promotion/Disease Prevention...99

Health Screening 100

High-Risk Behaviors 101

Lifestyle Choices..102

Self-Care 103

Techniques of Physical Assessment 103

Summing It Up 106

Practice Questions: Health Promotion and Maintenance 108

Answer Key and Explanations 110

5 Psychosocial Integrity 113

Overview...113

Abuse and Neglect 114

Behavioral Interventions 119

Coping Mechanisms 122

Crisis Intervention 124

Cultural Awareness/Cultural Influences on Health...126

End-of-Life Care 127

Family Dynamics 128

Grief and Loss 129

Mental Health Concepts 130

Religious and Spiritual Influences on Health 138

Sensory/Perceptual Alterations..139

Stress Management 142

Substance Use and Other Disorders and Dependencies....................................143

Support Systems...148

Therapeutic Communication...148

Therapeutic Environment...149

Summing It Up 150

Practice Questions: Psychosocial Integrity..152

Answer Key and Explanations 154

6 Physiological Integrity 157

Overview...157

Client Needs for Basic Care and Comfort...158

Assistive Devices..158

Elimination 162

Mobility/Immobility..165

Nonpharmacological Comfort Interventions..169

Nutrition and Oral Hydration 172

Personal Hygiene, Rest, and Sleep 179

Client Needs for Pharmacological and Parenteral Therapies....................181

Contraindications, Interactions, Side Effects, and Adverse Effects 182

Dosage Calculation..189

Medication Administration 194

Total Parenteral Nutrition (TPN) 201

Pharmacological Pain Management 203

Client Needs for Reduction of Risk Potential 204

Monitoring Changes in Client Condition 205

Diagnostic Tests and Laboratory Values..208

Potential for Alterations in Body Systems 216

Potential Complications from Diagnostic Tests, Treatments, and Procedures 218

Potential Complications from Surgical Procedures and Health Alterations 227

System-Specific Assessments and Therapeutic Procedures........................229

Client Needs for Physiological Adaptation..235

Alterations in Body Systems 236

Fluid and Electrolyte Imbalances 258

Hemodynamics 273

Illness Management..280

Pathophysiology and Medical Emergencies 283

Summing It Up...286

Practice Questions: Physiological Integrity 289

Answer Key and Explanations...291

PART IV: PRACTICE TESTS

Practice Test 2 295

Answer Sheet 295

Answer Key and Explanations..312

Practice Test 3 325

Answer Sheet 325

Answer Key and Explanations..341

PART V: APPENDICES

A   **State Boards of Nursing** 357

B   **Nursing Organizations** 367

C   **Websites of Interest**.. 369

Before You Begin

Peterson's *Master the™ NCLEX-RN®* is written for candidates hoping to pass the NCLEX-RN examination, given by National Council of State Boards of Nursing, Inc. (NCSBN®). This book gives you the most thorough review and test-like practice available, covering all the categories and subcategories tested on the exam.

WHO SHOULD USE THIS BOOK?

Peterson's *Master the™ NCLEX-RN®* is perfect for nurses who have six months or less of nursing experience and are interested in preparing to become a registered nurse. Use this book if you can answer "yes" to the following statements:

- You want to prepare on your own time and at your own pace, but you don't have time for a preparation program that takes weeks to complete.

- You want a guide that covers all the key points you need to know but doesn't waste time on topics you don't absolutely have to know for the exam.

- You want to avoid taking risks with this all-important exam by relying on "beat the system" guides that are long on promises but short on substance.

- You want a collection of practice NCLEX-RN exams that look like the tests you will actually take to pass the exam.

HOW THIS BOOK IS ORGANIZED

Peterson's *Master the™ NCLEX-RN®* is divided into four parts to help you understand the role of the registered nurse, the structure of the NCLEX-RN, and what you need to know to pass the NCLEX-RN examination and obtain licensure. Full-length practice tests are included to help test your knowledge and provide a basis for creating a study plan.

Part I (Chapter 1) gives you a quick overview of the important facts you need to know about the registered nurse profession, the current NCLEX-RN Test Plan, and the computer-adaptive testing environment.

Part II (Chapter 2) provides the first full-length practice test, a diagnostic test designed to help you identify those areas where you need to spend more time in your review sessions.

Part III (Chapters 3–6) reviews the following Client Needs categories and subcategories found on the current NCLEX-RN Test Plan:

1. Safe and Effective Care Environment

   ○ Management of Care

   ○ Safety and Infection Control

2. Health Promotion and Maintenance

3. Psychosocial Integrity

4. Physiological Integrity

   ○ Basic Care and Comfort

   ○ Pharmacological and Parenteral Therapies

   ○ Reduction of Risk Potential

   ○ Physiological Adaptation

Part IV (Practice Tests 2 and 3) includes two full-length practice tests that simulate the actual exam, so you're fully prepared for test day.

Part V (Appendix A–C) provides supplemental information on state boards of nursing and professional organizations, as well as websites you can check for health, education, and job information.

HOW TO USE THIS BOOK

Review **Part I** to familiarize yourself with the registered nurse profession, the array of career opportunities, and the career outlook. Part I will also provide you with the opportunity to review the NCLEX-RN Test Plan. Proven test-taking strategies and study techniques are provided along with our top 10 strategies for choosing the correct answer.

Take the **Diagnostic Test** in **Part II**. This full-length test is designed to replicate the types of questions you will find on the actual NCLEX-RN. We've provided detailed answer explanations for all answer choices so that you can review why an answer was correct or not correct. Utilize the **Diagnostic Test Assessment Grid** at the end of the chapter to help pinpoint what you know—and what you don't know. Your results provide you with a starting point to tailor your study plan.

Review the chapters in **Part III**. Each review chapter covers one of the client needs categories and its sub-categories in depth, reviewing all the major concepts you will need to know to pass the NCLEX-RN. Before you dive into a chapter, skim the bulleted overview, which lists the topics covered in the chapter. The over-view will allow you to quickly target the areas in which you are most interested. At the end of every review chapter, you will find 10 practice questions along with detailed answer explanations. Use these questions to test your understanding and further assess where you will need to focus your study plan.

Take the practice tests in **Part IV** under test-like conditions. As you finish each practice test, check your answers against the answer keys and read the explanation for each question you missed. If you have the time, read all the answer explanations—they're great for more in-depth NCLEX-RN review. You can use your results from these practice tests to identify your strengths and weaknesses, and then spend the rest of your time leading up to your exam reviewing the areas where you need the most improvement.

Reference the supplemental material in **Part V** as needed for more information on professional organizations and helpful websites to enhance your learning experience and expand your knowledge base.

Print or Online? You Decide!

In addition to the two online tests that are included with the purchase of this book, Peterson's now gives you the option to take the diagnostic and practice tests in *Peterson's Master the™ NCLEX-RN®* either on paper or online. Choose how you want to take them: on paper for a more traditional study approach, or online to simulate the actual NCLEX-RN test-taking experience, with automated timing, instant feedback, and scoring results. Take all the tests on paper, all online, or in a combination of the two. The choice is yours.

To access your free online tests, visit the following URL:

www.petersons.com/testprep/nclex/

Add the *NCLEX-RN Online Companion* to your cart and enter the coupon code **NCLEX1** at checkout.

SPECIAL STUDY FEATURES

Master the™ NCLEX-RN® is designed to be as user-friendly as it is complete. To this end, it includes several features to make your preparation more efficient.

Overview

Each chapter begins with a bulleted overview listing the topics that are covered in the chapter. This will allow you to quickly target the areas in which you are most interested.

Summing It Up

Each review chapter ends with a point-by-point summary that captures the most important information in the chapter. The summaries are a convenient way to review the main points one last time before the exam.

Notes and Tips

As you make your way through this guide, be on the lookout for the NOTE and TIP boxes. This bonus information is designed to draw your attention to valuable concepts and test-taking advice, as well as to highlight vital details about the NCLEX-RN exam format.

PROVEN STRATEGIES TO RAISE YOUR SCORE

In taking the NCLEX-RN exam, some strategies are more useful than others. The following tips will help you pass the exam.

1. Create a study plan and stick to it. The right study plan will help you get the most out of this book in the time that you have.

2. Review key test elements daily for several weeks before the exam. Reread the Test Plan to be sure that you understand the categories and subcategories, and reread the information about alternate test formats.

3. Complete all the exercises in this book. Doing so will help you recognize your areas of strength and discover which areas need improvement.

4. If possible, visit the test center before the day of the exam. This will help you become familiar with the location and how long it takes to travel there. On the day of the exam, leave plenty of time to get to the test center in case the buses/subways/trains are running late, the weather is bad, or parking your car is a problem.

5. Avoid cramming the night before the exam. This will only make you feel more nervous. It is not likely to help you learn enough to make a difference on your test score.

6. Relax the night before the test. Try to take your mind off the exam for a while. Go to a movie or hang out with a friend—but not with someone who will be taking the test with you.

7. Be sure to bring one acceptable form of identification to the test center. You will not be able to take the exam without the proper form of identification, and you will have to reregister and pay another examination fee.

8. Listen to what the test administrator tells you and pay attention to the tutorial. Don't worry, though, because you don't need to be a computer whiz to take the test.

9. Read every word of every question on the exam. Pay attention to details. They provide clues and help prevent you from selecting the wrong answer choice.

10. Don't spend too much time on any one question. You have up to six hours to complete your exam—but you still can't afford to spend too much time on any one question. Try to maintain a steady pace. Due to the computer-adaptive nature of the exam, it is more important to get the questions right so the exam is accurately assessing your abilities.

GIVE US YOUR FEEDBACK

Peterson's publishes a full line of books—test prep, education exploration, financial aid, and career preparation. Peterson's publications can be found at high school guidance offices, college libraries and career centers, and your local bookstore and library. In addition, you can find Peterson's products online at **www.petersons.com**.

We welcome any comments or suggestions you may have about this publication. Please call our customer service department at 800-338-3282 Ext. 54229 or send an email message to **custsvc@petersons.com**. Your feedback will help us make educational dreams possible for you—and others like you.

YOU'RE WELL ON YOUR WAY TO SUCCESS!

Remember that knowledge is power. Using Peterson's *Master the*™ *NCLEX-RN*® will help you become familiar with the kind of content that appears in the actual NCLEX-RN exam. We look forward to helping you obtain your RN license. Good luck!

PART I
THE REGISTERED NURSING PROFESSION AND THE NCLEX-RN®

CHAPTER 1 About the RN Profession and the NCLEX-RN®

About the RN Profession and the NCLEX-RN®

OVERVIEW

- **Registered Nurses and Their Career Outlook**
- **Nursing Education**
- **Licensure**
- **NCLEX-RN® Exam Basics**
- **Proven Test-Taking Strategies and Study Techniques**
- **NCLEX-RN® Test Plan**
- **Top 10 Strategies for Choosing the Correct Answer**
- **Summing It Up**

Congratulations on your journey to becoming a registered nurse! By picking up this book, you're making a commitment to prep hard, pass your NCLEX-RN exam, and start along the path toward the exciting, challenging, and vital career of nursing. This chapter will lay out the profession as a whole and will explain all you need to know about the NCLEX-RN exam.

REGISTERED NURSES AND THEIR CAREER OUTLOOK

According to the National Council of State Boards of Nursing (NCSBN), there are currently more than 4.8 million active registered nurses in the United States. Although the number of employed registered nurses per population in each state varies widely, professional nurses are the largest health care profession in the United States. According to the American Nurses Association (ANA), there will be more registered nurse jobs available through 2022 than for any other profession. The U.S. Bureau of Labor Statistics (2018) projects that 1.1 million new RNs will be needed to avoid a further shortage. The projected need for additional nurses is due to the increased emphasis on preventative care, increasing chronic conditions, and the overall demand for health care services from the aging population that is living longer and engaging in more active lives.

According to the U.S. Bureau of Labor Statistics, between May 2016 and May 2017, the majority of nurses earned an income ranging from $48,690 to $104,100 annually, with a median salary of $70,000 per year. This figure represents a 3.7% increase compared to the previous year. Factors that influence nursing salaries include specified areas of practice, employment environment, length of practice, and educational level. Nursing salaries also vary from state to state.

NURSING EDUCATION

Professional nursing education did not begin until 1860 in England, where nursing education was founded on the principles established by Florence Nightingale. In 1873, the first school of nursing established in the United States was based on those same principles. In the 1890s, nurses began organizing significant professional associations, including the organizations now known as the National League for Nursing and the American Nurses Association. During that period, state nursing associations were beginning to form and were instrumental in establishing and passing state registration acts. These acts intended to establish the legal title of the professional registered nurse (RN) and to provide a licensing system for the practice of nursing. Currently, prelicensure education includes accredited nursing programs that offer an associate degree, bachelor's degree, or master's degree. Admission requirements to a nursing program vary based on the academic institutional requirements.

LICENSURE

The requirements for eligibility to take the NCLEX-RN examination are determined by the state board of nursing for the state in which the candidate intends to practice. The examination the candidate will take to obtain licensure is developed by the NCSBN. The NCLEX-RN is a national examination that does not contain state-specific information.

A licensed RN can only practice in the state for which licensure has been obtained. For an RN to obtain licensure in another state, he or she must apply for endorsement by the desired state board of nursing. It is not necessary to retake the NCLEX-RN examination; however, requirements for licensure vary from state to state, so it is important to check with the specific state board of nursing.

A **compact license** (or **multistate license**) is terminology that refers to the Nurse Licensure Compact (NLC). The nurse included in an NLC has a primary license plus the ability to practice in all NLC states. To be eligible for the NLC, the nurse must declare a compact state as his or her legal residence. Nurses who reside in noncompact states may apply for licensure by endorsement, which limits practice to a single-state license. There is no limit to how many single-state licenses a nurse may hold.

An enhanced Nurse Licensure Compact (eNLC) was implemented on January 19, 2018, with 31 member states as of July 2019. The intent of the eNLC is to align licensing standards across participating states, allowing nurses to have one multistate license with the ability to practice in person or via telehealth in his or her home state as well as other eNLC states. See Appendix A for contact information for the boards of nursing for each state belonging to the eNLC. It is important to note that the board of nursing for each state has rules and regulations that define the scope of practice within that state.

NCLEX-RN® EXAM BASICS

The NCLEX-RN examination was developed to ensure the minimum knowledge, skills, and abilities necessary to deliver safe, effective nursing care were present at an entry level. Entry level is defined as six months or less of nursing experience. The examination is based on a test plan that serves as a blueprint outlining the content on which the candidate will be tested. The basic test plan for the NCLEX-RN is updated every three years to ensure the competencies that are measured are current.

After reviewing the requirements and eligibility to take the NCLEX-RN examination as determined by the board of nursing for the state in which the candidate intends to practice, all candidates should access the NCSBN's website (**www.ncsbn.org**) for the most up-to-date information regarding the NCLEX-RN exam.

The NCSBN website includes instructions for the application and registration process, designated testing locations, and the current NCLEX-RN Test Plan. The site will also tell you what to do to prepare before the exam, what to do the day of the exam, and what occurs after the exam.

Computer Adaptive Testing

An interactive system called **computer adaptive testing (CAT)** is used to administer the NCLEX-RN examination. CAT uses computer technology and measurement theory to provide a valid and reliable measurement of nursing competence. Each NCLEX-RN examination is unique because the technology can interactively select questions that match the candidate's ability based on the previous questions that have been answered. The chosen questions are classified by test plan category and level of difficulty. This testing process continues until the candidate's knowledge and skills meet the NCLEX-RN test plan requirements and until a pass or fail decision is made.

The NCLEX-RN test questions can range from 75 to 265 items. This number includes 15 items classified as pretest items, which are not scored. There is a maximum time limit of 6 hours for the examination; there is no minimum time limit. The allotted maximum time includes time allocated for the tutorial and sample items, as well as all optional breaks during the exam.

Test questions are presented one at a time on the computer screen. The item shown must be answered in order to proceed to the next. Once an answer is submitted, you will no longer have the ability to return to the previous item.

The overall duration for the NCLEX-RN examination is determined by the amount of correct and incorrect responses to the items. The computer-adaptive nature of the examination selects items based on your responses. Each item requires a varied amount of time to complete. A good rule of thumb is to spend 1–2 minutes on each test item to maintain an adequate pace throughout the exam.

The length of your examination is not an indication of a pass or fail result, as it is possible to fail regardless of the length of the examination. The decision for passing or failing the NCLEX-RN examination is governed in the following three ways:

1. The examination ends when it can be determined with 95% confidence that your performance is either above or below the passing standard, regardless of the number of items answered or the amount of testing time that has elapsed.

2. If your ability levels are very close to the passing standard, the computer will continue to administer items until the maximum number is reached. At this point, the 95% confidence rule is disregarded, and the final ability is estimated. If the final ability is above the passing standard, then you will pass, and if it is below, you will fail the exam.

3. If you run out of time and the computer has not determined with 95% certainty whether you have passed or failed, alternative criteria are used. If at least the minimum number of required items were answered, the computer looks at the last 60 ability estimates. This does not mean that you had to answer the last 60 questions correctly. Each ability estimate is based on all previous answers. If the last 60 ability estimates were consistently above the passing standard, you would pass. If your ability estimate drops below the passing standard even once in the previous 60 items, you will fail the exam.

PROVEN TEST-TAKING STRATEGIES AND STUDY TECHNIQUES

As mentioned previously, it is important to familiarize yourself with the information on the NCSBN's website (**www.ncsbn.org**). Remember when you demanded a study guide in nursing school before an exam? Similarly, the NCSBN has provided you with a detailed test plan. The test plan is there to help guide you into the role of a safe, competent nurse.

Your key to NCLEX-RN success lies in the effort that you put into your NCLEX-RN preparation. Devise a study plan, stay organized, study consistently, and begin reviewing for the NCLEX-RN early. It is essential that you make time daily to prepare for the examination in an environment that is conducive to test taking. Make sure your study environment is quiet. Before every study session you should be rested, well nourished, and comfortable. If possible, get into the habit of reviewing practice questions on the computer. Sticking to a structured study plan will make your test preparation effective and keep you focused on reaching your goal: passing the NCLEX-RN.

> **NOTE**
>
> Remember that the practice tests found in this book are also available online at **www.petersons.com/testprep/nclex**. Since the NCLEX-RN examination is administered on a computer, it's helpful to practice as much as possible on a computer.

To begin your NCLEX-RN test preparation, take the Diagnostic Test (Chapter 2), which is designed to assess your knowledge strengths and weaknesses. After scoring your test and reading the answer explanations, use the Diagnostic Test Assessment Grid (page 57) to help you pinpoint your trouble areas. If your test score indicates a need to focus on a specific subject area, your next step is to review that subject matter first.

After you have thoroughly reviewed the material, be sure to reinforce your understanding of the concepts presented in the chapters by answering the practice question sets. How well you do on the practice questions will help you gauge how effectively you are studying and retaining the information presented. Once you are feeling confident about the material you have reviewed, retest your knowledge using Practice Test 2, review the material again where needed, and follow the same process with Practice Test 3. Remember, these tests are accessible online, so not only can you practice with test-like questions, but you can also get comfortable taking a test on the computer.

> **TIP**
>
> The NCLEX-RN examination is not designed to assess your ability to memorize, but to determine your knowledge of the subjects and content areas. Take the time to review the content, test your abilities, identify what you need to review, and then review to reinforce what you already know.

When you review NCLEX-RN test questions, read every explanation to every answer, even if you selected the correct response. Doing so is a great way to reinforce what you know, identify remaining trouble areas, and clarify concepts that might still be a bit unclear. Take the time to jot down what you need to review, and then spend time doing so. Then, when you have completed your review of the material, answer more practice test questions to re-evaluate your knowledge. This drill-and-review approach will help you to sound the concepts deep into your memory; once you have the concepts well in mind, their application on the NCLEX-RN should come easily.

As stated earlier in the discussion about CAT testing, each item must be answered, or you will not be able to proceed to the next question. If you are unsure of the correct answer, **DO NOT** guess. Every time you answer an item, the computer re-estimates your ability. If you are unsure, reread the scenario to evaluate precisely what the question is asking of you and then begin eliminating wrong answers.

After you review the scenario, ask yourself the following questions:

- What exactly am I being asked to do?

- Where am I in the nursing process?

- At what level of Maslow's hierarchy of needs is the client?

- What is developmentally appropriate for the client?

- Is there a safety component?

Before eliminating answers, ask yourself the following questions:

- Is this reasonable and appropriate for the situation?

- Is this the safest choice for the client?

- Is this the most important thing that I can do for the client at this time?

If you are answering a multiple-choice question, choose the most comprehensive answer that encompasses all of the other choices that apply to the situation. If you are answering a multiple-response question, the answers are either true or false in relation to the scenario.

Your responses should put the client first rather than items such as tasks, paperwork, charting, or other members of the health care team. It is important to remember that the nursing profession is about the client. There is nothing else you should be doing other than taking care of the client to whom you are assigned.

> **TIP**
>
> Do NOT guess if you are unsure of the answer to a question. Evaluate what the question is asking of you, and then eliminate wrong answers. This approach will result in a more accurate CAT assessment of your abilities on the actual NCLEX-RN examination.

In addition, your answers should be based only on the question as provided to you; make sure you are not reading anything into the given situation or scenario. The NCLEX-RN scenario has provided you with exactly the information that you need to respond appropriately.

NCLEX-RN® TEST PLAN

All task statements in the 2019 NCLEX-RN Test Plan require that you apply the fundamental principles of clinical decision making and critical thinking to nursing practice. You will integrate concepts from the social sciences (psychology and sociology), biological sciences (anatomy, physiology, biology, and microbiology), and physical sciences (chemistry and physics).

Integrated Nursing Processes

Processes that are fundamental to the practice of nursing have been identified by the NCSBN and are integrated throughout the Client Needs categories and subcategories. The processes identified and defined by the NCSBN include those listed below.

- *Nursing Process* is a scientific, clinical reasoning approach to client care that includes assessment, analysis, planning, implementation, and evaluation.

- *Caring* involves the interaction of the nurse and client in an atmosphere of mutual respect and trust. In this collaborative environment, the nurse provides encouragement, hope, support, and compassion to help achieve desired outcomes.

- *Communication and Documentation* includes the verbal and nonverbal interactions between the nurse and the client, the client's family, and the other members of the health care team. Events and activities associated with client care are recorded in written and/or electronic records that demonstrate adherence to the standards of practice and accountability in the provision of care.

- *Teaching/Learning* refers to facilitating the acquisition of knowledge, skills, and abilities to promote a change in behavior.

- *Culture and Spirituality* involves the interaction of the nurse and the client (individual, family, or group, including significant others and populations), which recognizes and considers the client-reported, self-identified, unique, and individual preferences to client care, the applicable standard of care, and legal considerations.

In addition to using the nursing process, you will be expected to apply concepts such as caring, communication, documentation, teaching and learning, and culture and spirituality throughout the four major categories of the test plan.

The content of the NCLEX-RN Test Plan is organized into four major client needs categories. Two of the four categories are divided into subcategories, as shown in the following list.

Client Needs Categories and Subcategories

1. Safe and Effective Care Environment
   - Management of Care
   - Safety and Infection Control
2. Health Promotion and Maintenance
3. Psychosocial Integrity
4. Physiological Integrity
   - Basic Care and Comfort
   - Pharmacological and Parenteral Therapies
   - Reduction of Risk Potential
   - Physiological Adaptation

Safe and Effective Care Environment

This first major Client Needs category consists of two subcategories, each of which assesses your ability to promote favorable client outcomes by providing and directing nursing care that enhances the care delivery setting in order to protect clients and health care personnel.

Management of Care

This subcategory is designed to assess your ability to provide and direct nursing care that enhances the care delivery setting to protect the client and health care personnel.

MANAGEMENT OF CARE
Related Activity Statements from the *2017 RN Practice Analysis: Linking the NCLEX-RN® Examination to Practice*

- Integrate advanced directives into the client plan of care.
- Assign and supervise care of the client provided by others (e.g., LPN/VN, assistive personnel, other RNs).
- Organize your workload to manage time effectively.
- Practice and advocate for cost-effective care.
- Initiate, evaluate, and update the client plan of care.
- Provide education to clients and staff about client rights and responsibilities.
- Advocate for client rights and needs.
- Collaborate with interprofessional team members when providing client care.
- Manage conflict among clients and health care staff.
- Maintain client confidentiality and privacy.
- Provide and receive handoff of care reports on assigned clients.
- Use approved abbreviations and standard terminology when documenting care.
- Perform procedures necessary to safely admit, transfer, and/or discharge a client.
- Prioritize the delivery of client care.
- Recognize ethical dilemmas and take appropriate action.
- Practice in a manner consistent with a code of ethics for nurses.
- Verify the client receives appropriate education and consents for care and procedures.
- Receive and transcribe health care provider orders.
- Utilize resources to enhance client care (e.g., evidenced-based research, information technology, policies and procedures).
- Recognize limitations of yourself and others and utilize resources.
- Report client conditions as required by law (e.g., abuse/neglect, communicable disease).
- Provide care within the legal scope of practice.
- Participate in performance improvement projects and quality improvement processes.
- Assess the need for referrals and obtain necessary orders.

Related content includes, but is not limited to, the following:

- Advance directives/self-determination/life planning

- Advocacy

- Assignment, delegation, and supervision

- Case management

- Client rights

- Collaboration with interdisciplinary team

- Concepts of management

- Confidentiality/information security

- Continuity of care

- Establishing priorities

- Ethical practice

- Informed consent
- Information technology
- Legal rights and responsibilities
- Performance improvement (quality improvement)
- Referrals

Safety and Infection Control

This Safe and Effective Care Environment subcategory assesses your ability to protect clients and health care personnel from health and environmental hazards.

SAFETY AND INFECTION CONTROL
Related Activity Statements from the *2017 RN Practice Analysis: Linking the NCLEX-RN® Examination to Practice*

- Assess the client for allergies and intervene as needed (e.g., food, latex, environmental allergies).
- Protect the client from injury (e.g., falls, electrical hazards).
- Ensure proper identification of the client when providing care.
- Verify the appropriateness and accuracy of a treatment order.
- Participate in emergency response plans (e.g., internal/external disaster, bomb threat, community planning).
- Use ergonomic principles when providing care (e.g., safe client handling, proper lifting).
- Follow procedures for handling biohazardous and hazardous materials.
- Educate the client on safety issues.
- Acknowledge and document practice errors and near misses (e.g., incident report for medication error).
- Report any unsafe practice of health care personnel and intervene as appropriate (e.g., substance abuse, improper care, staffing practices).
- Facilitate the appropriate and safe use of equipment.
- Follow the security plan procedures (e.g., newborn nursery security, violence, controlled access).
- Apply principles of infection control (e.g., hand hygiene, aseptic technique, isolation, sterile technique, universal/standard precautions).
- Educate the client and staff regarding infection control measures.
- Follow requirements for the use of restraints.

Related content includes, but is not limited to, the following:

- Accident/error/injury prevention
- Emergency response plan
- Ergonomic principles
- Handling hazardous and infectious materials
- Home safety
- Reporting of incident/event/irregular occurrence/variance
- Safe use of equipment
- Security plan

- Standard precautions/transmission-based precautions/surgical asepsis
- Use of restraints/safety devices

Health Promotion and Maintenance

This second major Client Needs category assesses your ability to provide and direct the nursing care of the client that incorporates knowledge of expected growth and development, prevention and early detection of health problems, and strategies to achieve optimal health.

HEALTH PROMOTION AND MAINTENANCE
Related Activity Statements from the *2017 RN Practice Analysis: Linking the NCLEX-RN® Examination to Practice*

- Provide care and education for the newborn, infant, and toddler client from birth through 2 years old.
- Provide care and education for the preschool, school age, and adolescent client ages 3 through 17 years.
- Provide care and education for the adult client ages 18 through 64 years.
- Provide care and education for the adult client ages 65 years and over.
- Provide prenatal care and education.
- Provide care and education to an antepartum client or a client in labor.
- Provide postpartum care and education.
- Assess and educate clients about health risks based on family, population, and community characteristics.
- Assess the client's readiness to learn, learning preferences, and barriers to learning.
- Plan and/or participate in community health education.
- Educate the client about health promotion and maintenance recommendations (e.g., physician visits, immunizations).
- Perform targeted screening assessments (e.g., vision, nutrition).
- Educate the client about prevention and treatment of high-risk health behaviors (e.g., smoking cessation, safe sexual practices, needle exchange).
- Assess the client's ability to manage care in the home environment and plan care accordingly.
- Perform comprehensive health assessments.

Related content includes, but is not limited to, the following:

- The aging process
- Ante/intra/postpartum and newborn care
- Developmental stages and transitions
- Health promotion/disease prevention
- Health screening
- High-risk behaviors
- Lifestyle choices
- Self-care
- Techniques of physical assessment

Psychosocial Integrity

The third major Client Needs category assesses your ability to provide and direct nursing care that promotes and supports the emotional, mental, and social well-being of the client who is experiencing stressful events, as well as clients with acute or chronic mental illness.

PSYCHOSOCIAL INTEGRITY

Related Activity Statements from the *2017 RN Practice Analysis: Linking the NCLEX-RN® Examination to Practice*

- Assess the client for abuse or neglect and intervene as appropriate.
- Incorporate behavioral management techniques when caring for a client.
- Assess the client's ability to cope with life changes and provide support.
- Assess the potential for violence and use safety precautions.
- Incorporate client cultural practices and beliefs when planning and providing care.
- Provide end-of-life care and education to clients.
- Assess family dynamics to determine a plan of care.
- Provide care for a client who is experiencing grief or loss.
- Provide care and education for acute and chronic psychosocial health issues (e.g., addictions/dependencies, depression, dementia, eating disorders).
- Assess psychosocial, spiritual, and/or occupational factors affecting care and plan interventions.
- Provide care for a client experiencing visual, auditory, and/or cognitive distortions.
- Recognize nonverbal cues to physical and/or psychological stressors.
- Assess the client for substance abuse, dependency, withdrawal, or toxicities and intervene as appropriate.
- Use therapeutic communication techniques.
- Promote a therapeutic environment.

Related content includes, but is not limited to, the following:

- Abuse/neglect
- Behavioral interventions
- Coping mechanisms
- Crisis intervention
- Cultural awareness/cultural influences on health
- End-of-life care
- Family dynamics
- Grief and loss
- Mental health concepts
- Religious and spiritual influences on health
- Sensory/perceptual alterations
- Stress management
- Substance use and other disorders and dependencies
- Support systems

- Therapeutic communication
- Therapeutic environment

Physiological Integrity

The fourth major Client Needs category consists of four subcategories that assess your ability to promote physical health and wellness by providing care and comfort, reducing client risk potential, and managing health alterations.

Basic Care and Comfort

This subcategory is intended to assess your ability to provide comfort and assistance in the performance of activities of daily living.

BASIC CARE AND COMFORT

Related Activity Statements from the *2017 RN Practice Analysis: Linking the NCLEX-RN® Examination to Practice*

- Assist the client to compensate for a physical or sensory impairment (e.g., assistive devices, positioning, compensatory techniques).
- Assess and manage clients with an alteration in elimination.
- Perform irrigations (e.g., of bladder, ear, eye).
- Perform skin assessment and/or implement measures to maintain skin integrity and prevent skin breakdown.
- Apply, maintain, or remove orthopedic devices.
- Implement measures to promote circulation (e.g., active or passive range of motion, positioning, and mobilization).
- Assess the client for pain and intervene as appropriate.
- Recognize complementary therapies and identify potential contraindications (e.g., aromatherapy, acupressure, supplements).
- Provide nonpharmacological comfort measures.
- Monitor the client's nutritional status.
- Provide nutrition to the client through tube feedings.
- Evaluate client intake and output, and intervene as needed.
- Assess and/or intervene in the client's performance of activities of daily living.
- Perform postmortem care.
- Assess the client's sleep/rest pattern and intervene as needed.

Related content includes, but is not limited to, the following:

- Assistive devices
- Elimination
- Mobility/immobility
- Nonpharmacological comfort interventions
- Nutrition and oral hydration
- Personal hygiene
- Rest and sleep

Pharmacological and Parenteral Therapies

This subcategory assesses your ability to provide care related to the administration of medications and parenteral therapies.

PHARMACOLOGICAL AND PARENTERAL THERAPIES

Related Activity Statements from the *2017 RN Practice Analysis: Linking the NCLEX-RN® Examination to Practice*

- Administer blood products and evaluate client response.
- Assess central venous access devices.
- Perform calculations needed for medication administration.
- Evaluate client response to medication.
- Educate the client about medications.
- Prepare and administer medications using the rights of medication administration.
- Review pertinent data prior to medication administration (e.g., contraindications, lab results, allergies, potential interactions).
- Participate in the medication reconciliation process.
- Titrate the dosage of medication based on assessment and ordered parameters.
- Handle and maintain medication in a safe and controlled environment.
- Evaluate the appropriateness and accuracy of the medication order for the client.
- Handle and/or administer high-risk medications.
- Monitor intravenous infusions and maintain the site.
- Administer medications for pain management.
- Handle and/or administer controlled substances within regulatory guidelines.
- Administer parenteral nutrition and evaluate the client's response.

Related content includes, but is not limited to, the following:

- Adverse effects/contraindications/side effects/interactions
- Blood and blood products
- Central venous access devices
- Dosage calculation
- Expected actions/outcomes
- Medication administration
- Parenteral/intravenous therapies
- Pharmacological pain management
- Total parenteral nutrition (TPN)

Reduction of Risk Potential

This subcategory assesses your ability to reduce the likelihood that clients will develop complications or health problems related to existing conditions, treatments, or procedures.

> **REDUCTION OF RISK POTENTIAL**
> Related Activity Statements from the *2017 RN Practice Analysis: Linking the NCLEX-RN® Examination to Practice*
>
> - Assess and respond to changes and/or trends in the client's vital signs.
> - Perform diagnostic testing (e.g., electrocardiogram, oxygen saturation, glucose monitoring).
> - Monitor the results of diagnostic testing and intervene as needed.
> - Obtain blood specimens (e.g., venipuncture, venous access device, central line).
> - Obtain specimens other than blood for diagnostic testing (e.g., wound, stool, urine).
> - Insert, maintain, or remove a nasal/oral gastrointestinal tube.
> - Insert, maintain, or remove a urinary catheter.
> - Insert, maintain, or remove a peripheral intravenous line.
> - Maintain a percutaneous feeding tube.
> - Apply and/or maintain devices used to promote venous return (e.g., antiembolic stockings, sequential compression devices).
> - Use precautions to prevent injury and/or complications associated with a procedure or diagnosis.
> - Evaluate the client's responses to procedures and treatments.
> - Recognize trends and changes in the client's condition and intervene as needed.
> - Perform focused assessments.
> - Educate the client about treatments and procedures.
> - Provide preoperative or postoperative education.
> - Provide preoperative care.
> - Manage the client during a procedure with moderate sedation.
> - Manage the client following a procedure with moderate sedation.

Related content includes, but is not limited to, the following:

- Changes/abnormalities in vital signs

- Diagnostic tests

- Laboratory values

- Potential for alterations in body systems

- Potential for complications of diagnostic tests/treatments/procedures

- Potential for complications from surgical procedures and health alterations

- System-specific assessments

- Therapeutic procedures

Physiological Adaptation

This subcategory assesses your ability to manage and provide care for clients with acute, chronic, or life-threatening physical health conditions.

PHYSIOLOGICAL ADAPTATION

Related Activity Statements from the *2017 RN Practice Analysis: Linking the NCLEX-RN® Examination to Practice*

- Assist with invasive procedures (e.g., central line, thoracentesis, bronchoscopy).
- Implement and monitor phototherapy.
- Maintain optimal temperature of the client.
- Monitor and care for clients on a ventilator.
- Monitor and maintain devices and equipment used for drainage (e.g., surgical wound drains, chest tube suction, negative pressure wound therapy).
- Perform and manage care of the client receiving peritoneal dialysis.
- Perform suctioning.
- Perform wound care and/or dressing change.
- Provide ostomy care and/or education (e.g., tracheal, enteral).
- Provide pulmonary hygiene (e.g., chest physiotherapy, incentive spirometry).
- Provide postoperative care.
- Manage the care of the client with a fluid and electrolyte imbalance.
- Monitor and maintain arterial lines.
- Manage the care of a client with a pacing device.
- Manage the care of a client on telemetry.
- Manage the care of a client receiving hemodialysis or continuous renal replacement therapy.
- Manage the care of a client with an alteration in hemodynamics, tissue perfusion, and/or hemostasis.
- Educate the client regarding an acute or chronic condition.
- Manage the care of a client with impaired ventilation/oxygenation.
- Evaluate the effectiveness of the treatment plan for a client with an acute or chronic diagnosis.
- Perform emergency care procedures.
- Identify pathophysiology related to an acute or chronic condition.
- Recognize the signs and symptoms of client complications and intervene.

Related content includes, but is not limited to, the following:

- Alterations in body systems
- Fluid and electrolyte imbalances
- Hemodynamics
- Illness management
- Medical emergencies
- Pathophysiology
- Unexpected response to therapies

Exam Layout

The percentage of test questions assigned to each Client Needs category and subcategory of the NCLEX-RN Test Plan is based on the results of the *Report of Findings from the 2017 RN Practice Analysis: Linking the NCLEX-RN® Examination to Practice* (NCSBN, 2018) and expert judgment provided by members of the NCLEX-RN Examination Committee. The following reflects the distribution of content from each category and subcategory.

NCLEX-RN TEST PLAN BREAKDOWN	
Client Needs Categories and Subcategories	Percentage of Items from Each Category/Subcategory
Safe and Effective Care Environment • Management of Care • Safety and Infection Control	 17–23% 9–15%
Health Promotion and Maintenance	6–12%
Psychosocial Integrity	6–12%
Physiological Integrity • Basic Care and Comfort • Pharmacological and Parenteral Therapies • Reduction of Risk Potential • Physiological Adaptation	 6–12% 12–18% 9–15% 11–17%

What to Expect on the Exam

The NCLEX-RN exam uses consistent language and universal terminology that is appropriate for an entry-level nurse. The exam is not focused on specific areas of nursing. Remember, the NCLEX-RN exam is a computer adaptive test and the items are selected based on your ability. The exam adheres to the test plan's content area percentages, so the items fall across all difficulty levels to cover all of the areas of the test plan. You may receive a question that seems to be very similar to a question received earlier in the examination. There are a variety of reasons for this, but do not assume this has occurred because a previous similar item was answered incorrectly. Just continue to select the answer for each question that you believe to be correct.

All of the items on the exam are written at an application or higher level of cognitive ability, which will require you to utilize problem solving skills to select the correct answer. According to the NCSBN, the items to which you will respond come in various formats. There is no established percentage of questions that will be in an alternative format. Again, the computer selects items based only on your ability.

The use of common terminology is important to provide consistency in the language for the test taker. Therefore, it is essential to become familiar with the terminology used throughout the NCLEX-RN examination. The following is a terminology list with the definitions that have been obtained from the 2019 NCLEX-RN Test Plan.

- **Client:** Individual, family, or group that includes significant others and populations
- **Prescription:** Orders, interventions, remedies, or treatments ordered or directed by an authorized primary health care provider

- **Primary Health Care Provider:** Member of the health care team (usually a medical physician or other specialty [e.g., surgeon or nephrologist], nurse practitioner, etc.) licensed and authorized to formulate prescriptions on behalf of the client

- **Unlicensed Assistive Personnel (UAP):** Any unlicensed personnel trained to function in a supportive role, regardless of title, to whom a nursing responsibility may be delegated.

Need-to-Know Pharmacology

The NCSBN does not have a specific list of medications available to study. However, for consistency, the NCLEX-RN exam primarily uses generic medication names only, and some items may refer to the classification of medications. Therefore, it is important to familiarize yourself with the generic names of the medications and have a basic understanding of the classifications for commonly used prescriptions.

On a positive note, the prefixes and suffixes of generic drugs tend to follow a pattern that will make it easier to review and remember them. An understanding of their purpose, expected action, route of administration, antidotes, adverse effects, contraindications, side effects, and interactions will keep your client safe.

Units of Measurements and Laboratory Values

The NCLEX-RN exam items currently include a combination of international systems of units (SI) and imperial measurement options used in the nursing profession, so the unit of measurement presented in the item will be familiar to the candidate. According to the 2019 NCLEX-RN Test Plan, you must be able to identify the following laboratory values:

- ABGs (pH, PO_2, PCO_2, SaO_2, HCO_3)
- BUN
- Cholesterol (total)
- Creatinine
- Glucose
- Glycosylated hemoglobin (HgbA1c)
- Hematocrit
- Hemoglobin
- INR
- Platelets
- Potassium
- PT
- PTT
- aPTT
- Sodium
- WBC

Item Formats

The NCLEX-RN examination includes a variety of item formats, including:

- Multiple-choice

- Multiple-response (select more than one correct answer from a given list)

- Fill-in-the-blank calculation

- Hot spots (click on the correct spot on a given image)

- Exhibits

- Ordered-response items (sort a given list of items into the correct order)

- Audio and graphic items

All item types may include multimedia, such as charts, tables, graphics, and audio. All answers to alternative items will be scored either as right or wrong—there is no partial credit given.

TOP 10 STRATEGIES FOR CHOOSING THE CORRECT ANSWER

1. Familiarize yourself with the information on the National Council of State Boards of Nursing website (**www.ncsbn.org**). Everything that you need to understand—from registering for the exam to the structure of the exam—is available to you online.

2. Do not forget that the NCLEX-RN is a test to measure the competencies needed to ensure public protection and to assess your ability to perform safely and effectively as a newly licensed entry-level RN. Therefore, you must be familiar with the use of prioritization techniques. Pay attention to the words used in the questions. Bolded words in the questions such as **best, most, essential, first, priority, immediately, highest**, and **initial** are a signal that this a priority question. All of the answers will be correct; however, only one will reflect the first thing you need to do. Using the nursing process, ABC's (airway, breathing, and circulation), and Maslow's hierarchy of needs will help you answer priority questions. When choosing an answer to a priority question, address the physiological needs of the client first. If the physiological needs are met, examine the item for underlying safety issues. Using this same systematic approach can help you eliminate incorrect answer choices in any question format.

3. When you are taking your NCLEX-RN examination, the only client you are caring for is the one on your screen and all of the prescriptions you need are available. The only time you will notify the health care provider is after you have implemented a step in the nursing process and have determined that there is absolutely nothing you can do as a nurse to help the client. Do not notify the health care provider for expected signs and symptoms of a disease. Again, you will only notify the health care provider if the client is experiencing signs and symptoms of potential complications associated with the disease and there is nothing you can do to help them. Remember, your job is to keep the client safe!

4. Use your clinical imagination! When you open a question, visualize yourself right there preparing to care for your assigned client. Avoid choosing answers based on what you did in clinical or at work. There are many correct ways of caring for a client, but you need to make sure you do it the NCLEX way. The NCLEX-RN is based on research-based, evidence-based practice.

5. Make sure you understand what the question is asking of you before you look at the answer choices. After answering the question, recheck the stem of the question to make sure you answered exactly what you were being asked to do. In other words, do not read into the question.

6. When you are being asked to perform an intervention for a client, always choose the safest and least invasive choice first. This will lead to a correct NCLEX-RN exam answer.

7. When encountering answers that are similar, go back and reread the question. Change the question into a true or false statement, look at each answer, and ask yourself if this is true or false.

8. Do not panic if you cannot answer a question. You made it through nursing school, so tell yourself you can do this! Even if something seems unfamiliar, you still have the necessary knowledge to answer the question. Go back to your fundamental understanding of essential subject matter and use the general principles to help you think critically. Remember the concepts from the bodies of knowledge the NCSBN assumes you can integrate into your care? They include social sciences (psychology and sociology), biological sciences (anatomy, physiology, biology, and microbiology), and physical sciences (chemistry and physics). Use these principles to answer the question.

9. Use the nursing process in each clinical scenario. Identify which step of the process the question requires you to use. The nursing process should always be followed in a systematic order to address the client's needs. The acronym ADPIE (Assessment, Diagnosis, Planning, Implementation, and Evaluation) will help you remember the systematic order of the nursing process. For example, if an intervention is implemented, you will then evaluate the outcome.

10. Pay attention to negative keywords because they offer a limited solution. Negative keywords are important to identify before choosing an answer. Words such as *all*, *everyone*, *every*, *ever*, *must*, *none*, *never*, *complete*, and *not only* are very limiting; they are not highly applicable in real practice. When these words are used, it implies there are no other options or exceptions.

SUMMING IT UP

- There are currently over 4.8 million active registered nurses. The U.S. Bureau of Labor Statistics projects that 1.1 million new RNs will be needed through 2022 to avoid a further shortage because of the increased emphasis on preventative care, increasing chronic conditions, and the overall demand for health care services from the aging population.

- Between May 2016 and May 2017, the majority of nurses earned an income ranging from $48,690 to $104,100 annually, with a median salary of $70,000 per year.

- The NCLEX-RN is a national examination that does not contain state-specific information; however, a licensed RN can only practice in the state where the licensure has been obtained. To obtain licensure in another state, the RN must apply for endorsement by the desired state's board of nursing. Requirements for licensure vary from state to state.

- A **compact license** or **multistate license** refers to the **Nurse Licensure Compact (NLC)**. The **enhanced Nurse Licensure Compact (eNLC)**, implemented January 19, 2018, allows nurses to have one multistate license with the ability to practice in person or via telehealth in his or her home state as well as other eNLC states.

- The NCLEX-RN examination measures the minimum knowledge, skills, and abilities to deliver safe, effective nursing care at an entry level, defined as six months of nursing experience or less. All NCLEX-RN candidates should access the NCSBN's website (**www.nccbn.org**) for the most up-to-date information regarding the exam.

- An interactive system called **computer adaptive testing (CAT)** will be used to administer the examination.

- All task statements in the *2019 NCLEX-RN Test Plan* require that you apply the fundamental principles of clinical decision making and critical thinking to nursing practice. You will integrate concepts from the following:
  - Social sciences (psychology and sociology)
  - Biological sciences (anatomy, physiology, biology, and microbiology)
  - Physical sciences (chemistry and physics).

- Processes that are fundamental to the practice of nursing will be integrated throughout the Client Needs categories and subcategories, including the nursing process, caring, communication and documentation, teaching and learning, and culture and spirituality.

- The content of the NCLEX-RN Test Plan is organized into the following four major Client Needs categories:
  1. Safe and Effective Care Environment (26–38% of exam items)
  2. Health Promotion and Maintenance (6–12% of exam items)
  3. Psychosocial Integrity (6–12% of exam items)
  4. Physiological Integrity (38–62% of exam items)

- The NCLEX-RN exam uses consistent language and universal terminology that is appropriate for an entry-level nurse and is not focused on specific areas of nursing. All of the NCLEX-RN items are written at an application or higher level of cognitive ability, which will require you to utilize problem solving skills to select the correct answer.

- The items you will respond to come in various formats, including the following:
  - Multiple-choice
  - Multiple-response (where you will select more than one correct answer from a given list)
  - Fill-in-the-blank calculation
  - Hot spots (where you will have to click on the correct spot of a given image)
  - Exhibits
  - Ordered-response items (where you will have to sort a given list of items into the correct order)
  - Audio and graphic items

PART II
DIAGNOSING STRENGTHS AND WEAKNESSES

CHAPTER 2   Practice Test 1: Diagnostic Test

ANSWER SHEET: PRACTICE TEST 1: DIAGNOSTIC TEST

1. ① ② ③ ④
2. ① ② ③ ④
3. ① ② ③ ④
4. ① ② ③ ④
5. ① ② ③ ④
6. ① ② ③ ④
7. ① ② ③ ④
8. ① ② ③ ④
9. ① ② ③ ④
10. ① ② ③ ④
11. ① ② ③ ④
12. ① ② ③ ④
13. ① ② ③ ④
14. ① ② ③ ④ ⑤ ⑥
15. ① ② ③ ④
16. ① ② ③ ④
17. ① ② ③ ④
18. ① ② ③ ④
19. ① ② ③ ④ ⑤ ⑥
20. ① ② ③ ④
21. ① ② ③ ④
22. ① ② ③ ④
23. ① ② ③ ④
24. ① ② ③ ④ ⑤ ⑥
25. ① ② ③ ④

26. ① ② ③ ④
27. ① ② ③ ④
28. ① ② ③ ④
29. ① ② ③ ④
30. ① ② ③ ④ ⑤ ⑥
31. ① ② ③ ④
32. ① ② ③ ④
33. ① ② ③ ④
34. ① ② ③ ④
35. ① ② ③ ④
36. ① ② ③ ④
37. ① ② ③ ④
38. ① ② ③ ④
39. ① ② ③ ④ ⑤ ⑥
40. _____
41. ① ② ③ ④ ⑤ ⑥
42. ① ② ③ ④
43. ① ② ③ ④
44. ① ② ③ ④
45. ① ② ③ ④
46. ① ② ③ ④
47. ① ② ③ ④
48. ① ② ③ ④
49. ① ② ③ ④
50. ① ② ③ ④

51. ① ② ③ ④
52. _____
53. ① ② ③ ④
54. ① ② ③ ④
55. ① ② ③ ④
56. ① ② ③ ④ ⑤ ⑥
57. ① ② ③ ④
58. ① ② ③ ④
59. ① ② ③ ④
60. ① ② ③ ④ ⑤ ⑥
61. ① ② ③ ④
62. ① ② ③ ④
63. ① ② ③ ④
64. ① ② ③ ④
65. ① ② ③ ④
66. ① ② ③ ④
67. ① ② ③ ④
68. ① ② ③ ④ ⑤ ⑥
69. ① ② ③ ④ ⑤ ⑥
70. _____
71. ① ② ③ ④
72. ① ② ③ ④ ⑤ ⑥
73. ① ② ③ ④
74. ① ② ③ ④
75. ① ② ③ ④

76. ① ② ③ ④
77. ① ② ③ ④ ⑤ ⑥
78. ① ② ③ ④
79. ① ② ③ ④
80. ① ② ③ ④
81. ① ② ③ ④
82. ① ② ③ ④ ⑤ ⑥
83. ① ② ③ ④
84. ① ② ③ ④
85. ① ② ③ ④ ⑤ ⑥
86. ① ② ③ ④
87. ① ② ③ ④
88. _____
89. ① ② ③ ④
90. ① ② ③ ④
91. ① ② ③ ④ ⑤ ⑥
92. ① ② ③ ④
93. _____
94. ① ② ③ ④
95. ① ② ③ ④
96. ① ② ③ ④
97. ① ② ③ ④
98. ① ② ③ ④
99. ① ② ③ ④
100. ① ② ③ ④ ⑤ ⑥

Answer Sheet

Practice Test 1: Diagnostic Test

100 Questions – 150 minutes

> **Directions:** This test matches the current NCSBN NCLEX-RN test plan. You may encounter the following types of questions:
>
> 1. **Multiple-choice** questions that will have only one correct answer.
> 2. **Multiple-answer** questions that will have more than one correct answer.
> 3. **Fill-in-the-blank** questions that will require math calculations.
> 4. **Hot spot** questions, where you will mark a very specific location on an image.
>
> Each item will require you to perform critical thinking. It is important that you identify exactly what the question is asking before moving on to the answer choices. For multiple-choice and multiple-response questions, read all the answer choices, choose the best answer(s), and fill in the corresponding circle(s) on the answer sheet. Take care to not just pick the first answer that makes sense. For fill-in-the-blank questions, use the appropriate math calculation and fill in the correct answer in the blank provided. For hot spot questions, follow the directions provided in the question to indicate the correct answer. An answer key and explanations follow the practice test.

1. The nurse caring for a postoperative client activates the rapid response team after noting the following ECG rhythm. While waiting for the team to arrive, which is the nurse's **priority** action?

   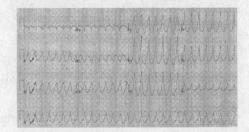

   1. Apply oxygen.
   2. Check the pulse.
   3. Check the leads.
   4. Obtain a defibrillator.

2. Where should the nurse anticipate observing a capture on the ECG tracing of a client with a pacemaker?

   1. Prior to the P wave
   2. Following the QRS wave
   3. Prior to the U wave
   4. Following the Q wave

3. When monitoring a client who has received atropine preoperatively, which adverse effect should the nurse anticipate?

   1. Bradycardia
   2. Hypertension
   3. Urinary retention
   4. Muscle weakness

Diagnostic Test

4. A client tells the nurse she felt insulted during group therapy. Which response by the nurse reflects therapeutic communication?

   1. "You really should have spoken up for yourself."

   2. "Give me an example of what was said that upset you."

   3. "I would not worry about how other people act toward you."

   4. "The next time that occurs remove yourself from the situation immediately."

5. A client in the first trimester of pregnancy states to the nurse, "My husband and I have been trying to have a family, but he does not seem interested in the pregnancy." Which response should the nurse provide to the client?

   1. "Some men are not comfortable expressing their emotions."

   2. "Your husband may be feeling self-doubt about taking on the role of a father."

   3. "Your husband will become more focused as the birth of the baby approaches."

   4. "Not all men are focused on pregnancy, but will bond with the baby after birth."

6. Which action taken by a client using a cane requires nursing intervention?

   1. The client's elbow is flexed 30 degrees.

   2. The client holds the cane on the strong side.

   3. The client moves their weak leg past the cane.

   4. The client moves the cane followed by the strong leg forward.

7. Which classification of laxative should be of **most** concern to the nurse when administering to a client with kidney disease?

   1. Osmotic

   2. Stimulant

   3. Surfactant

   4. Bulk-forming

8. A client tells the nurse he would like to create a health care by proxy. Which information will the nurse share with the client?

   1. "It is best to appoint one person to prevent conflict."

   2. "I recommend you have an alternative person for your health care proxy."

   3. "I recommend that you create a living will instead of a health care proxy."

   4. "It is best to create a durable power of attorney to ensure your affairs are taken care of."

9. Which type of precaution will the nurse implement for the client suspected of having bacterial meningitis?

   1. Contact

   2. Droplet

   3. Airborne

   4. Isolation

10. The nurse is providing preoperative care for a client scheduled for the repair of a detached retina. Which should the nurse include in the plan of care?

    1. Apply a shield over the client's eyes.

    2. Decrease environmental lighting.

    3. Restrict the movement of the client's head.

    4. Instruct the client to ask for assistance with ambulation.

11. The nurse turning a client with a new chest tube dislodges the tube. Which **immediate** action should the nurse take?

    1. Place a gloved hand over the insertion site.

    2. Obtain petroleum gauze and place it over the site.

    3. Ask the client to inhale before putting gauze over the site.

    4. Ask the client to exhale before placing a gloved hand over the site.

12. The nurse is providing education for a client scheduled for a myringotomy. Which statement made by the client indicates an understanding of the information?

    1. "I will drink through a straw for the first few weeks."
    2. "I will avoid bending over for the next three weeks."
    3. "I will report any drainage to my health care provider."
    4. "I will avoid blowing my nose with my mouth open."

13. Which factor should the nurse understand has a direct effect on how well blood and fluid leave the chest through a chest tube?

    1. Intrathoracic pressure
    2. Amount of suction applied
    3. Adequate water seal chamber
    4. Number of collection chambers

14. Which should the nurse anticipate including in the care plan for a client the first 24 hours post thyroidectomy? **Select all that apply.**

    1. Suction oral secretions as necessary.
    2. Use pillows to support the head and neck.
    3. Loosen the neck dressing as the swelling increases.
    4. Keep emergency thoracentesis equipment readily available.
    5. Empty the drain for a moderate amount of serosanguinous drainage.
    6. Have the client place both hands behind the neck before coughing.

15. The nurse is providing education for an obstetrical client scheduled for a one-hour glucose screening. Which information should the nurse include in the instructions?

    1. Avoid eating or drinking 8 hours prior.
    2. Pour the drink over ice to prevent nausea.
    3. Do not make any dietary changes before the screening.
    4. Avoid restricting your exercise several days before the screening.

16. Which seating arrangement should the nurse use to promote communication when interviewing a client?

    1. Sit side by side with the client.
    2. Create a face-to-face interview setting.
    3. Place a desk between the nurse and the client.
    4. Have the client sit in the room and the nurse sit by the door.

17. The nurse is caring for a client experiencing a narcotic overdose. Which arterial blood gas findings should the nurse associate with the condition of the client?

    1. pH 7.41, $PaCO_2$ 44, HCO_3 21
    2. pH 7.28, $PaCO_2$ 62, HCO_3 30
    3. pH 7.25, $PaCO_2$ 74, HCO_3 20
    4. pH 7.35, $PaCO_2$ 34, HCO_3 28

18. Which statement made by a client with diabetes who is performing foot care at home should be of **most** concern to the nurse?

    1. "I rub the dry areas of my feet with lotion."
    2. "I keep the calluses on my feet filed down."
    3. "I have turned down the water heater to 105°."
    4. "I bought warm slippers to wear around the house."

Diagnostic Test

Diagnostic Test

19. Which factors are associated with an **increased** risk of aspiration for a client receiving enteral feedings? **Select all that apply.**

　1. Administering higher volumes of tube feedings

　2. Administering high bolus feeding volumes

　3. Administering a feeding when the gastric residual volume is low

　4. Failing to instill the aspirated stomach contents back into the tube

　5. Observing feeding contents in a client's mouth when performing oral care

　6. Decreasing the feeding rate while placing the head of bed flat to reposition the client

20. The nurse is providing education for the treatment of engorgement during lactation suppression for a postpartum client. Which information should the nurse include?

　1. Apply ice or cold packs to the breasts for 15 minutes every hour.

　2. Apply warm compresses to the breasts for 15 minutes every hour.

　3. Massage the tissue of the breasts in a downward motion for five minutes every hour.

　4. Express some of the milk to relieve breast engorgement for a few minutes every hour.

21. Which assessment finding should the nurse anticipate for the client who requires a front wheel walker for ambulation?

　1. Activity intolerance

　2. Decreased upper motor strength

　3. Inability to bear weight on one leg

　4. Muscle weakness in the lower extremities

22. The nurse is reviewing the NST of a client at 39 weeks gestation. Which interpretation should the nurse report to the health care provider?

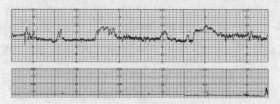

　1. Positive

　2. Reactive

　3. Negative

　4. Nonreactive

23. The nurse has provided education for a client with late-stage rheumatoid arthritis about nonpharmacological interventions for comfort. Which statement made by the client indicates an understanding of the information?

　1. "I will use ice packs to prevent inflammation."

　2. "I will perform my finger and hand exercises after the application of ice."

　3. "I will use heat packs when I experience any inflammation of my joints."

　4. "I will take a hot shower in the morning to help relieve the stiffness of my joints."

24. Which changes in electrolytes should the nurse anticipate for a client experiencing hypoparathyroidism? **Select all that apply.**

　1. Calcium 7.8 mEq/dL

　2. Sodium 138 mEq/L

　3. Vitamin D 10 ng/mL

　4. Potassium 4.2 mEq/L

　5. Phosphorous 5.4 mg/dL

　6. Magnesium 1.2 mEq/L

25. Prior to administering a dose of heparin, the nurse notes the client has an aPTT of 58 seconds. Which action should the nurse take?

    1. Hold the dose.
    2. Document the finding.
    3. Administer the heparin.
    4. Administer protamine sulfate.

26. A client receiving palliative care services has experienced increased pain and weight loss. Which action will the nursing case manager take to resolve the problem?

    1. Seek a referral.
    2. Reassess the situation.
    3. Hold an interprofessional conference.
    4. Offer options from which the client can choose.

27. Which type of intravenous fluid should the nurse anticipate being prescribed for a client who is experiencing excessive vomiting?

    1. 0.9% sodium chloride
    2. 0.45% sodium chloride
    3. 5% dextrose in lactated Ringer's
    4. 5% dextrose in 0.45% sodium chloride

28. During which part of the nursing process will the nurse case manager determine the eligibility of a client for hospice care?

    1. Planning
    2. Diagnosis
    3. Evaluation
    4. Assessment

29. Which describes the process of client advocacy when implementing an intervention?

    1. Reassurance
    2. Reformulation
    3. Exchanging information
    4. Generation of alternatives

30. The nurse is preparing to evaluate the laboratory results of a client with diabetes insipidus. Which findings should the nurse associate with the disorder? **Select all that apply.**

    1. BUN 29 mg/dL
    2. Specific gravity 1.035
    3. Creatinine 0.5 mg/dL
    4. Serum sodium 147 mg/dL
    5. Serum uric acid 8.0 mg/dL
    6. Serum potassium 5.1 mg/dL

31. Which describes the nurse advocating for a client after evaluation of treatment?

    1. Affirming the outcome
    2. Prioritizing the next action
    3. Gathering further client data
    4. Making decisions about planned treatment

32. The nurse is preparing to scan the bladder of a postoperative client. Which education should the nurse include **before** the procedure?

    1. "This will allow me to visualize the position of your bladder."
    2. "This procedure will require a couple of readings for accuracy."
    3. "I will be able to estimate the volume of urine your bladder can hold."
    4. "I will move the scanner over your pubic bone to measure the urine in the bladder."

33. The nurse has provided education for a client scheduled for a renal scan requiring the intravenous administration of a radioisotope. Which statement made by the client indicates an understanding of the procedure?

   1. "I will not eat anything after midnight."
   2. "I may receive other prescriptions during the procedure."
   3. "I will make sure that I do not drive for at least 24 hours."
   4. "I should avoid close contact with others for the first 24 hours."

34. The nurse manager is preparing to discuss misuse of chemical restraints with staff. Which intentional tort will the nurse refer to during the discussion?

   1. Battery
   2. Assault
   3. Negligence
   4. False imprisonment

35. The nurse has received a verbal report during the handoff of a client with a new assessment finding of orthostatic hypotension. Which statement made by the nurse providing the report should be of **most** concern to the nurse?

   1. "I have instructed the client to remain in bed."
   2. "I have not discussed this finding with the client."
   3. "I am trying to get a hold of the health care provider."
   4. "I still need to document the assessment in the clients record."

36. A client asks the nurse why she has to have a nasogastric tube placed before for a partial gastrectomy. Which **primary** information should the nurse provide?

   1. It prevents aspiration of stomach contents.
   2. It prevents an electrolyte imbalance post procedure.
   3. It prevents the gastric contamination of the peritoneal cavity.
   4. It provides a route to administer nutrition after the procedure.

37. When discussing client information, which action should the nurse implement to maintain the client's privacy?

   1. Use the client's initials only.
   2. Refer to the client by diagnosis.
   3. Avoid discussion in a public domain.
   4. Discuss the client using a room number.

38. Upon admission to the hospital, the nurse has provided a client with his rights. Which statement made by the client indicates further teaching is required?

   1. "I understand that not all risks of treatment may be known."
   2. "I have a right to all the information related to my diagnosis."
   3. "I have to right to know what the consequences are if I refuse treatment."
   4. "I can be provided with long-term financial implications of my treatment."

39. Which tasks **cannot** be delegated by the registered nurse to the licensed practical nurse (LPN)? **Select all that apply.**

   1. Flush a client's PICC line.
   2. Measure a client for crutches.
   3. Administer IV pain medication.
   4. Obtain a blood sample from a central line.
   5. Administer medications through an NG tube.
   6. Monitor a client receiving a blood transfusion.

40. The nurse is preparing to place five electrodes on a client to obtain an ECG. Where
should the nurse put the brown lead? **Draw
an arrow to the correct position.**

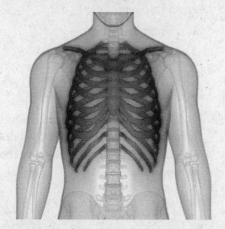

41. The nurse is assessing a client undergoing
hyperbaric oxygen therapy for carbon monoxide poisoning. Which assessment findings
are **most** concerning? **Select all that apply.**

    1. Tinnitus
    2. Vomiting
    3. Headache
    4. Irritability
    5. Tachypnea
    6. Muscle weakness

42. A client with schizophrenia states to the
nurse, "I don't want to live anymore." Which
category of symptom will the nurse document the client as experiencing?

    1. Positive
    2. Negative
    3. Affective
    4. Cognitive

43. Which action should the nurse recognize
is considered as the physical restraint of a
client?

    1. Placing a splint on a client's wrists
    2. Tucking a client in bed to confine
movement
    3. Immobilization of an infant during a
procedure
    4. Placing a helmet on a toddler at risk for
seizures

44. A postpartum client scheduled to receive a
rubella vaccine tells the nurse she is worried
her newborn will be exposed to the vaccine
through breastfeeding. Which response
should the nurse provide to the client?

    1. "The vaccine is not a live-attenuated
virus."
    2. "The vaccine will not be secreted in the
breast milk."
    3. "The virus in the vaccine is not commu-
nicable in breast milk."
    4. "The infant will receive passive immu-
nity through breastfeeding."

45. The nurse is preparing to provide education
for a client prescribed sertraline. Which
information will the nurse include in the
discussion?

    1. Drowsiness
    2. Weight loss
    3. Sexual dysfunction
    4. Potential for abuse

46. Which assessment finding should the nurse
be **most** concerned about for the client who
has had a tracheostomy?

    1. Increased air is needed to maintain cuff
pressure.
    2. Food particles are seen in the tracheal
secretions.
    3. The tracheal tube pulsates in synchrony
with the heartbeat.
    4. The client does not receive the set tidal
volume on the ventilator.

Diagnostic Test

47. Which technique should the nurse include in the tracheal suctioning of the client?
    1. Add saline solution to the trach before suctioning.
    2. Initiate suction and begin withdrawing the catheter.
    3. Keep the suction length to a maximum of 10–15 seconds.
    4. Verify that the source of suction is between 60–130 mmHg.

48. For which should the nurse monitor the client when suctioning an artificial airway?
    1. Dyspnea
    2. Bradycardia
    3. Blood pressure fluctuation
    4. Decreased oxygen saturation

49. The nurse is preparing to position a client for postural drainage; the client has diminished breath sounds in the upper anterior lobes. In which position should the nurse place the client?
    1. Right lateral Trendelenburg
    2. Leaning forward at a 45° angle
    3. Supine with pillows under knees
    4. Prone with pillows under the lower extremities

50. The nurse is preparing to initiate intravenous therapy for a client who requires blood administration. Which should the nurse consider **prior** to the treatment?
    1. Choose a vein that feels cord-like.
    2. Initiate the therapy in the most distal site.
    3. Choose a vein that is deepest in the tissue.
    4. Initiate the treatment with a 16-gauge catheter.

51. The nurse has unsuccessfully placed a 22-gauge peripheral catheter in the client's dorsal vein in the left arm. Into which vein should the nurse insert the catheter on the second attempt?
    1. Ulnar
    2. Radial
    3. Median
    4. Cephalic

52. From which anatomical location should the nurse anticipate obtaining a blood draw for an adult client? **Draw an arrow to the correct position.**

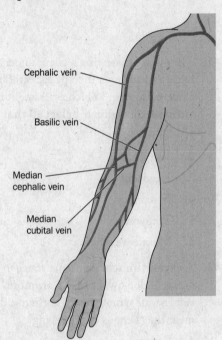

53. Which information will the nurse include to promote voiding for the client experiencing urinary retention?
    1. Offer fluids before voiding.
    2. Decompress the bladder manually.
    3. Pour cool water over the perineum.
    4. Encourage the intake of cranberry juice.

54. A client on a psychiatric unit experiencing delusions states to the nurse, "I am afraid someone is going to come into this unit and get me." Which **immediate** response should the nurse provide the client?

    1. "Let's go sit together in the dayroom."
    2. "You are safe, the unit doors are locked."
    3. "Would you like to go sit in the seclusion room?"
    4. "Who do you think is going to come into the unit?"

55. Which statement made by the licensed practical nurse (LPN) should be of concern to the nurse?

    1. "I can place the urinary catheter into the client."
    2. "I will start the gastrostomy tube feeding on the client."
    3. "I can take the phone orders from the health care provider."
    4. "I will go perform the care on the client's tracheostomy tube."

56. Which actions can the nurse delegate to the UAP for the client who has a bronchoscopy? **Select all that apply.**

    1. Obtain the vital signs.
    2. Collect a sputum sample.
    3. Assess the client's gag reflex.
    4. Check the dressing for drainage.
    5. Assist the client with repositioning.
    6. Remind the client to breathe deeply and cough.

57. Which statement made by a client scheduled for cerebral angiography should the nurse be **most** concerned about?"

    1. "I am very thirsty."
    2. "I feel very nauseated."
    3. "I have not eaten for 8 hours."
    4. "I am nervous about having an IV."

58. The nurse is reviewing seizure precautions with the parents of a young child with epilepsy. Which statement made by the parent indicates further education is required?

    1. "I will make sure my child leaves the bathroom door unlocked."
    2. "I will keep my child out of the bathtub and encourage showers."
    3. "I will make sure someone is in the swimming pool with my child."
    4. "I will make sure my child does not play on high playground equipment."

59. Which assessment is used to evaluate the vision of a newborn?

    1. Red reflex
    2. Accommodation
    3. Light perception
    4. Peripheral vision

60. Prior to delegating a task to a UAP, which rights should the nurse consider? **Select all that apply.**

    1. Task
    2. Person
    3. Supervision
    4. Competence
    5. Circumstance
    6. Communication

61. Which incident should a nurse who is employed by a Joint Commission-accredited hospital anticipate being reported as a sentinel event?

    1. A client threatening the staff with violent behavior
    2. A client who commits suicide two days after discharge
    3. A client admitted to the health care facility with botulism
    4. A client who has acquired a stage two pressure ulcer after admission

Diagnostic Test

Diagnostic Test

62. Which client condition should the nurse be **most** concerned about for the client scheduled for a diagnostic test using an iodinated contrast agent?

1. An adult with a history of epilepsy
2. An adult experiencing acute pancreatitis
3. An adult experiencing nausea and vomiting
4. An adolescent client with irritable bowel syndrome

63. The nurse has instructed the client on the use of an automatic epinephrine injector. Which statement indicates the client understands the information?

1. "I will keep two injectors readily available."
2. "I will call 911 before I inject the epinephrine."
3. "I will remove my pants prior to injecting it into my thigh."
4. "I will come to the emergency department if the drug is not effective."

64. The nurse reviewing the laboratory report of a client's cerebral fluid notes that the color was found to be orange. Which should the nurse associate with the findings?

1. Protein
2. Bacteria
3. Bilirubin
4. Red blood cells

65. Which type of auditory test will the nurse use when performing hearing screening tests for young children?

1. Play audiometry
2. Pure tone audiometry
3. Behavioral audiometry
4. Auditory brainstem response

66. Which client is a **priority** for the nurse to assess?

1. A 48-year-old client being treated with chemotherapy for lung cancer who reports shortness of breath over the past three days.
2. A 36-year-old client with type 1 diabetes who has had vomiting and diarrhea for the past three days.
3. A 28-year-old male admitted with generalized abdominal pain, nausea, and vomiting for the past three days.
4. A 22-year-old female experiencing urinary frequency, hematuria, and urinary retention for the past two days.

67. Which type of contraception should the nurse recommend as the **most** effective for a breastfeeding client?

1. Condoms
2. Diaphragm
3. Progestin injection
4. Hormonal contraceptive ring

68. Which statements made by the nurse reflect an understanding of spiritual support for a client? **Select all that apply.**

1. "My client practices a specific religion so I will offer to notify her spiritual leader."
2. "My client does not have a religious preference, but I will offer to notify the chaplain."
3. "I am concerned that my dying client will not accept the services of the hospital chaplain."
4. "My client's family has asked me to notify the leader of their church to come see the client."
5. "I will reschedule the social worker's visit because my client is performing a spiritual ritual."
6. "I have notified the chaplain because my client has expressed a great deal of spiritual distress."

69. Which symptoms should the nurse anticipate for a client experiencing opioid withdrawal? **Select all that apply.**

    1. Meiosis
    2. Yawning
    3. Euphoria
    4. Hypotension
    5. Slurred speech
    6. Bone and muscle pain

70. The nurse is using a visual aid while providing education for a client who is scheduled to
have an intracranial pressure monitor placed.
Which location should the nurse identify
as the placement of the tip of the catheter?
Draw an arrow to the correct location.

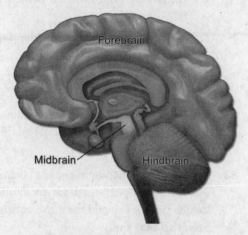

71. A client newly diagnosed with HIV asks the
nurse why the ELISA screening tested negative several months prior. Which response
should the nurse provide?

    1. "The ELISA has a high false negative."
    2. "The HIV viral load was insignificant."
    3. "Your body had not produced
       antibodies."
    4. "The testing sample used was
       inadequate."

72. Which will the nurse include when maintaining a neutral standing posture to avoid
injury? **Select all that apply.**

    1. Flexed knees
    2. Back straight
    3. Wrists flexed
    4. Elbows locked
    5. Feet hip-width apart
    6. Shoulders thrust back

73. Which client will the nurse assess **last**?

    1. A client with a severe headache, stiff
       neck, and a temperature of 101.8°F
    2. A client reporting chest discomfort over
       the past two hours and a sudden onset
       of shortness of breath
    3. A client currently receiving chemother-
       apy for breast cancer with a temperature
       of 102.6°F
    4. A client with a sudden onset of chest
       palpitations, heart rate of 96, and blood
       pressure of 128/74

74. The nurse is preparing to administer an
injection to a client. Which activity places
the nurse at risk for musculoskeletal injury?

    1. Lowering the side rail
    2. Lowering the client's bed
    3. Placing the feet facing the client's bed
    4. Keeping the arms below the shoulders

75. The nurse is assessing a client who has had
arterial revascularization of a left lower
extremity for severe claudication. With
which finding should the nurse be **most**
concerned?

    1. Redness
    2. Edema
    3. Warmth
    4. Aching

76. Which pain scale should the nurse use to assess a two-year-old postoperative child?

    1. Oucher scale
    2. FLACC scale
    3. Wong Baker's faces
    4. Visual analog scale

77. Which information should the nurse include in the general assessment of the client? **Select all that apply.**

    1. Age
    2. Height
    3. Weight
    4. Gender
    5. Mobility
    6. Medications

78. A client asks the nurse how skeletal traction can prevent pain. Which response should the nurse provide?

    1. "Traction keeps the pins in place."
    2. "Traction prevents muscle spasms."
    3. "Traction prevents compartment syndrome."
    4. "Traction keeps the extremity immobilized."

79. A family member tells the nurse that he does not want the client to know that the diagnosis is terminal. Which response should the nurse provide?

    1. "I will have to review the client's living will and durable power of attorney."
    2. "I understand your concern, but I cannot withhold information from the client."
    3. "I will need to review the health care by proxy to identify the health care surrogate."
    4. "I will contact the health care provider and ethics committee to review your request."

80. A client tells the nurse he did not understand anything about the treatment the health care provider discussed. Which action should the nurse take?

    1. Request a consult from the ethics committee.
    2. Provide verbal and written educational material.
    3. Inform the health care provider of the client's concern.
    4. Encourage the client to have a family member present during any discussion.

81. Which information should the nurse include in the teaching for a client with an ileostomy?

    1. "Empty the pouch when it is one-third full."
    2. "Notify the health care provider if the stoma is reddened."
    3. "The time between eating gas-forming foods and flatulence is 6–8 hours."
    4. "Cleanse the skin around the stoma with antiseptic wipes before replacing the bag."

82. The nurse is preparing to assess a client who is experiencing stimulant intoxication. Which findings should the nurse anticipate? **Select all that apply.**

    1. Paranoia
    2. Insomnia
    3. Irritability
    4. Chest pain
    5. Dilated pupils
    6. Mental alertness

83. The nurse is caring for a client who is experiencing hypertension, angina, and dysrhythmias. Which prescription will the nurse anticipate administering?

    1. Enalapril
    2. Diltiazem
    3. Nifedipine
    4. Propranolol

84. Which of the below is the **primary** reason cancer goes undiagnosed in older adults more often than in younger adults?

    1. The older adult is less likely to be screened.
    2. The older adult is at a higher risk for cancer.
    3. The older adult has limited access to health care.
    4. The older adult may not recognize the symptoms.

85. Which laboratory results should be of **most** concern to the nurse prior to administering an aldosterone antagonist to a client with heart failure? **Select all that apply.**

    1. aPTT
    2. Platelets
    3. Sodium
    4. Potassium
    5. Serum creatinine
    6. Blood urea nitrogen

86. A client's IV pump begins to sound an unexplained alarm. Which **initial** action will the nurse take?

    1. Reset the IV pump.
    2. Remove the IV pump.
    3. Assess the pump for damage.
    4. Troubleshoot the IV pump.

87. The nurse has provided education to a client and his wife about the signs and symptoms of the early stages of Alzheimer's disease. Which statement made by the client's wife indicates an understanding of the information?

    1. "I can expect my husband to sleep more throughout the day."
    2. "My husband will need help choosing clothes for the proper season."
    3. "My husband will have difficulty retrieving correct words for things."
    4. "I can expect my husband to experience changes in his ability to walk."

88. The nurse is reinforcing education for the parents of an infant scheduled for the repair of the foramen ovale. **Draw an arrow to identify which area of the heart will be repaired.**

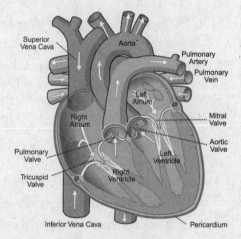

By Wapcaplet - Own work, CC BY-SA 3.0, https://commons.wikimedia.org/w/index.php?curid=830253

89. The nurse has provided safety education for the client with a halo vest. Which statement indicates the client requires additional education?

   1. "I can shave the hair around the pin sites."

   2. "I will use support under my head at night."

   3. "If a pin loosens, I will apply pressure to the pin."

   4. "I will notify my health care provider if my weight changes."

90. Following a horizontal evacuation plan, where will the nurse evacuate the clients following a fire?

   1. Move the clients out of the facility.

   2. Transfer the clients to the floor below.

   3. Move the clients to the next smoke compartment.

   4. Transfer the clients into another unit on the same floor.

91. Which will the nurse include when discussing factors that contribute to a false low blood pressure with assistive personnel? **Select all that apply.**

   1. Deflating the cuff too slowly

   2. Using a cuff that is too narrow

   3. Arm position above the heart level

   4. Noise in the surrounding environment

   5. Stethoscope not directly placed over the artery

   6. Blood pressure taken while the client's legs are crossed

92. Which should the nurse consult to obtain a description of an authoritative statement of the duties of the registered nurse?

   1. State Board of Nursing Practice Act

   2. Standards of Professional Nursing Practice

   3. Health care facility's policy and procedures

   4. National Council of the State Boards of Nursing

93. The nurse is preparing to assess a client with a newly placed percutaneous endoscopic gastrostomy (PEG) tube. Which anatomical location should the nurse anticipate assessing? **Draw an arrow to the correct location.**

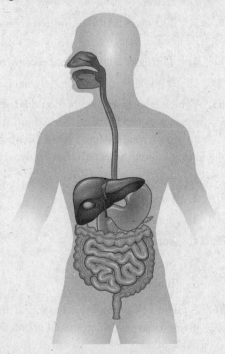

94. Which therapeutic assessment finding should the nurse anticipate for a client with heart failure who is receiving an angiotensin II receptor blocker?

   1. Decreased angina

   2. Decreased blood pressure

   3. Increased activity tolerance

   4. Increased oxygen saturation

95. The nurse is preparing to administer supplemental oxygen to a client with unstable COPD. Which mask should the nurse anticipate using?

1.

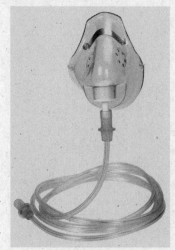

2.

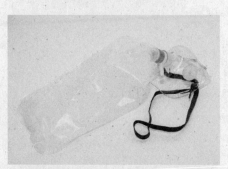

3.

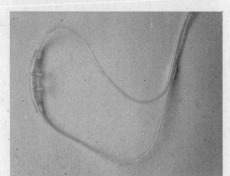

By ICUnurses - Own work, CC BY-SA 4.0, https://commons.wikimedia.org/w/index.php?curid=34382459

4.

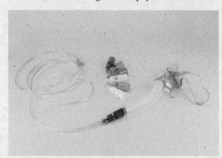

96. The educator has reviewed the principles of surgical asepsis with a nurse. Which statement made by the nurse indicates further teaching is required?

1. "Avoid tossing sterile objects into the sterile field."
2. "Two inches of the border is considered nonsterile."
3. "Sterile forceps can be used to place sterile items on the field."
4. "When pouring water, hold the bottle two inches above the receptacle."

97. Which statement made by a family member of a client who has died three months prior should be of **most** concern to the nurse?

1. "I still feel so empty."
2. "I am tired of the anger that keeps coming up."
3. "I cannot find gratification in anything that I do."
4. "I feel bad that I did not spend more time with him."

98. Which therapeutic effect will the nurse anticipate for a client with diabetes insipidus who has been prescribed desmopressin?

1. Resolved hypertension
2. Improved cardiac output
3. Regulated water excretion
4. Normalized blood glucose

99. The nurse has provided education for a client who has been prescribed 10 mg of loratadine daily for seasonal allergies. Which statement made by the client indicates further teaching is required?

1. "I don't have to take this medication with food."
2. "I may feel a bit dizzy after taking the medication."
3. "I will avoid driving until I know how this medication affects me."
4. "I will take this medication an hour prior to going outside."

Diagnostic Test

100. With which assessment findings should the nurse associate the ECG rhythm? **Select all that apply.**

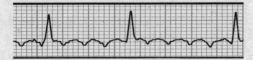

1. Dyspnea
2. Confusion
3. Chest pain
4. Flushed skin
5. Hypertension
6. Peripheral edema

Diagnostic Test

ANSWER KEY AND EXPLANATIONS

1. 2	23. 4	43. 2	62. 3	81. 1
2. 2	24. 1, 3, 5, 6	44. 3	63. 1	82. 4, 5, 6
3. 3	25. 3	45. 3	64. 4	83. 2
4. 2	26. 3	46. 3	65. 2	84. 1
5. 3	27. 1	47. 3	66. 2	85. 4, 5, 6
6. 3	28. 4	48. 2	67. 3	86. 2
7. 1	29. 1	49. 3	68. 2, 5	87. 3
8. 2	30. 1, 4	50. 2	69. 2, 6	88. Arrow points to atrial septum (right atrium)
9. 2	31. 1	51. 4	70. The intracranial pressure catheter tip is placed in the lateral ventricle of the brain	
10. 3	32. 2	52. Arrow points to crevice of elbow between the median cephalic and the median basilic vein.		89. 3
11. 1	33. 2			90. 3
12. 2	34. 4			91. 3, 4, 5
13. 2	35. 2		71. 3	92. 2
14. 1, 2, 5, 6	36. 3		72. 1, 2	93. Arrow points to stomach
	37. 3		73. 4	
15. 3	38. 1	53. 1	74. 2	
16. 1	39. 1, 3, 4	54. 2	75. 4	94. 3
17. 2		55. 3	76. 2	95. 4
18. 2	40. Arrow points to 4th intercostal space, right sternal border	56. 1, 2, 5, 6	77. 2, 3, 5	96. 2
19. 2, 5, 6		57. 2	78. 2	97. 3
20. 1		58. 2	79. 2	98. 3
		59. 3	80. 3	99. 2
21. 2	41. 1, 4	60. 1, 2, 3, 5, 6		100. 1, 2, 3
22. 4	42. 3	61. 2		

1. **The correct answer is 2.** Ventricular tachycardia is a ventricular dysrhythmia that is life threatening. The client's pulse should be assessed immediately before any other intervention. Applying oxygen (choice 1), checking the leads (choice 3), and obtaining a defibrillator (choice 4) are all actions that would occur after the nurse has checked the pulse. A client with ventricular tachycardia may be stable or unstable with a pulse and will require oxygen, an antidysrhythmic,

and cardioversion. While it is a good idea to check the leads to ensure the capture is correct, it is not the first priority. If the client has no pulse, the client requires CPR, defibrillation, epinephrine (vasopressor), and an antidysrhythmic.

2. **The correct answer is 2.** The pacing stimulus delivered by the pacemaker is depicted by a spike on the ECG tracing that follows depolarization of a P wave, indicating atrial depolarization, or a QRS complex indicating

Answers Diagnostic Test

ventricular depolarization. The pattern of spikes depicted on the ECG is referred to as a capture.

3. **The correct answer is 3.** Adverse reactions of atropine include urinary retention and tachycardia. Atropine decreases oral and respiratory secretions, treats sinus bradycardia, heart block, and bronchospasms, refraction, and uveitis.

4. **The correct answer is 2.** Asking the client to provide an example of what upset her is an example of therapeutic communication. Telling the client she should have spoken up for herself (choice 1) sends a disapproving message and may make the client defensive. Informing the client she should not worry about how others act towards her (choice 3) devalues her feelings. Instructing the client to remove herself from the situation immediately the next time it occurs (choice 4) is a nontherapeutic technique of giving advice and devalues the client's concerns.

5. **The correct answer is 3.** The focusing phase of the father usually begins in the last trimester of the pregnancy. Usually during this time, the father becomes more actively involved as he discusses his role in labor and prepares for parenthood. The inability of the client's husband to express emotions (choice 1) or experience self-doubt about the role of fatherhood (choice 2) are assumptions. Telling the client that not all men are focused on pregnancy, but will bond with the baby after birth (choice 4) is inaccurate. Fatherhood is experienced throughout the pregnancy.

6. **The correct answer is 3.** The client is using the wrong leg to move forward. When using a cane, the client will move the cane forward six inches in front and six inches to the side of the strong leg, followed by the moving the weak leg toward the cane and then move the strong leg past the cane (choice 4). The client should be holding the cane on the strong side (choice 2). When the client holds the cane, the elbow is flexed at a 30° angle (choice 1).

7. **The correct answer is 1.** A client with renal disease receiving an osmotic laxative is at risk for magnesium accumulating to toxic levels, as well as other electrolyte imbalances. Osmotic laxatives are hyperosmotic, which causes a substantial amount of water loss. These laxatives can result in electrolyte imbalances, as they draw nutrients and other contents out with the water.

8. **The correct answer is 2.** A health care by proxy allows another individual to make medical decisions in the event the client is unable to do so. Choice 1 is not the best information to share with the client because in case the delegated decision-maker is unavailable in an emergency, at least one or more alternates should be named. A living will is specific to what the client wants to receive and is not a document that allows others to make medical decisions, so choice 3 is not a recommendation the nurse should make. Similarly, the nurse should not recommend a document, such as a power of attorney in choice 4, unless there is a specific understanding of what the client would prefer. A durable power of attorney allows a person to make legal decisions for the client other than just medical decisions.

9. **The correct answer is 2.** A client suspected of having bacterial meningitis requires droplet precautions in addition to standard precautions. Contact (choice 1) and airborne precautions (choice 3) will not provide protection against meningitis. *Isolation precaution* (choice 4) is a general term used for infection control precautions, which include standard and transmission-based precautions.

10. **The correct answer is 3.** Before the repair of a detached retina, it is essential to prevent further tearing or detachment, so the client's head movement should be restricted. It is only necessary to apply a shield or patch over the affected eye to prevent movement. Using a shield over both eyes (choice 1) places the client at risk for sensory deprivation and can increase anxiety. Decreasing environmental

lighting (choice 2) can be dangerous and puts a client at risk for falls. The client's movement should be restricted; the client should not be ambulatory (choice 4).

11. **The correct answer is 1.** Before calling for help, the nurse will immediately place a gloved hand over the insertion site. If the nurse did not witness the chest tube removal, there is a risk that the client might accumulate trapped air in the pleural space. In this situation, choice 4 should be the immediate action for the nurse to take. The nurse will request the client to exhale forcefully, and before the next inhalation, place a gloved hand over the site (if there is no petroleum gauze immediately available). Asking the client to inhale before covering the site (choice 3) places the client at risk for tension pneumothorax. Leaving the client to obtain petroleum gauze to put over the site (choice 2) delays emergency care.

12. **The correct answer is 2.** The client making the statement in choice 2 understands the information the nurse has provided. The client should not bend over for the following three weeks to avoid increasing middle ear pressure, which may disrupt the surgical site. Further education may be necessary if the client makes the statements in choices 1, 3, and 4. The client should be instructed to avoid drinking through a straw because the increased pressure may disrupt the surgical site. Some drainage is an expected finding for the first few days post-surgery. The client will be instructed to change the dressing every 24 hours and immediately report excessive drainage. The client will be instructed to avoid blowing his or her nose with the mouth closed to prevent an increase in the pressure.

13. **The correct answer is 2.** The amount of suction applied is a factor that affects how well blood and fluid leave the chest through a chest tube. Other factors include the length of the tubing and the inner diameter of the tube. Intrathoracic pressure (choice 1) refers to pressure in the pleural cavity. When

changes in pressure occur, these changes are reflected as fluctuations or tidaling in the water seal chamber. The purpose of the water seal chamber (choice 3) is to allow air to exit and prevent air from flowing into the pleural space. The number of collection chambers (choice 4) does not affect how well blood and fluid leave through the chest tube.

14. **The correct answers are 1, 2, 5, and 6.** Oral secretions may need to be suctioned following a thyroidectomy. A pillow is used to support the head and neck after surgery, and the client should avoid neck extension because it may disrupt the surgical site. The client may experience a moderate amount of serosanguinous drainage in the first 24 hours. The client will place both hands behind their neck before coughing to support the neck and reduce tension on the suture line. If the dressing around the neck becomes too tight (choice 3), this may be an indication of a complication that could impede the airway. The client should immediately be assessed for hemorrhage or any respiratory compromise and the health care provider notified immediately. Emergency tracheostomy equipment (not thoracentesis equipment as choice 4 indicates) should be kept immediately available.

15. **The correct answer is 3.** It is not necessary to make any dietary changes before the screening. It is not required that the client avoid eating or drinking 8 hours before the glucose screening, so choice 1 is incorrect information. The solution will become diluted if poured over ice, so choice 2 is incorrect. Choice 4 would be information to relay to a client who requires the second step of the testing. In this case, the client should be instructed to avoid restricting both diet and exercise several days before the test.

16. **The correct answer is 1.** Sitting side by side with the client provides a less intense interview setting by allowing the client to look away comfortably. A face-to-face interview setting (choice 2) allows for the client or the nurse to look away from each other without

discomfort, but could hinder open communication. A desk placed between the nurse and the client during the interview (choice 3) creates a barrier. The nurse should not position herself in a way that may make the client feel trapped in the room (choice 4).

17. **The correct answer is 2.** Respiratory depression is associated with a narcotic overdose. Respiratory acidosis occurs when the client becomes hypoxic as is reflected by a pH 7.28, $PaCO_2$ 62, and HCO_3 30. The pH is acidotic, the $PaCO_2$ is above the normal range (indicating an acidotic condition), and the bicarbonate is elevated as a result of trying to resolve the acidic condition.

18. **The correct answer is 2.** The nurse should be most concerned if the client indicates he will file the calluses on his feet. The client should not try to treat the calluses on his own; rather he should be instructed to contact the health care provider. A lotion (choice 1) can be used on dry areas of the feet, but the nurse should clarify that the client should avoid putting the lotion in between the toes. The statement in choice 3 should not concern the nurse as the water temperature should be no higher than 105° to prevent burns. Similarly, the nurse should not be concerned with the client wearing slippers around the house as the protective covering could help prevent injury.

19. **The correct answers are 2, 5, and 6.** High bolus feeding volumes and feeding contents in a client's mouth are both associated with an increased risk of aspiration for a client receiving enteral feedings. When placing the head of the bed flat for repositioning, the tube feedings should be turned off to decrease the risk of aspiration. Higher volumes of tube feedings (choice 1) and administration of a feeding when the gastric residual volume is low (choice 3) are not associated with an increased risk for aspiration. Failure to instill the aspirated contents back into the tube (choice 4) can result in an electrolyte imbalance.

20. **The correct answer is 1.** Engorgement occurs during the suppression of lactation and results in discomfort. To help relieve the discomfort the client can be instructed to apply ice or cold packs to the breasts for 15 minutes every hour. The client should avoid any breast stimulation (choice 3), using warm compresses (choice 2), or expressing milk (choice 4), as this will stimulate the let-down reflex, resulting in milk production.

21. **The correct answer is 2.** A client with a front-wheel walker requires support during ambulation, but lacks upper motor strength to pick up a walker and move it forward. The client must be able to bear weight on both legs (choice 3) to safely use a walker with front wheels. A client with an activity intolerance (choice 1) may require a four-wheel walker with a seat to allow for frequent rest during ambulation. A walker with wheels is not used for clients with weakness in the lower extremities (choice 4).

22. **The correct answer is 4.** A nonreactive NST will be reported to the health care provider. An NST that is reactive after 32 weeks gestation reflects a fetal heart rate acceleration of 15 beats for 15 seconds above the baseline twice within a 20-minute window. A reactive NST (choice 2) is a reassuring finding. The terms *positive* (choice 1) and *negative* (choice 3) describe the results for an oxytocin challenge test also known as a contraction stress test.

23. **The correct answer is 4.** A hot shower in the morning can relieve pain and stiffness for a client with late-stage rheumatoid arthritis. If a client makes the statements in choices 1, 2, and 3, then further education may be needed. Ice packs are used to treat inflammation, but do not prevent it. Hand and finger exercises should be performed after warmth is applied to the joints.

24. **The correct answers are 1, 3, 5, and 6.** Changes in electrolytes for a client with hypoparathyroidism include decreased calcium, vitamin D, and magnesium, and an

increase in phosphorous. The sodium (choice 2) and potassium (choice 4) levels are not affected.

25. **The correct answer is 3.** The aPTT is within an acceptable range, so the nurse should administer the heparin. The normal range of aPTT is 25–35 and, when treated with heparin therapy, will be 1.5 to 2 times the normal control values. The nurse should not hold the dose (choice 1) and the finding can be documented (choice 2), but the prescription needs to be administered. Administering protamine sulfate (choice 4) is unnecessary.

26. **The correct answer is 3.** A focus of the nurse case manager is the coordination of care using a collaborative approach to provide and coordinate health care services for a client. The client experiencing pain and weight loss requires collaboration between interdisciplinary team members to address the clinical findings, which can be best addressed by having a conference with the appropriate health care professionals. A referral (choice 1) is not an initial intervention prior to communicating with the health care team. Reassessment (choice 2) occurs after the plan of care has been established, outcomes have been identified, and the interventions have been implemented. The client will be included in the collaboration, but prior to meeting with the health care team, there are no options (choice 4) to offer the client.

27. **The correct answer is 1.** Lost volume is replaced with fluids that are isotonic to plasma volume, such as 0.9% sodium chloride. These solutions increase extracellular fluid volume due to fluid loss. Hypotonic solutions such as 0.45% sodium chloride (choice 2) are used to replace intracellular fluid loss. Hypertonic solutions such as 5% dextrose in 0.45% sodium chloride (choice 4) and 5% dextrose in lactated Ringer's (choice 3) pull fluid into the vascular system, thereby increasing the vascular volume.

28. **The correct answer is 4.** The nurse case manager will determine the eligibility of the client for hospice care during the assessment. From a case management perspective, the nurse will prioritize the problems and identify resources (choice 1) according to the client's clinical condition. The nurse will identify the problem during the diagnosis (choice 2). The evaluation period (choice 3) offers the nurse the opportunity to measure goal attainment.

29. **The correct answer is 1.** Reassurance reflects client advocacy during the implementation process. Reformulation (choice 2) is advocacy displayed during the evaluation process. Exchanging information (choice 3) is part of the advocacy process that occurs during the client assessment and diagnosis. Generating alternatives (choice 4) reflects nursing advocacy, which occurs in the planning process.

30. **The correct answers are 1 and 4.** For a client with diabetes, normal ranges for the laboratory values are as follows:

    - Blood urea nitrogen (BUN): 18–21 mg/dL
    - Serum creatinine: 0.8–1.3 mg/dL
    - Sodium: 135–145 mEq/L
    - Uric acid: 3.5–7.5 mg/dL
    - Potassium: 3.5–5 mEq/L
    - Urine specific gravity: 1.010–1.030

    Diabetes insipidus results in severe dehydration due to the volumes of dilute urine that are excreted by the client. Laboratory results will reveal an elevated BUN, creatinine, serum sodium, and low specific gravity and serum potassium.

31. **The correct answer is 1.** Affirmation of the outcome reflects nursing advocacy for the client. Nursing advocacy occurs throughout the nursing process. Prioritizing the next action (choice 2) occurs during the planning of treatment, gathering further client data (choice 3) occurs during the assessment period, and making decisions about planned treatment (choice 4) is an example of advocacy during implementation.

Answers Diagnostic Test

32. **The correct answer is 2.** A bladder scanner is a noninvasive method used to estimate a client's bladder volume. The nurse should let the client know before the procedure that at least two readings are recommended to obtain an accurate estimate. The intent of the bladder scanner is not to visualize a bladder (choice 1) or estimate the amount of urine a bladder can hold (choice 3). The bladder scanner is placed one inch above the symphysis pubic bone (choice 4) and held still so an accurate reading can be obtained.

33. **The correct answer is 2.** Furosemide or captopril may be administered to improve the visual assessment of the renal blood flow and function of the kidney. Further education by the nurse would be needed for the statements made in choices 1, 3, and 4. The procedure does not require the client to be NPO. There is no sedation for the procedure, so the client's driving ability will not be affected. Since the isotope used for the scan is eliminated within 24 hours of receiving it and is not radioactive, it is not necessary for the client to avoid contact with others.

34. **The correct answer is 4.** Medication misused as a chemical restraint is false imprisonment. Battery (choice 1) is the actual touching or harm of another individual. Assault (choice 2) involves intentional threats or gestures associated with the harm of another individual. Negligence (choice 3) is an unintentional tort involving a failure to provide care at the level that a reasonably competent and skilled health care professional would provide under similar circumstances that results in the injury or death of a client.

35. **The correct answer is 2.** Failure to inform the client of a finding and follow up with appropriate teaching can result in the injury or death of the client and is an example of malpractice. Instructing the client to remain in bed (choice 1), attempting to notify the health care provider (choice 3), and a delay

in documenting assessment findings (choice 4) are not as concerning as failure to inform the client.

36. **The correct answer is 3.** The primary reason the NGT is inserted and connected to suction is to prevent the gastric secretions from contaminating the peritoneum during the procedure. The nasogastric tube is left in place afterward to prevent accumulated secretions from being aspirated and to put pressure on the surgical incision. An increase in gastric secretions places the client at risk for vomiting (choice 1), thus creating the potential for an electrolyte imbalance (choice 2). Nutrition will not be administered through the nasogastric tube (choice 4) post partial gastrectomy.

37. **The correct answer is 3.** The nurse will avoid discussing client information in a public domain to maintain client confidentiality. The client can still be identified using initials (choice 1), diagnosis (choice 2), and room number (choice 4).

38. **The correct answer is 1.** If the client indicates he understands that not all risks of treatment may be known, then further teaching by the nurse is required. The client has a right to full disclosure and information regarding the risks of any treatment or procedure. No further teaching is needed for statements 2, 3, and 4. The client has the right to all of the information related to their diagnosis as well as the short- and long-term financial implications of treatment. The client also has a right to know the consequences if treatment is refused.

39. **The correct answers are 1, 3, and 4.** An LPN cannot access or flush any type of central line, administer intravenous pain prescriptions, or obtain a blood sample from a central line. The LPN may measure the client for crutches (choice 2), administer medications through an NG tube (choice 5), and monitor a client receiving a blood transfusion (choice 6).

40. **The correct answer is shown below.** The brown lead is placed in the fourth intercostal space, right sternal border.

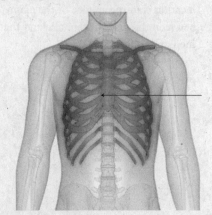

41. **The correct answers are 1 and 4.** The client undergoing hyperbaric oxygen therapy for carbon monoxide poisoning is at risk for oxygen toxicity. Assessment findings associated with oxygen toxicity include tinnitus and irritability. Vomiting, headache, tachypnea, and muscle weakness are symptoms of carbon monoxide poisoning.

42. **The correct answer is 3.** Affective symptoms reflect emotions such as hopelessness and suicidality. Positive symptoms (choice 1) are psychotic behaviors such as hallucinations and delusions. Negative symptoms (choice 2) refer to a decrease or absence of normal function, which includes avolition and anhedonia. Cognitive symptoms (choice 4) are reflected by a subtle or obvious impairment in thinking, such as poor solving problem skills and poor memory.

43. **The correct answer is 2.** Tucking a client into bed tight enough to confine movement is considered a physical restraint. Placing splints on a client's wrists (choice 1), immobilizing an infant during a procedure (choice 3), and placing a helmet on a toddler at risk for seizures (choice 4) are considered safety precautions.

44. **The correct answer is 3.** The nurse should let the client know that the rubella vaccine is not communicable in breast milk, although it is a live-attenuated virus (choice 1), which

can be found in breast milk (choice 2). A rubella vaccine does not provide passive immunity to the infant (choice 4).

45. **The correct answer is 3.** A client taking an SSRI such as sertraline may experience sexual dysfunction, insomnia, and weight gain. Antidepressants such as an SSRI do not have a potential for misuse.

46. **The correct answer is 3.** A tracheal tube that pulsates in synchrony with the heartbeat is indicative of a trachea–innominate artery fistula and is a medical emergency. The continued pressure from the malpositioned tube causes necrosis and erosion of the innominate artery. Increased air that is needed to maintain a cuff pressure (choice 1), food particles noted in the tracheal secretions (choice 2), and a client who is not receiving the set tidal volume on the ventilator (choice 4) are significant findings that need to be corrected; but none are the finding of most concern.

47. **The correct answer is 3.** The client should not be suctioned for longer than 10–15 seconds to avoid causing respiratory distress. Saline solution (choice 1) should not be used during the initial suctioning, so the secretions can be assessed, but may be needed with additional suctioning. The catheter should be withdrawn only 1–2 cm to ensure the catheter is not against the mucosal tissue before initiating suctioning, but removal of the catheter does not begin at this time (choice 2). The suction source should be set between 80–120 mmHg to avoid mucosal trauma and hypoxemia, rather than being set at 60–130 mmHg (choice 4).

48. **The correct answer is 2.** Vagal stimulation and bronchospasm can occur when passing the catheter through the airway and suctioning. Bradycardia is a symptom of vagal stimulation for which suctioning should be stopped immediately and the client hyperventilated. Dyspnea (choice 1), blood pressure fluctuations (choice 3), and decreased oxygen saturation (choice 4) are symptoms of

impaired gas exchange caused by secretions in the airway.

49. **The correct answer is 3.** A client requiring drainage of the anterior upper lobes will be positioned supine with pillows under the knees. A client who requires drainage of the right lower lobe will be positioned right laterally in Trendelenburg (choice 1). A client requiring drainage of the posterior upper lobes is positioned leaning forward at a 45-degree angle (choice 2). A client requiring drainage of the lower lateral and posterior lobes is positioned prone (choice 4).

50. **The correct answer is 2.** The intravenous therapy should be initiated in the most distal site. A vein that feels hard or cord-like (choice 1) should be avoided. Veins closest to the surface of the skin should be chosen. Veins that are deep in the tissue (choice 3) have arteries and nerves that lie parallel to them that can become damaged, and infiltration may go undetected. It is not necessary to use a 16-gauge venous catheter (choice 4) for a blood transfusion. A 16-gauge venous catheter is used only for trauma or surgical clients who require rapid fluid resuscitation.

51. **The correct answer is 4.** The venous catheter can be placed in the cephalic vein. The ulnar, radial, and median veins are not appropriate sites to insert a peripheral catheter.

52. **The correct answer is shown below.** The initial attempt to obtain a blood sample should be in the antecubital space. The location is in the crevice of the elbow between the median cephalic and the median basilic vein.

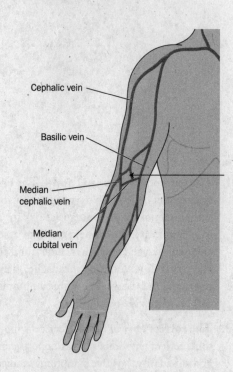

Cephalic vein

Basilic vein

Median cephalic vein

Median cubital vein

53. **The correct answer is 1.** Offering fluids prior to voiding ensures the client is adequately hydrated to maintain diluted urine and stimulate the micturition reflex. Cool water (choice 3) may cause muscle constriction resulting in urinary retention. Neither decompressing the bladder manually (choice 2) nor drinking cranberry juice (choice 4) are used to promote voiding.

54. **The correct answer is 2.** The nurse will immediately reassure the client that he is safe. Asking the client to sit in the dayroom (choice 1) does not provide the reassurance of safety. The seclusion room (choice 3) is not intended to be used to help a client feel safe. Asking the client who he thinks will come into the unit (choice 4) will increase the client's stress level and may perpetuate the client's delusion.

55. **The correct answer is 3.** The scope of the LPN's practice does not include taking phone orders from health care providers. The LPN may insert a urinary catheter (choice 1), initiate a gastrostomy tube feeding (choice 2), and perform routine care of a tracheostomy tube (choice 4).

56. **The correct answers are 1, 2, 5, and 6.** The UAP can obtain the vital signs, collect a sputum sample, assist the client with repositioning, and remind the client to deep breath and cough. The nurse is responsible for assessments, which include the client's gag reflex (choice 3) and the dressing for drainage (choice 4).

57. **The correct answer is 2.** A client receiving a cerebral angiography will be positioned in a supine position that places the client at risk for aspiration if vomiting occurs during the procedure. The client should be kept NPO and will have an IV inserted to inject the contrast media and provide hydration. The client's other comments will not interfere with the procedure.

58. **The correct answer is 2.** If a parent indicates that she will keep the child out of the bathtub and encourage showers, then the nurse needs to further educate the parent that a young child can bathe with supervision. The statements in choices 1, 3, and 4 are accurate and no further education is needed.

59. **The correct answer is 3.** Light perception is used to test vision in a newborn. Light perception testing is done by shining a light into the eyes and noting the response to the light. Assessment of the red reflex (choice 1) is used to screen for visual pathology of the eye, but does not test vision. Accommodation (choice 2) and peripheral vision (choice 4) are assessed in children old enough to cooperate.

60. **The correct answers are 1, 2, 3, 5, and 6.** Prior to delegating a task to a UAP, the rights the nurse will consider include the right task, person, supervision, circumstance, and communication. Competence (choice 4) is not considered to be a client right, as competence is established by licensing and certification.

61. **The correct answer is 2.** Suicide of any client receiving care, treatment, and services in a staffed around-the-clock care setting or within 72 hours of discharge must be reported as a sentinel event. A client threatening staff (choice 1) is not reportable. Botulism (choice 3) is required to be reported to the CDC. A stage 3 or 4 pressure ulcer after admission to the health care facility must be reported as a sentinel event, but a stage 2 pressure ulcer (choice 4) does not require reporting.

62. **The correct answer is 3.** The client experiencing nausea and vomiting is at risk for dehydration. When iodinated contrast agents are used, dehydration places the client at risk for kidney damage. A history of epilepsy (choice 1), acute pancreatitis (choice 2), or irritable bowel syndrome (choice 4) is not the finding of most concern.

63. **The correct answer is 1.** The statement in choice 1 indicates that the client clearly understands that at least two drug-filled injectors need to be available in case more than one is necessary. The client is instructed to inject the epinephrine and then call 911, not the other way around as choice 2 indicates. Choice 3 is incorrect because epinephrine can be injected through the pants, avoiding seams and pockets. After using epinephrine for an allergic reaction, the client should go to the nearest hospital for monitoring, not go to the ER if the drug is ineffective as choice 4 indicates.

64. **The correct answer is 4.** An orange appearance of cerebral spinal fluid is associated with red blood cells. An elevated protein (choice 1) may be related to a hazy color. Bacteria (choice 2) is not associated with any specific color of fluid. Cerebral spinal fluid that is yellow is associated with bilirubin (choice 3).

65. **The correct answer is 2.** Pure tone audiometry is used for hearing screening in young children. The audiometer produces sounds at different volumes and pitches and the child is asked to respond in a certain way when the tone is heard through earphones. Play audiometry (choice 1) is used for toddlers, behavioral audiometry (choice 3) is used for infants, and auditory brainstem response (choice 4) is used for newborns' hearing screens.

66. **The correct answer is 2.** The client with type 1 diabetes who has had vomiting and diarrhea for the past three days is at high risk for diabetic ketoacidosis and requires immediate evaluation. The client being treated with chemotherapy for lung cancer experiencing shortness of breath over a three-day period (choice 1); a client with generalized abdominal pain, nausea, vomiting, and diarrhea (choice 2); and the client with urinary frequency, hematuria, and urinary retention (choice 4) are not priority assessments.

67. **The correct answer is 3.** A progesterone injection is the most effective birth control for a client who is breastfeeding. The progesterone injection has a typical failure rate of 4%, whereas condoms (choice 1) have a 13% failure rate, the diaphragm (choice 2) has a 17% failure rate, and the hormonal contraceptive ring (choice 4) has a 7% failure rate.

68. **The correct answers are 2 and 5.** Spiritual care is not specifically associated with religious beliefs, and all clients should be offered spiritual support. The nurse will cultivate an uninterrupted environment in which a client can perform spiritual rituals. The nurse will respect the client's right to decline a hospital chaplain's services (choice 3). The nurse should not notify a spiritual leader solely based on the knowledge that the client practices a specific religion (choice 1). A chaplain is notified (choice 6) after permission from the client has been obtained, regardless of the family's request (choice 4) unless the client is no longer able to make decisions for himself.

69. **The correct answers are 2 and 6.** Symptoms associated with opioid withdrawal include yawning and bone and muscle pain. Meiosis (choice 1), euphoria (choice 3), hypotension (choice 4), and slurred speech (choice 5) are symptoms of opioid intoxication, rather than withdrawal.

70. **The correct answer is shown below.** The intracranial pressure catheter tip is placed in the lateral ventricle of the brain to provide a measurement of the pressure of the cerebral spinal fluid.

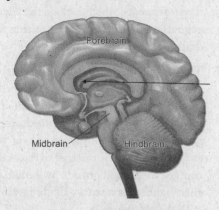

71. **The correct answer is 3.** The ELISA is a screening tool used to measure the antibodies produced in response to HIV. The antibodies cannot always be detected immediately after infection. Choice 1 is an incorrect response because the ELISA does not have a high false negative. The ELISA measures antibodies, not viral loads so choice 2 is an incorrect response too. Choice 4 is not the best response because the testing sample is not the most likely reason the screening was inaccurate.

72. **The correct answers are 1 and 2.** The nurse will stand with knees flexed and back straight. The wrists should be straight, elbows unlocked and slightly flexed, feet shoulder-width apart, and the shoulders rolled forward.

73. **The correct answer is 4.** The client who will be assessed last is the client with chest palpitations, heart rate of 96, and blood pressure of 128/74. This client's vital signs are not unstable, and the symptoms described are

associated with anxiety. The febrile client with a severe headache and stiff neck (choice 1) is exhibiting symptoms of meningitis, which can result in rapid deterioration. The client with chest discomfort and a sudden onset of shortness of breath (choice 2) may be experiencing myocardial ischemia. The febrile client receiving chemotherapy (choice 3) is at high risk for neutropenia and infection.

74. **The correct answer is 2.** Lowering the bed requires the nurse to bend over, risking injury to the back. The side rail (choice 1) is lowered to avoid reaching over. The nurse's feet should be facing the client's bed (choice 3) to avoid overreaching or twisting the back, and the arms should be kept below the shoulder line (choice 4).

75. **The correct answer is 4.** Aching pain is the most concerning finding in this case, as it may indicate that a blockage of the graft has occurred. Redness (choice 1), edema (choice 2), and warmth (choice 3) are expected findings after the restoration of the arterial circulation.

76. **The correct answer is 2.** The FLACC scale is a behavioral pain measuring tool used to assess postoperative children from ages two months to seven years. The Oucher scale (choice 1), Wong Baker's faces (choice 3), and visual analog scale (choice 4) are self-reporting pain scales that are inappropriate to use for a two-year-old child.

77. **The correct answers are 2, 3, and 5.** Included in a general survey are the client's height, weight, and mobility. The client's age (choice 1), gender (choice 4), and medication information (choice 6) are obtained during the health history assessment.

78. **The correct answer is 2.** The purpose of traction includes stabilization and realignment of bones and prevention of muscle spasms. Muscle spasms can cause misalignment of the bone, which results in pain. Traction is not intended to keep the pins in place (choice 1) nor to immobilize the entire extremity (choice 4). Traction cannot prevent compartment syndrome (choice 3).

79. **The correct answer is 2.** The client has a right to know the diagnosis and prognosis in order to make informed decisions about treatments. Neither a durable power of attorney (choice 1), health care by proxy (choice 3), nor the ethics committee (choice 4) are used as a means to withhold information from a client.

80. **The correct answer is 3.** The nurse will inform the health care provider of the client's concern. The nurse can provide the client education to help him understand the information (choice 2), but the nurse's role is not to obtain informed consent. The nurse is responsible for the verification of informed consent, witnessing the consent, and confirming the client has sufficient knowledge about his treatment. The health care provider must provide the client the information that is necessary for the client to make treatment decisions. The ethics committee (choice 1) is used to facilitate decision making in ethical situations. The client has the right to understand his treatment and should not have to have another person present to help him understand the information unless he chooses to do so (choice 4).

81. **The correct answer is 1.** The nurse should include in the teaching that emptying the pouch when it is one-third full will prevent the bag from dislodging the seal. The information in choice 2 doesn't make sense because a stoma should be pink or reddened. Choice 3 is incorrect because the time between eating gas-forming foods and flatulence for a client with an ileostomy is 2–4 hours, not 6–8. Choice 4 is also incorrect because premoistened wipes that contain alcohol should be avoided as they may affect skin barrier adherence.

82. **The correct answers are 4, 5, and 6.** Signs and symptoms of stimulant intoxication include chest pain, dilated pupils, and mental alertness. Paranoia (choice 1),

Answers Diagnostic Test

Answers Diagnostic Test

insomnia (choice 2), and irritability (choice 3) are symptoms associated with stimulant withdrawal.

83. **The correct answer is 2.** Diltiazem is a calcium channel-blocker that acts on the arterioles and heart to treat hypertension, angina, and dysrhythmias. Enalapril (choice 1) is an ACE inhibitor used in the treatment of heart failure. Nifedipine (choice 3) is used to treat hypertension and angina, but is not effective for dysrhythmias. Propranolol (choice 4) is a nonselective beta-adrenergic agonist used to treat dysrhythmias.

84. **The correct answer is 1.** Cancer often goes undiagnosed or is discovered in the later stages in the older adult because the older adult is less likely to be screened. A higher risk factor (choice 2), limited access to health care (choice 3), and the ability to recognize symptoms of cancer (choice 4) are not primary reasons cancer often goes undiagnosed in the older adult.

85. **The correct answers are 4, 5, and 6.** Aldosterone antagonists are potassium-sparing diuretics and should not be administered to clients with impaired kidney function or elevated serum potassium. The client's potassium, serum creatinine, and blood urea nitrogen must be monitored. The aPTT (choice 1), platelets (choice 2), and sodium (choice 3) are not the most important laboratory results to evaluate prior to the administration of an aldosterone antagonist.

86. **The correct answer is 2.** If an unexplained alarm sounds, the IV pump will be removed to prevent client injury from occurring. Following the health care facility's policy and procedure, the IV pump will be removed and evaluated for safety. Resetting (choice 1) or troubleshooting (choice 4) the pump are not appropriate actions. The pump will be sent to the proper department for further assessment (choice 3).

87. **The correct answer is 3.** Clients in the early stages of Alzheimer's disease will experience difficulty retrieving words that were once familiar. A client who sleeps more during the day (choice 1) and experiences changes in the ability to walk (choice 4) is demonstrating symptoms associated with the late stage of Alzheimer's disease. A client in the middle stages of Alzheimer's disease will require assistance with choosing clothing that is appropriate for the season (choice 2).

88. **The correct answer is shown below.** A patent foramen ovale is an opening in the atrial septum allowing blood to pass between the right and left atrium. Usually, the foramen ovale closes at birth when the blood pressure rises in the left side of the heart. If it does not close, this places a client at risk for a stroke, transient ischemic attacks, and a heart attack.

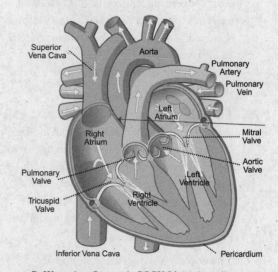

By Wapcaplet - Own work, CC BY-SA 3.0, https://commons.wikimedia.org/w/index.php?curid=830253

89. **The correct answer is 3.** The client should not apply pressure to a pin if it becomes loose. If a pin becomes loosened, the client is instructed to avoid excessive movement and immediately notify the health care provider. The statements in choices 1, 2, and 4 indicate the client needs no additional education. The client can shave the hair around the pin

sites. The client should not place any type of support under her head at night, but can use pillows for back support. Changes in weight can affect the fitting of the vest.

90. **The correct answer is 3.** When horizontally evacuating the clients, they will be moved to an adjacent safe smoke compartment on the same floor. The clients are not moved out of the facility (choice 1), transferred to the floor below (choice 2), or transferred to another unit (choice 4).

91. **The correct answers are 3, 4, and 5.** Factors that contribute to a false low blood pressure include positioning the client's arm above the heart, noise in the surrounding environment, and the stethoscope not directly placed over the client's artery. Deflating the cuff too slowly (choice 1), using a cuff that is too narrow (choice 2), or taking a blood pressure while the client's legs are crossed (choice 6) will result in a false high reading.

92. **The correct answer is 2.** The American Nurses Association's Standards of Professional Nursing Practice are authoritative statements of the duties that all registered nurses are to perform competently. The state boards of nursing (choice 1) are responsible for regulating the nursing practice as well as outlining the standards for safe nursing care and issuing licenses to practice nursing within a designated jurisdiction. Policy and procedures (choice 3) are resources that provide information about how nursing care is to be delivered. The NCSBN (choice 4) is an independent, not-for-profit organization through which nursing regulatory bodies act and consult together on matters of common interest and concern that affect public health, safety, and welfare, including the development of nursing licensure examinations.

93. **The correct answer is shown below.** A PEG tube is inserted through the abdominal wall and directly into the stomach. The PEG tube is used as a long-term feeding option that bypasses the mouth and swallowing mechanisms.

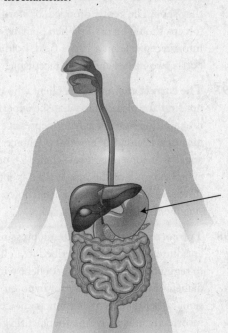

94. **The correct answer is 3.** Angiotensin II receptor blockers reduce the symptoms of heart failure and improve left ventricular function, resulting in an increased activity tolerance. Angiotensin II receptor blockers are not used to decrease angina (choice 1) or decrease blood pressure (choice 2) or to increase oxygen saturation (choice 4).

95. **The correct answer is 4.** The venturi mask is the only mask for which the amount of oxygen can be controlled. A client with COPD has chronic hypercapnia and requires controlled oxygen therapy to prevent further deterioration.

96. **The correct answer is 2.** Further education is needed to clarify that a one-inch border of a sterile field (not a two-inch border) is considered nonsterile. The statements in the other answer choices are accurate. Sterile objects should not be tossed on the field, they should be gently dropped, or sterile forceps should be used. When pouring water into a receptacle on a sterile field, hold the bottle two inches above the receptacle.

97. **The correct answer is 3.** A client who cannot find any pleasure in what she experiences is exhibiting signs of a major depressive disorder. Feelings of emptiness (choice 1), anger that comes and goes (choice 2), or expressed guilt of the lack of time spent with the deceased when he was alive (choice 4) are statements associated with grief.

98. **The correct answer is 3.** Desmopressin is an antidiuretic hormone prescribed to a client to regulate water excretion. A client with diabetes insipidus is at risk for hypotension, rather than hypertension as choice 1 incorrectly indicates. The therapeutic goal when administering desmopressin is not to improve cardiac output, so choice 2 is incorrect. Desmopressin does not regulate blood glucose levels, so choice 4 is not a therapeutic effect the nurse can anticipate.

99. **The correct answer is 2.** Loratadine is a second generation nonsedating H_1 antagonist used to treat seasonal allergies. If the client states that she expects to feel a bit dizzy after taking the medication, then further teaching is required. Dizziness should be immediately reported to the health care provider. The statements in choices 1, 3, and 4 are accurate and no further teaching is required. Loratadine can be taken with or without food. Loratadine may cause very little or no sedation; however, the client should avoid driving or other activities that require alertness until the response to the prescription is known. Loratadine should be taken 1–3 hours prior to the exposure to known allergies.

100. **The correct answers are 1, 2, and 3.** Atrial flutter can cause a decrease in cardiac output resulting in dyspnea, confusion, and chest pain. Decreased cardiac output is not characterized by flushed skin (choice 4), hypertension (choice 5), or peripheral edema (choice 6).

DIAGNOSTIC TEST ASSESSMENT GRID

Now that you've completed the diagnostic test and read through the answer explanations, you can use your results to target your studying. The following table shows you exactly where you can find thorough coverage for each client needs category. Find the question numbers from the diagnostic test that gave you the most trouble and highlight or circle them below. The chapters with the most markings are your ideal starting points on your preparation journey.

Client Needs Category	Question Number	Chapter Reference
Safe and Effective Care Environment	8, 9, 26, 28, 29, 31, 34, 35, 37, 38, 39, 43, 55, 56, 58, 60, 61, 66, 68, 72, 73, 74, 79, 80, 86, 89, 90, 92, 96	Chapter 3
Health Promotion and Maintenance	5, 15, 20, 44, 59, 65, 67, 77, 84, 91	Chapter 4
Psychosocial Integrity	4, 16, 42, 54, 69, 82, 87, 97	Chapter 5
Physiological Integrity	1, 2, 3, 6, 7, 10, 11, 12, 13, 14, 17, 18, 19, 21, 22, 23, 24, 25, 27, 30, 32, 33, 36, 40, 41, 45, 46, 47, 48, 49, 50, 51, 52, 53, 57, 62, 63, 64, 70, 71, 75, 76, 78, 81, 83, 85, 88, 93, 94, 95, 98, 99, 100	Chapter 6

What question type gave you the most trouble?

☐ Safe and Effective Care Environment

☐ Health Promotion and Maintenance

☐ Psychosocial Integrity

☐ Physiological Integrity

Chapters to focus on first: _____

PART III
NCLEX-RN® REVIEW

CHAPTER 3   Safe and Effective Care Environment

CHAPTER 4   Health Promotion and Maintenance

CHAPTER 5   Psychosocial Integrity

CHAPTER 6   Physiological Integrity

Safe and Effective Care Environment

OVERVIEW

- **Client Needs for Management of Care**
- **Case Management**
- **Client Rights**
- **Concepts of Management**
- **Information Security and Confidentiality**
- **Legal Rights and Responsibilities**
- **Client Needs for Safety and Infection Control**
- **Handling Hazardous and Infectious Materials**
- **Reporting of Incident/Event/Irregular Occurrence/Variance**
- **Safe Use of Equipment**
- **Home Safety**
- **Summing It Up**
- **Practice Questions: Safe and Effective Care Environment**
- **Answer Key and Explanations**

Nurses promote the achievement of client outcomes by providing and directing nursing care to enhance the delivery of health care and to protect clients and health care personnel. This chapter will cover the most important points that you need to know for questions in the Safe and Effective Care Environment category.

CLIENT NEEDS FOR MANAGEMENT OF CARE

The focus of the NCLEX-RN Management of Care subcategory is to assess the nurse's role in the promotion of client outcomes by providing and directing nursing care. The nursing focus is intended to enhance the care delivery setting and protect both the client and health care personnel. This chapter will highlight the nurse's legal and ethical role in the coordination of client care and collaboration with other members of the health care team to provide safe, cost-effective care while promoting optimum wellness and advocating for the client's rights. A client's rights include privacy, safety, and the ability to participate in all treatment decisions that affect his or her physical, mental, and spiritual well-being.

Chapter 3

CASE MANAGEMENT

Registered nurses who manage the care of clients provide education, obtain resources for the client, and monitor costs using a multidisciplinary approach to maintain the client's highest level of wellness in health care, community, and home care settings. Nursing case management involves creating and altering care plans that are individualized based on diagnosis, treatments, and the client's ability to care for him- or herself. Ongoing monitoring of a client using a case management model further allows the nurse to ensure that the client is receiving the appropriate level of care, that the interdisciplinary team members are effective, and that the client has the necessary materials and equipment, all the while advocating for cost-effective care.

Assignment, Delegation, and Supervision

To organize the workload and manage time effectively, the nurse responsible for the care of the clients may assign or delegate tasks to other health care workers, such as an LPN/VN, assistive personnel, or another RN. The act of **assignment** is defined by the NCSBN as, "The performance of designated nursing activities/tasks by a licensed nurse or certified nursing assistant that are consistent with the scope of practice of a licensed nurse or the role description of a certified nursing assistant; the distribution of work that each staff member is responsible for during a given work period." The act of **delegation** is defined by the NCSBN as, "Transferring to a competent individual the authority to perform a specific nursing task in a selected situation. The nurse retains the responsibility and accountability for the tasks."

Before delegating anything, it is imperative the nurse is knowledgeable about the practice act in the state where he or she is licensed. Furthermore, when considering the tasks or assignments to be delegated, each decision must observe the five "rights" of delegation, remembering that anything that involves critical decision making or nursing judgment cannot be delegated.

The five rights of delegation are as follows:

1. **Right task:** Is the task appropriate and centered on the client's needs based on the competency of personnel to whom it is assigned? Can the task be delegated legally? Is the task within the scope of practice of the delegatee? Do facility policies and procedures support the delegation?

2. **Right circumstances:** Are the resources, proper equipment, and the right supervision available? Is the client stable?

3. **Right person:** Do the assigned personnel have the ability and experience to perform the task using competent, prudent judgment and decision making?

4. **Right communication:** Have you, the RN, effectively communicated the tasks to be performed and the concerns that should be reported?

5. **Right supervision:** Have you, the RN, evaluated the task for correct completion? Have you evaluated the effectiveness of the delegatee's use of time management?

Collaboration with the Interdisciplinary Team

The nurse uses effective communication and planning when managing and coordinating client care with other disciplines. Using the four C's of effective communication reduces the chance for miscommunication that places the client at risk for ineffective treatment or injury. The nurse who uses the four C's provides clear, concise, correct, and complete communication. Through collaboration with interdisciplinary team members and client conferences, the health care team can participate in the ongoing review of the client's plan of care. The nurse also serves as a resource—based on his or her particular area of expertise—for other staff members to promote optimal quality care.

Performance Improvement (Quality Improvement)

The registered nurse is expected to have a clear understanding of and actively participate in performance improvement or quality assurance activities that are in place to measure and improve quality of care, client safety, client outcomes, and resource utilization. While participating in performance improvement or quality assurance projects, current evidence-based research and other references will be integrated into the process. Following the health care facility's policy and procedures, the nurse reports all potential and actual safety occurrences to the risk management department to help prevent future incidents or minimize the damage that has occurred.

Referrals

All clients will be assessed for actual or potential problems that require interdisciplinary care, such as a referral within the health care system or community. Collaboration with the health care provider may be necessary to obtain referrals that require a prescription. All communication and requests for referrals are completed based on the health care facility's policies and procedures, as well as carefully maintaining the client's right to privacy using only the required documents.

CLIENT RIGHTS

Patient bills of rights, such as the Patient's Bill of Rights set by the American Hospital Association (AHA) in 1973 and revised in 1992, exist to protect clients. The AHA Patient's Bill of Rights addresses the expectations that health care facilities, providers, and employees must uphold. Other essential bills of rights include those that specifically address the rights of clients with mental health conditions or who are receiving hospice care.

General areas addressed in the Patient's Bill of Rights include the following:

- Safety
- Privacy
- Refusal of treatment
- Access to medical records
- Access to emergency services
- Filing a complaint or grievance
- Dignity, respect, and nondiscrimination
- Choice of providers and health care plans
- The right to examine and receive an explanation of billing
- Information regarding diagnosis, treatment, and prognosis
- Confidentiality of health care information; information disclosure
- Receiving comprehensive information to make decisions about treatments

Client responsibilities are also included in the Patient's Bill of Rights. These responsibilities explain the expectations the health care provider has of the client, including the following:

- Provide accurate and complete information regarding current and past health, hospitalizations, and treatments

- Report unexpected changes in the client's condition to the health care provider

- Convey a clear understanding and comprehension of the plan of action

- Follow treatment plans and keeping appointments

- Accept financial responsibility

Nursing can further advocate and protect the client's rights by providing staff with education to help ensure that all members of the health care team support the client.

Advance Directives/Self-Determination/Life Planning

Federal law requires that all health care facilities, as well as other designated service providers, offer and provide written instruction regarding the use of advance directives. Nurses play a crucial role in educating and promoting the client's use of advance directives and ensuring they are integrated into the plan of care. The ANA's *Code of Ethics for Nurses with Interpretive Statements* requires nurses to provide education about advanced care planning and to be able to discuss the different types of advance directives with the client or family. The nurse can further support this initiative by encouraging completion of the document.

Advocacy

Advocacy entails protecting the safety and rights of the client, respecting the client's decisions, and promoting the discussion of treatment options and participation in treatment decisions. When nurses provide comprehensive education to their clients, they are empowering clients to actively participate in their care and enabling them to make decisions about their treatment plans. The nurse is responsible for utilizing the health care team as a resource to promote the advocacy of the client. Members of the health care team include interpreters, chaplains, social workers, those identified in the chain of command, or any professional who is needed to promote the wellness, safety, and rights of the client.

Informed Consent

Informed consent reflects the client's autonomy to accept or decline treatment after being informed of the risks and benefits of the offered treatment, as well as any alternative treatment options. Information for treatment is provided by the primary health care provider or the member of the health care team performing the treatment. Verbal and written consent, as well as any further written information, should be provided to the client in his or her spoken language. It is essential for the nurse to recognize that the client understands the information, and the nurse advocates accordingly on the client's behalf if there are any concerns. The client must not only understand the components of the informed consent, but must also voluntarily agree to treatment without coercion. Exceptions to informed consent include a life-threatening emergency, a voluntarily waived consent, and incapacitation. The essential components of informed consent include the following:

- The treatment or procedure

- Discussion of HIPAA laws

- The right to refuse treatment

- Alternative(s) to the treatment

- The necessity for the treatment

- Dissemination of client information

- Risks and benefits of the treatment

- Expected outcomes of the treatment

- Benefits and risks of alternative treatment

- The health care provider performing the treatment

When obtaining informed consent, the nurse must ascertain that the client is competent and of legal age, and can therefore provide consent. The nurse is responsible for verifying that the client has signed the consent and has sufficient knowledge to make a decision.

Generally, children under 18 years of age require parental or guardian permission for treatment; however, this age limitation varies from state to state. Although informed consent regarding minors is state-based, any legally emancipated minor may provide informed consent as long as he or she is able to give informed consent. Depending on state law, a minor may be considered emancipated if one of the following applies:

- Married (is or was legally married)

- Lives separately and is independent of parental support

- Emancipated by court order

- A current or former member of the Armed Forces

CONCEPTS OF MANAGEMENT

When managing the care of a client, the nurse coordinates the client's care by planning the strategies and evaluating outcomes that are necessary for optimal client wellness. It is important that the nurse understand the roles and responsibilities of all available interdisciplinary health care team members. In understanding each role, the nurse can effectively manage the care of the team and any conflict that may occur, as well as integrate the appropriate discipline into the client's plan of care.

Continuity of Care

Communication with other health care team members includes the use of the client's records, referrals, and transfer forms. The nurse will collaborate and communicate with other members of the health care team to provide a safe transition of care with the use of a facility-approved communication tool. Only abbreviations and standard terminology approved by the health care facility are used when communicating verbally or documenting in the client records. When the nurse receives a client for admission, the formulation of the plan of care is immediately initiated. All transfers and discharges also require nursing communication and coordination with a focus on maintaining the safety of the client. Any unresolved issues throughout the process will be addressed by the nurse using the proper chain of communication.

Establishing Priorities

The nurse applies concepts from the social, biological, and physical sciences to establish nursing priorities for interventions when caring for multiple clients. The individual client's care plan is also revised as needed to measure and evaluate client outcomes.

Ethical Practice

Ethical nursing practice should be reflective of the ANA's *Code of Ethics for Nurses with Interpretive Statements* (often referred to simply as "the code"). Following the health care facility's policy, the nurse will communicate concerns about ethical issues that affect both staff and clients. A priority goal during an ethical issue is to attempt to resolve the ethical dilemma or any conflict involving the client or health care team members. All outcomes of the interventions aimed to promote ethical practice and resolve conflict are evaluated for an appropriate and effective resolution.

INFORMATION SECURITY AND CONFIDENTIALITY

Information technology is used to capture, transmit, and store the health care data of a client. The benefits of information technology include, but are not limited to, enhanced communication, client safety, standardized care, computerized order entry, accessibility of up to date information, and efficient coordination of care.

When using electronic technology, the nurse is responsible for documenting information accurately, thoroughly, and in a timely manner, and—just as importantly—ensuring a client's prescriptions have been received, reviewed, and processed. Information technology provides the nurse with the opportunity to access evidence-based practice research and policies and procedures to safely and effectively care for the client. Clients can also be directed to reliable sources of health care information by the nurse.

The nurse has a professional, legal, and ethical responsibility to protect the client's rights to privacy and confidentiality. Medical records and client information should be protected and secured as mandated by the Health Insurance Portability and Accountability Act of 1996 (HIPAA); the HIPAA Privacy Rules; and the health care facility's policies, procedures, and regulations. Therefore, a client's medical records can only be accessed on a "need-to-know" basis by those providing indirect and direct care. HIPAA and the HIPAA Privacy Rule require each health care facility to provide employee regulations that reflect the law.

The HIPAA Security Rule requires "appropriate administrative, physical and technical safeguards to ensure the confidentiality, integrity, and security of electronic protected health information." The nurse has a legal obligation to intervene immediately if the client's health care records are breached by anyone, including visitors, family members, or other health care workers.

LEGAL RIGHTS AND RESPONSIBILITIES

Following the health care facility's policy and procedures, the registered nurse is directly responsible for safeguarding a client's valuables and personal property. When the client is admitted or transferred to a department, the nurse will obtain detailed documentation of items to be safeguarded, as well as ensuring that all items are returned upon discharge.

Based on the laws of the Nurse Practice Act, nurses are legally accountable for their practice, which includes only accepting assignments that adhere to the state practice act and are clearly within their scope of practice. An essential part of the nursing role in avoiding legal concerns is to provide education to staff, clients, and family members about their legal rights and responsibilities. When presenting this information, it is important to remember that the client always has the right to refuse any treatment. When ensuring that a client understands the treatment plan, the nurse is legally obliged to adhere to the federal and state mandates, as well as the health care facility's policies and procedures, when agreeing to serve as an interpreter for staff or a primary health care provider.

Federal and state laws require nurses to report suspected child abuse and neglect, medical neglect of children and the elderly, and elder abuse in the community or in nursing homes. Other mandated events that are to be reported include, but are not limited to, violence with weapons, some communicable diseases, unsafe practice by a health care provider, and suspected or known substance abuse by another health care worker.

CLIENT NEEDS FOR SAFETY AND INFECTION CONTROL

The focus of the NCLEX-RN Safety and Infection Control subcategory is to assess the nurse's judgment in protecting clients and health care personnel from both health and environmental hazards. Potential harmful situations include allergies, falls, electrical injury, failure to correctly identify a client while providing care, implementation of inappropriate or inaccurate treatment orders, failure to provide proper client education on safety issues, and the improper use of restraints.

The nurse can help prevent injury to a client and staff through participation in emergency response plans, application of proper ergonomic principles, safe use of equipment, and adherence to the security and emergency response plan. When safety issues arise or an adverse event occurs, the nurse has a duty to intervene as appropriate, acknowledge and document practice errors and near misses, and to report any unsafe practice of health care personnel. When implementing and adhering to proper measures for infection control, it is important that the nurse handle biohazardous waste and hazardous materials according to policies and procedures, apply the principles of infection control throughout all client and environmental encounters, and participate in the education of the clients and staff regarding the measures of infection control.

Accident/Error/Injury Prevention

A safe health care environment is based on the nurse's knowledge, skills, and ability to identify safety risks and implement the proper interventions to prevent accidents, errors, and injury to clients and other health care personnel. Maintaining a safe environment not only requires the identification of potential safety issues but necessitates the correction of any situation associated with a safety hazard. When the nurse recognizes any potential hazard, it should be immediately removed, and the finding reported according to the health care facility's policy and procedures.

The nurse is accountable for the proper verification of all clients. A National Patient Safety Goal identified by The Joint Commission (TJC) requires the use of two patient identifiers before providing any client care, treatment, or service. The two acceptable identifiers are determined by the health care facility and are found in the policy and procedures. Examples of acceptable identifiers include the client's full name, date of birth, medical record number, or other person-specific identifiers.

Allergy safety begins with the initial assessment of the client and continues throughout treatment using judicious ongoing monitoring of the client and the environment. Part of preventing injury to a client is the integration of allergies into the nursing plan of care. These allergies may include, but are not limited to, food, latex, environmental triggers, and medications.

A client's age, developmental stage, lifestyle, cognition, mental status, mobility, and sensory perception deficits are some of the factors that are taken into consideration when creating an environment of safety. An example of preventing injury based on a developmental risk factor is the correct use of infant and child car seats. Motor vehicle accidents are one of the major contributing factors to the injury and death of infants and children.

Altered sensory perception, cognition, mental status, or mobility may interfere with a client's ability to signal or communicate with a staff member. The nurse's inability to respond in a timely manner to a client who cannot communicate significantly increases the client's risk for falls and injury. The unresponsiveness of the nurse is not intentional; it is due to the nurse's lack of awareness of the client's need for assistance. When planning safe care for this client, an appropriate room assignment should be considered, such as placing the client closest to the nurse's station. Safe room assignments should always be considered when caring for clients with any identified conditions, including those who require seizure precautions to help prevent accidents or injury.

Other risk factors that place the client at risk for injury include incontinence, disease states, medications, and faulty equipment. Faulty equipment or inappropriate use of equipment can result in significant injury or death to a client or health care personnel.

When caring for a client, the nurse has a professional, legal, and ethical obligation to fully understand and review the treatments, procedures, and prescriptions for appropriateness and accuracy. When questions arise, the nurse will seek clarification through collaboration with the health care provider or interdisciplinary team members who are involved in the prescribed treatment. Carrying out treatments, procedures, and administering prescriptions that the nurse does not fully understand is a safety hazard and places the client at risk for injury or death.

Another consideration for accident, error, and injury prevention includes maintaining the integrity of the client's musculoskeletal system through proper body alignment, positioning, and safe client handling. The client may also require a specific exercise routine to be integrated into the plan of care to maintain musculoskeletal functioning.

Standard Precautions/Transmission-Based Precautions/Surgical Asepsis

The CDC identifies the first tier of infection control as **standard precautions**. Standard precautions are the minimum infection control practices that are applied to all clients regardless of their unconfirmed or confirmed infectious status. The role of safeguarding clients from infectious diseases rests largely on nursing. Adhering to the recommended precautions and recognizing sources of infection are key to prevention. Sources of infection are not always the clients or staff. Client care areas, floors, IV poles, beds, mobile equipment, and bed railings are just some potential sources of infection.

Understanding and actively practicing the use of standard precautions will help prevent and control the transmission of microorganisms among clients and health care workers. Standard precautions are used to prevent the transmission of diseases that may be acquired through contact with blood, body fluids, or other unrecognizable sources.

Standard precautions include the following:

- Use of personal protective equipment (PPE)
- Sharps safety
- Hand hygiene
- Respiratory hygiene
- Safe injection practices
- Sterile instruments and devices
- Cleanliness and disinfection of environmental surfaces

Transmission-based precautions are the second tier of infection control. These precautions are used in addition to standard precautions when there is a suspected or known infection. Each type of precaution requires a specific kind of isolation as well as PPE.

Precautions include the following:

- **Contact precautions:** Used for clients with known or suspected infections that represent an increased risk for contact transmission. Clients with conditions such as open wounds, MRSA, VRE, RSV, or diarrheal illness require contact isolation.

- **Droplet precautions:** Implemented for clients known or suspected to be infected with pathogens transmitted by respiratory droplets that are generated by coughing, sneezing, or talking. Clients with conditions such as pneumonia, whooping cough, bacterial meningitis, or influenza require droplet precautions.

- **Airborne precautions:** Implemented for clients known or suspected to be infected with pathogens transmitted by the airborne route. Clients with conditions such as measles, chickenpox, or tuberculosis require airborne precautions.

When applying the principles of infection control the nurse will use either **aseptic technique** or **clean technique**, depending on the clinical situation. Aseptic technique should always be used to minimize the risk of contaminating an invasive device or during an invasive procedure. When using an aseptic technique or monitoring another health care worker performing a procedure for a client that requires aseptic technique, the nurse is responsible for evaluating whether the technique is performed correctly.

TJC identifies the difference between aseptic and clean technique as follows:

Aseptic Technique

- Utilization of barriers: sterile gloves, gowns, drapes, mask

- Client preparation and equipment: antiseptic skin preparation; sterile instruments, equipment, and devices

- Environmental controls: keeping doors closed and minimizing traffic in and out of operating rooms; excluding unnecessary personnel during procedures

- Contact guidelines: sterile-to-sterile contact

Clean Technique

- Utilization of barriers: appropriate hand hygiene, clean gloves

- Client preparation and equipment: prevent direct contamination of supplies and materials

- Environmental controls: routine cleaning of the client's environment

- Contact guidelines: sterile-to-sterile rule does not apply

The health care facility's policies and procedures for infection control will be used by the nurse to understand and utilize the proper measures to address the potential infectious risks to staff and clients. For example, when caring for an immunocompromised client, the primary goal is to protect the client from potential infections. Protecting the immunosuppressed client requires that the nurse include precautions strictly adhering to transmission-based precautions in the client's plan of care.

By monitoring the accuracy and effectiveness of infection control precautions implemented by staff members, the nurse has the opportunity to protect the client and provide staff education as needed. By providing staff education about infection control for a client, the nurse can significantly reduce the risk of transmitting harmful microorganisms. Infection control measures such as handwashing and respiratory etiquette should also be included in client education to help prevent the transmission of microorganisms. Other nursing responsibilities include following the state laws for reporting communicable diseases to the proper authorities, such as the public health department and the CDC.

Emergency Response Plan

The overall organization of client care in an emergency response plan is based on the principles of **triage**. The nurse is responsible for triaging clients during an internal or external disaster. Triage requires the ability to think both rapidly and critically, and to accurately assess clients using a decision-making process. Decision-making processes are based on the health care facility's emergency response plan and its policy and procedures. Models that may be used are three- or five-tiered systems or color-coded tags for classification of the acuity of clients.

TJC requires that all health care facilities create an emergency response plan that includes conducting risk assessments, establishing policy and procedures, providing annual training, and conducting emergency drills. Since nurses are responsible for the clients in the health care facility, it is imperative that they participate in all phases of the planning for the emergency response plan.

Security Plan

In order to effectively and efficiently maintain client and staff safety, the nurse must be familiar with client triage, as well as the health care facility's security plan and evacuation policy, procedures, and protocols. Emergent situations require critical thinking, rapid clinical decision making, and effective communication on the part of the nurse. Through involvement and training in the security plan, the nurse will gain an understanding of prevention and his or her role during an emergent situation.

Awareness of and familiarity with the security plan will enable the nurse to effectively and safely participate in both external and internal emergent situations. Some examples of external emergencies for which the nurse should be prepared include natural disasters; mass casualties; chemical, biological, or radiological attacks; infectious disease emergencies; and community violence. Internal emergencies that may occur include infant abduction, violence, fire, bomb threats, or active shooting. Participation in security planning enables the nurse to provide input into the use of security measures, such as special badges in secured areas, alarmed doors, alarmed client wrist bands to prevent infant abductions, mock emergency disaster drills, security breaches, areas that require closed-circuit monitoring, and visiting policies.

HANDLING HAZARDOUS AND INFECTIOUS MATERIALS

Hazardous materials are substances that can harm humans or the environment. Nurses will handle hazardous and infectious materials such as radioactive material, chemicals, gases, or drugs. The Occupational Safety and Health Administration (OSHA) requires hazardous materials to be identified by a Safety Data Sheet (SDS) label. Information that is helpful to document on an SDS label includes the following:

- Chemical ingredients
- All hazards regarding the chemical
- Safe handling storage and incompatibilities
- Potential for fire or explosion and how to properly extinguish if it occurs
- Emergency procedures, protective equipment, and proper methods of containment and cleanup
- First-aid measures, important effects, acute and delayed symptoms, and required treatment
- Identification of the product including recommended use, restrictions of use, and emergency contact information for the manufacturer or distributor

TJC has adopted the OSHA regulations requiring that all flammable and combustible medical gases be placed in approved safety containers, specifically labeled and color-coded based on the gas they contain. When handling flammable, combustible material, it is important that the nurse follow the specific regulations for the use, handling, and storage of both portable gas systems as well as the centralized medical gas system. Knowing the location for the centralized gas shut-off valves can prevent injury during an emergency, as can the nurse's familiarity with his or her specific role during an emergency.

Handling infectious materials that include blood, tissue, body fluid, and secretions requires the nurse to be familiar with the following basic safety principles:

- Hand hygiene
- Special precautions
- Standard precautions
- Proper use of gloves
- Transmission precautions
- Proper use of PPE
- Single-client use of disposable items and equipment
- Proper handling and transferring of blood, body fluid, and tissue specimens
- Proper disposal of contaminated supplies, such as instruments and linens
- Proper disposal of sharps and syringes in the health care facility and community
- Proper identification of infectious materials such as color-coded waste receptacles or biohazard bags

The SDS and the health care facility's policies and procedures provide explicit instructions on proper handling, transfer, and disposal of biohazardous and hazardous materials. It is essential for the nurse to be able to identify all biohazardous, flammable, and infectious materials to prevent unnecessary exposure to self, other health care workers, and the client. All staff and clients who are at risk for exposure to any hazardous or infectious materials should be adequately educated on the techniques for safe handling and disposal.

Whenever there is a known risk to external ionizing radiation (x-rays and gamma rays) or internal radiation (brachytherapy) exposure, nurses will adhere to the principle of **ALARA (as low as reasonably achievable)**. ALARA means that even if the dose is small enough to have no direct benefit, it should be avoided.

Radiation safety principles to be followed include the following:

- **Time:** Reduce the time of exposure.
- **Distance:** Increase the distance between you and the radiation source.
- **Shielding:** Use lead or a lead equivalent to shield yourself from x-rays and gamma rays.

Special additional radiation precautions are taken for clients receiving brachytherapy. **Brachytherapy** is an implant therapy in which a sealed source of radioactivity is implanted in a body cavity close to the tumor and left in place for a period of time. Additional precautions include, but are not limited to, the following:

- Placing the client in a private room
- Wearing a dosimeter when caring for the client
- Minimizing time spent in the client's room
- Preventing all pregnant women from entering the room
- Keeping all supplies ready and available in the client's room

- Wearing appropriate PPE when coming in contact with contaminated objects or fluids
- Following the health care facility's policy and procedures for handling dislodged implanted devices
- Instructing all visitors to remain at least six feet away from the client and limiting visitation time to one hour or less over a 24-hour period

REPORTING OF INCIDENT/EVENT/IRREGULAR OCCURRENCE/VARIANCE

The purpose of reporting any incident, event, irregular occurrence, or variance is to provide a system for prompt investigation and immediate action as appropriate to rectify the situation. When reporting an incident, the report should contain complete factual data adhering to the health care facility's policy and procedures and use of the proper chain of command. Reporting of all occurrences allows the risk management and quality improvement departments to effectively take action and to track and identify trend data over time to create a safe and accountable health care environment.

Terms that the nurse must be familiar with include the following:

- **Incident:** unusual occurrence that causes unanticipated harm to another
- **Risk:** anything that could potentially cause harm
- **Variance:** deviation from the standard of practice or routine care

The nurse must recognize common reportable instances, such as medical incidents, unintended additional treatments, wrong or missed scheduled treatments, loss or damage of personal property, unsafe practice, employee or health care provider substance abuse, unsafe staffing patterns, improper care, and environmental potential or actual risks.

Issues that require occurrence reporting include, but are not limited to, the following:

- **Defects:** an imperfection of a machine or device that poses a risk or harm to the client or employees
- **Errors:** unintentional mistakes such as administering the wrong medication
- **Near miss:** an event or incident that could have resulted in an accident, injury, or illness, but did not, either through chance or timely intervention
- **Sentinel event:** an unexpected occurrence involving death or serious physical or psychological injury, or the risk thereof. Serious injury specifically includes loss of a limb or function. The phrase "or the risk thereof" includes any process variation for which a recurrence would carry a significant chance of a serious adverse outcome.

SAFE USE OF EQUIPMENT

Maintaining client and health care staff safety requires proper training before using any equipment, selection of appropriate equipment, inspection of the equipment, and education of clients about safe use. Some examples of standard equipment that may be used by nurses include stretchers, client lifts, oxygen, and intravenous pumps. Equipment that may pose a safety hazard for a client includes includes, but is not limited to, oxygen, wheelchairs, canes, crutches, and walkers. Equipment that is past due for inspection for preventative maintenance, has frayed electrical cords, or has loose or missing parts is hazardous and may cause injury. Any equipment suspected of being unsafe or subject to malfunctions should be immediately removed from the client care area and reported to the appropriate personnel following the health care facility's policy and procedure.

Ergonomic Principles

Prevention of injury to a client requires the nurse's self-awareness of ergonomic principles. Proper use of muscles to maintain body alignment and posture will promote proper body mechanics for safe client handling and prevention of self or client injury. All client care planning should take place after the nurse has assessed the client's ability to balance and transfer, as well as any requirement for assistive devices. The nurse's knowledge of ergonomic principles ensures the client is correctly positioned in the proper body alignment to promote wellness and prevent reparative stress injuries.

Use of Restraints/Safety Devices

TJC has standards that limit the use of physical and chemical restraints in health care settings. Before considering the use of restraints, it is important for the nurse to implement preventative measures.

Preventative measures include the following:

- Distraction
- Redirecting the client
- De-escalation strategies
- Use of bed or chair alarms
- Offering client activities
- Promptly addressing the client's needs
- Assessing the need for food, fluids, and comfort
- Having a staff/family member sit with the client

If restraints are required to maintain the safety of the client or staff, the least restrictive restraint is chosen. Restraints are used only in emergency situations and not on an "as needed" basis. The health care facility's policy and procedures provide guidelines for obtaining a prescription for restraints. The facility's policy and procedures also direct staff on the use and removal of restraints and convey the nurse's responsibility while caring for a client requiring restraints.

Some of the nursing responsibilities to be carried out within specific time frames while the client is restrained include the following:

- Toileting
- Hydration
- Range of motion
- Psychological needs
- Offer of fluids and food
- Skin checks for breakdown
- Circulatory checks in the extremities
- Assessment of mental status including behavior and cognition

The nurse's overall goal is to keep the client safe while at all times maintaining his or her dignity and to remove the restraints as soon as the client is assessed to be safe from self-harm or harm to others.

HOME SAFETY

Because most accidents occur in the home, it is essential for the nurse to perform a comprehensive **home safety assessment**. The assessment is based on the client's pathophysiology and will help identify environmental risks for injury as well as possible fire hazards in the home. Factors within the home that increase the client's risk for injury include, but are not limited to, the following:

- Clutter
- Steep steps
- Throw rugs
- Fire hazards
- Extension cords
- Uneven flooring
- Unstable furniture
- Unsanitary conditions
- Improper food storage
- Frayed electrical cords
- Poor lighting (too bright or too dim)

Other considerations for safety include the client's use of required health care equipment in the home. Equipment such as monitors, respiratory equipment, and ambulatory equipment are a few examples of home health devices that should be considered when assessing and implementing safety education and home modification.

When collaborating with the client and family, the nurse will assess for the understanding of the client's condition and knowledge of side effects of medications as well as other potential factors that may cause injury. Any health care equipment used in the home that requires client and family teaching will be evaluated for proper use by the nurse through observed return demonstration. Verification of the availability of protective equipment, such as a sharps containers or gloves and any other necessary safety equipment, is also included in the care plan.

SUMMING IT UP

- The nurse responsible for the care of the clients may assign or delegate tasks to other health care workers to organize the workload and manage time effectively. The **five "rights" of delegation** are as follows:

  1. Right task

  2. Right circumstances

  3. Right person

  4. Right communication

  5. Right supervision

- The nurse communicates with other health care team members to provide a safe transition of care and applies concepts from the social, biological, and physical sciences to establish nursing priorities for interventions when caring for multiple clients.

- General areas addressed in the **AHA Patient Bills of Rights** include the following:

  - Safety

  - Privacy

  - Refusal of treatment

  - Access to medical records

  - Access to emergency service

  - Filing a complaint or grievance

  - Dignity, respect, and nondiscrimination

  - Choice of providers and health care plans

  - The right to examine and receive an explanation of billing

  - Information regarding diagnosis, treatment, and prognosis

  - Confidentiality of health care information

  - Information disclosure

  - Receiving comprehensive information to make decisions about treatments

- Federal law requires that all health care facilities, as well as other designated service providers, offer and provide written instruction regarding the use of **advance directives**. The American Nurses Association (ANA) requires nurses to provide education about **advanced care planning** and to be able to discuss the different types of advance directives.

- **Advocacy** entails protecting the safety and rights of the client, respecting the client's decisions, and promoting the discussion of treatment options and participation in treatment decisions.

- **Informed consent** reflects the client's autonomy to agree or decline treatment after being informed of the risks, benefits, and alternatives of the offered treatment. The nurse must recognize that the client understands the information and advocates accordingly on his or her behalf if there are any concerns.

- Ethical nursing practice should reflect the ANA's *Code of Ethics for Nurses with Interpretive Statements*.

- **Information technology** is used to capture, transmit, and store the health care data of a client.

- Registered nurses are directly responsible for safeguarding clients' valuables and personal property and are also legally accountable for their practice—which includes only accepting assignments that adhere to the state practice act and are clearly within their scope of practice. RNs are also accountable for actively participating in quality assurance, proper verification of all clients, and prevention of injury to clients and staff.

- The overall organization of client care in an emergency response plan is based on the principles of **triage**. Nurses are responsible for triaging clients during disasters, which requires the ability to think critically and accurately assess clients.

- Nurses are responsible for **reporting** any incident, event, irregular occurrence, or variance. RNs are also responsible for the following:

  - Taking any appropriate action to rectify a situation

  - Using equipment safely

  - Having a clear understanding of the health care facility's security plan

  - Understanding and actively practicing the use of standard precautions to help prevent and control the transmission of microorganisms among clients and health care workers

  - Using restraints and other safety devices appropriately

- Nurses must be aware of **ergonomic principles** to prevent client injuries, handle hazardous and infectious materials safely, and assess a client's pathophysiology to identify environmental risks for injury.

PRACTICE QUESTIONS: SAFE AND EFFECTIVE CARE ENVIRONMENT

Directions: The following are examples of the types of questions you will encounter on the NCLEX-RN exam. Read each question carefully and choose the best answer unless otherwise directed. Check your answers against the answer key and explanations that follow.

1. A client is discussing his advance directive with the nurse. Which statement made by the client indicates an understanding of the document?
   1. "I would like my organs donated if something happens to me."
   2. "My son can make decisions about my health care if I am unable."
   3. "I just do not want to be resuscitated if something happens to me."
   4. "It is important my son have access to my medical records if I become seriously ill."

2. A client discharged from the hospital tells the nurse she can no longer afford her prescriptions for treatment. Which is the best action for the nurse to take?
   1. Contact a community social worker.
   2. Contact the client's insurance company.
   3. Request a generic version from the pharmacy.
   4. Research an alternative treatment for the client.

3. The nurse observes an upset family member reading a terminally ill client's electronic health care record. Which **initial** action should the nurse take?
   1. Contact the security department.
   2. Notify the risk management department.
   3. Check the client's records for a power of attorney.
   4. Escort the family member away from the computer.

4. Which task(s) should the nurse delegate to assistive personnel? **Select all that apply.**
   1. Culture a surgical incision.
   2. Collect a sputum specimen.
   3. Assist a client who is receiving bladder training.
   4. Remain with a client who is on suicide precautions.
   5. Obtain vital signs for a client who is due to receive digoxin.
   6. Apply a cold application to the swelling of a client's injured area.

5. Which nursing action describes the commitment of assault?
   1. Administering an injection that a client refused
   2. Failure to administer the proper dosage of a prescription
   3. Administering prescriptions to keep a client from waking at night
   4. Telling a client he will be restrained if he refuses a physical assessment

6. Which **initial** action should the nurse take to decrease the rate of catheter-associated urinary tract infections that have occurred on the unit?
   1. Provide staff education.
   2. Consult with the infection control nurse.
   3. Initiate a performance improvement activity.
   4. Review the records of the clients with infections.

7. The nurse in a client unit observes smoke coming from under the door of the supply room. Which **initial** action should the nurse take?

1. Extinguish the fire.
2. Evacuate the clients.
3. Activate the fire alarms.
4. Assess the source of the smoke.

8. Which should the nurse include in the assessment of an adult client's mobility before transfer?

1. Range of motion
2. Weight and height
3. Cognitive functioning
4. Physical therapy consult

9. A nurse is preparing to add an instrument to a sterile field. After opening the package, what technique should the nurse employ?

1. Hold the packaging and instrument over the middle of the sterile field.
2. Drop the instrument close to the edge of the field.
3. Apply sterile gloves and place the instrument on the field.
4. Stand as close as possible to the sterile field and drop the instrument close to an open space.

10. The nurse has provided education about home meal preparation for a client receiving chemotherapy. Which statement made by the client indicates further teaching is required?

1. "I will make sure my refrigerator is set below 40 degrees."
2. "I will peel the fruits and vegetables before eating them."
3. "I will eat any cooked meat within 24 hours of refrigeration."
4. "I will use a disinfectant to clean my kitchen countertops after each use."

ANSWER KEY AND EXPLANATIONS

1. 1	3. 4	5. 4	7. 2	9. 3
2. 1	4. 2, 3, 4, 6	6. 3	8. 1	10. 2

1. **The correct answer is 1.** A living will contains end-of-life decisions such as organ donation, so the statement in choice 1 best indicates the client's understanding of his advance directive. Choice 3 indicates that the client is referring to a DNR. It is not necessary to have an advance directive or living will to request a DNR status. The client can convey this directive to the health care provider so a DNR prescription can be documented in the medical record. A DNR prescription is needed with each hospital admission and should be reviewed and renewed per institutional policy. The statements in choices 2 and 4 indicate that the client is referring to a durable power of attorney for health care that would allow another (in this case, his son) to make medical decisions on his behalf and will also allow for his son to access his medical records if the client is unable to make any health care decisions.

2. **The correct answer is 1.** It is important to utilize advocacy resources appropriately. Contacting a community social worker is the best action for the nurse to take. A social worker is aware of many resources that can assist the client in obtaining her prescriptions that are necessary for treatment. It is not appropriate for the nurse to contact the insurance company (choice 2). Any change in the prescription (choice 3) must be through the prescriber. Alternative treatments (choice 4) should be discussed with the health care provider and the client.

3. **The correct answer is 4.** The nurse has a legal obligation to protect the privacy of the client and must correct the situation immediately by not allowing the violation to continue. The nurse should escort the family member away from the computer. Contacting the security department, if necessary (choice 1) notifying the risk management department (choice 2), and checking the client's records for a power of attorney (choice 3) are actions that would occur after the initial action to protect the client's privacy.

4. **The correct answers are 2, 3, 4, and 6.** The tasks listed in choices 3, 4, and 6 can all be delegated to assistive personnel. Assistive personnel can also collect a sputum specimen (choice 2), but only if the specimen is obtained by noninvasive means. The RN should not delegate assessing the surgical incision (choice 1) and obtaining the culture as well as monitoring the apical pulse (choice 5) before administering the digoxin.

5. **The correct answer is 4.** Telling a client he will be restrained if he refuses a physical assessment is an assault. Administering an injection that a client refused (choice 1) reflects the act of battery. Failure to administer the proper dosage of a prescription (choice 2) is negligence. Administering prescriptions to keep a client from waking at night (choice 3) is a form of false imprisonment.

6. **The correct answer is 3.** The goal of performance improvement is to improve the client outcomes of care, and is mandated by external regulating and credentialing agencies. The initiation of a performance improvement activity includes working collaboratively, a possible review of the records, and staff education.

7. **The correct answer is 2.** The initial step is to rescue anyone in immediate danger by following the instructions for the vertical or

horizontal evacuation of the clients. After the evacuation, the alarm should be activated (choice 3). If the smoke and fire are identified (choice 4) and contained, then efforts to extinguish the fire (choice 1) can begin.

8. **The correct answer is 1.** The range of motion should be included in the assessment before transferring the client. The client's weight and height (choice 2) and cognitive functioning (choice 3) do not specifically affect mobility. A physical therapy consult (choice 4) is not necessary for a routine assessment of mobility.

9. **The correct answer is 3.** When adding an instrument to a sterile field, the nurse should open the package, apply sterile gloves, and place the instrument on the field. The other answer choices can potentially disrupt the sterile items and contaminate the area.

10. **The correct answer is 2.** It is not necessary to peel all fruits and vegetables. Some fruits and vegetables may be washed with soap and water. The temperature of the refrigerator should be kept below 40°F (choice 1). Refrigerated cooked meat (choice 3) should be eaten within 3 to 4 days. Kitchen countertops should be disinfected (choice 4) after use.

Health Promotion and Maintenance

Chapter 4

- Newborn Care
- Transitions
- Prevention

- Assessment

- Practice Questions: Health Promotion and Maintenance

- Answer Key and Explanations

The focus of the NCLEX-RN Health Promotion and Maintenance category is to assess the nurse's ability to provide and direct nursing care for the client that incorporates knowledge of expected milestones for physical, emotional, social, and cognitive growth and development. Understanding these domains is useful in the prevention and early detection of health problems and will help guide the nurse in creating strategies to achieve optimal wellness.

THE AGING PROCESS

While multiple theories can be applied to nursing practice, Erik Erikson's stages of psychosocial development and Jean Piaget's cognitive development theory are widely used in nursing when assessing psychosocial and cognitive development. Each developmental period described by Erikson represents a stage or **maturational crisis** that must be completed to achieve a healthy personality and successful interactions with others. Examples of maturational crises that occur throughout development include events such as adolescence, marriage, parenthood, midlife, or retirement.

Just as a maturational crisis may happen, a **situational crisis** may occur throughout the stages of development. A situational crisis is an event such as pregnancy, loss of a job, the death of a spouse, or physical illness.

While not associated with growth and development, the effect of an **adventitious crisis** is important to recognize when caring for a client or family. An adventitious crisis is an unexpected tragedy that includes both natural and man-made disasters, such as an earthquake or a plane crash. The sudden, unplanned nature of the crisis often results in long-term psychological effects.

Piaget's theory of the stages of cognitive development is descriptive of a child's ability to understand concepts based on the child's developmental age.

Physical development is included in all assessments from newborn throughout adolescence. These assessments provide the nurse with the opportunity to educate the family and caregivers about the social, emotional, language/communication, cognitive, and physical development of their children. The Center for Disease Control publishes a "Milestone Checklist" the nurse can provide for the family to help monitor the overall age-appropriate development of a child. By engaging clients and their families in understanding the changes that occur throughout the lifespan, the nurse can establish a strong foundation to promote the health and wellness of the client and family.

The nurse's role throughout the lifespan includes the promotion of client and community wellness through education. Before providing care and education, health risks are assessed based on the family, population, and community. When promoting wellness, the nurse will perform comprehensive health assessments and screenings and promote the prevention of and offer treatment for high-risk health behaviors. The results of the evaluation of the client's ability to care for himself or herself in the home environment are integrated into the plan of care. When providing education, the nurse will take into consideration the client's readiness for learning, learning preferences, and any barriers to learning.

Many physical, psychosocial, and cognitive age-related changes occur throughout a client's lifespan. Natural, expected, or unexpected changes may arise in relation to illness. The nurse will assess the coping skills of the client and family throughout these changes. Providing clients and families with anticipatory guidance to prepare for these changes will help promote understanding and identify ways to cope with change.

Newborn Assessment

When providing care throughout the lifespan, the nurse will provide client and family care based on the client's age. When caring for a newborn, the assessment begins with a review of maternal health, pregnancy, labor, and delivery. The neonatal period ranges from birth to 28 days old, with the first major transition in life occurring from birth through the first 6–8 hours of life. This period is considered a transition from intrauterine to extrauterine life. Immediately after birth, the newborn must make many physiological adaptations that involve the heart rate, respiratory rate, and temperature regulation.

In the immediate period after birth, the nurse will use the **Apgar score** to describe the physiological state of a newborn during the transition after birth. Developed by anesthesiologist Virginia Apgar in 1952, the factors assessed by the Apgar score are represented by an acronym based on the last name of its inventor:

- **A:** Appearance, specifically skin color
- **P:** Pulse (heart rate)
- **G:** Grimace (reflex irritability)
- **A:** Activity (muscle tone)
- **R:** Respiratory effort

Each category has a maximum score of 2 and a minimum of 0. The higher the score, the more physiological stabile the newborn. The score is calculated at one and five minutes, and every five minutes after that for up to 20 minutes if the score is less than 7 at five minutes. Scores of 0–3 indicate severe distress, 4–6 means moderate difficulty, and 7–10 indicates minimal or no difficulty adjusting to extrauterine life.

At birth, the newborn is assessed to determine estimated gestational age using the **New Ballard Score**. This tool assesses the neurological and physical criteria to estimate the gestational age of the newborn. The New Ballard Score is accurate only within plus or minus two weeks of the expected date of delivery and is used to assign gestational age only when there is no reliable obstetrical information or there is a significant discrepancy between the obstetrically defined gestational age and the findings upon physical examination. The criteria used for the New Ballard Score are listed below.

Criteria used to assess physical maturity include the following:

- Skin

- Lanugo

- Plantar surface

- Breast

- Ear/eye

- Genitals (gender specific)

Criteria for neuromuscular maturity include the following:

- Posture

- Square window

- Arm recoil

- Popliteal angle

- Scarf sign

- Heel to ear

The scores assigned in each category range from –1 to 5. All scores are added together to determine the gestational age of the newborn. Scores can range from –10 to 50, and a lower score correlates with prematurity (born before 37 weeks gestation), whereas a higher score is associated with postmaturity (born after 42 weeks gestation).

Further newborn evaluation includes, but is not limited to, the following:

- **Axillary temperature:** 36.5–37.5°C (97.7–99.5°F)

- **Respiratory rate:** 30–60 breaths/minute

- **Apical pulse:** 110–160 beats/minute

- **Systolic blood pressure:** 60–80 mmHg, diastolic blood pressure 40–50 mmHg

- **Mean arterial pressure (MAP):** approximately the same as the newborn's gestational age

- **Birth weight:** 2,500–4,000 g (5.5–8.8 lbs.)

- **Length:** 18–22 inches (46–56 cm)

- **Head circumference:** 33–35 cm (normally 2 cm larger than chest circumference)

- **Chest circumference:** 31–33 cm

- **General appearance:** muscle tone, posture, general activity, consciousness, size

- **Behavior:** alert, quiet, crying, lethargic (Brazelton behavioral scale most frequently used)

- **Skin:** color, edema, turgor, nails, vernix, lanugo, physiological jaundice, Mongolian spots, birthmarks, nevus flammeous, telangiectatic nevi petechiae, café au lait, and port wine stains. Other common findings after birth include acrocyanosis, mottling, harlequin sign, erythema toxicum, and skin tags. The umbilical cord/clamp is assessed with an expected finding of a three-vessel cord.

- **Head:** appearance, fontanels (should be flat), the presence of molding, overriding sutures, caput succedaneum, cephalohematoma, forceps or vacuum markings

- **Neck:** appearance, range of motion, clavicles

- **Face:** symmetry

- **Eyes:** red reflex, color

- **Ears:** pinna alignment with outer canthus of eyes, placement, malformations, startle reflex

- **Nose:** nasal patency

- **Mouth:** intact palate, tongue, sucking and rooting reflex, moist mucous, Epstein's pearls

- **Chest:** synchronous chest movement, symmetrical nipples

- **Heart:** apical pulse, heart sounds

- **Lungs:** breath sounds, breathing pattern

- **Abdomen:** shape, bowel sounds

- **Genitalia:**
  - Female: edema of labia majora and minora, vaginal discharge of bloody mucus
  - Male: urinary meatus, rugae on the scrotum, palpable testes

- **Anus:** inspected for patency, any urine or stool noted

- **Back:** trunk incurvature, intact spine

- **Pulses:** brachial and femoral

- **Extremities:** posture, flexion, tone, the range of motion, palmar and plantar creases, number of fingers and toes, grasp, Moro and Babinski reflexes, length of legs, creases in posterior thighs, and Ortolani's maneuver to assess for hip dislocation

The nurse will also obtain parental permission and provide education for additional newborn procedures. This includes prescriptions routinely administered to a newborn after birth, such as erythromycin for eye prophylaxis; vitamin K to promote clotting; and, before discharge, a hepatitis B vaccination. Routine newborn blood testing includes blood type and Rh, newborn screenings for metabolic disorders, and—if indicated—a total serum bilirubin or Coombs test. Noninvasive procedures included in routine care are a hearing screening and a transcutaneous bilirubin measurement.

Additional newborn education provided to the parents includes the following:

- Holding

- Bathing

- Skin care

- Dressing

- Nutrition

- Diapering

- Suctioning

- Positioning

- Care of nails

- Stooling/voiding

- Umbilical cord care

- Feeding breast/bottle

- Health care provider visits

- Circumcision care (if applicable)

- Infection control; prevention of illness

- Indications to immediately notify the provider

Additional education provided to parents includes anticipatory guidance for safety concerns related to safe sleep, medicine, home environment, secondhand smoke, car seats, shaken baby syndrome, water, and lead poisoning.

Assessment of Infants

When the newborn period ends, infancy begins. The period of infancy lasts from 4 weeks to 1 year of age. Examination of an infant who is not able to sit alone is conducted with the infant laying on an examination table with the parent in full view. When the infant can sit, it is preferable to examine the infant on the parent's lap. The infant may be completely undressed; however, a diaper is left on a male until ready to examine the genital area. All auscultation is performed while the infant is quiet, and the reflexes are assessed proceeding in a head-to-toe fashion along with the rest of the examination.

Nursing care of the infant includes a physical exam and an assessment of the following:

- Sleep

- Nutrition

- Oral health

- Elimination

- Immunizations

- Family system

- Developmental surveillance

- Psychosocial/behavioral assessment

- Developmental screening at 9 months

- Measurement of length/weight, head circumference

- Lab tests—hematocrit and hemoglobin at 12 months of age

- Vital signs obtained in the following order: respirations, apical pulse, blood pressure (if applicable), and temperature

Additional education provided to parents includes safety issues related to home environment, toys, water, car seats, and potential lead poisoning.

Assessment of Toddlers

Infancy ends at 1 year of age, and the toddler stage begins. The toddler stage is considered to span from 1–3 years of age. When caring for a toddler, the primary goal of the nurse is to reduce the toddler's stress and anxiety and cultivate a nurse-child-parent relationship of trust and respect. Allowing time for preparation prior to any exam is very useful in decreasing stress and anxiety when interacting with a toddler. It is essential to enable the child to sit or stand near the parent. Nursing interventions, such as providing the child time to play and get acquainted with the nurse or letting the child inspect the equipment are techniques to decrease a toddler's stress and anxiety.

Before the exam, all initial physical contact should be minimal and equipment introduced slowly. During the examination, the child can be placed prone or supine in the parent's lap. Throughout the assessment, playful techniques such as counting fingers or toes can be included while inspecting the body areas and praising the child for cooperative behavior. Integrating any method to decrease the child's anxiety level will improve the accuracy of the assessment. Any traumatic procedures such as venipuncture or injection will be performed at the very end of the examination. Prior to the assessment of the toddler, the parent can help remove the outer clothing. Underwear should not be removed until the area is ready to be assessed. All auscultation, palpation, or percussion is performed when the toddler is quiet. If the toddler is not cooperative, the procedure will be completed quickly.

Nursing care of the toddler includes assessment of all general physiological systems as well as evaluation of the following:

- Oral health
- Elimination
- Sleep/activity
- Family system
- Nutritional intake
- Current immunizations
- Developmental milestones
- Height and weight plot on a growth chart
- Vital signs obtained in the following order: respirations, apical pulse, blood pressure (if applicable), and temperature

Additional evaluations include developmental, psychosocial, behavioral, and autism screenings (at 9 and 18 months of age), and a BMI screening at 24 months of age.

Further education provided to parents includes anticipatory guidance, such as discussing family parenting, feeding, and exposure to media; and discussing safety issues related to home environment, passenger safety, water safety, choking, and lead poisoning.

Assessment of Preschool Children

The period of preschool is considered to be 3–5 years of age. Preschoolers have a very active and vivid imagination, and therefore, before performing any assessment, it is important the nurse use sensory terms whenever possible to explain what is going to occur. Using games and imagination and encouraging the child to express feelings will help the nurse gain cooperation. Other nursing interventions include allowing the child to handle the equipment and using simple terms to explain what will be done with the equipment and why. At this age, a child still prefers to have the parents close by. The child is capable of undressing him- or herself, and it is essential to provide a gown and respect the need for privacy, as well as to allow the child to wear his or her underpants. When the child is cooperative, the nurse will proceed in a head-to-toe fashion; if the child is uncooperative, the nurse should refer to the guidelines used to assess a toddler.

During the assessment, the nurse can begin teaching the child in simple terms about the function of the body and care that is required. The assessment will include general physiological systems as well as evaluation of the following:

- Nutrition
- Oral health
- Elimination
- Height/weight
- Family system
- Immunizations
- Vision screening
- Body mass index
- Hearing screening
- Behavioral assessment
- Psychosocial assessment
- Developmental surveillance
- Vital signs, including blood pressure

Further education provided to parents includes anticipatory guidance related to feeding, development, use of media, water safety, strangers, riding-toy safety, passenger safety, and lead poisoning.

Assessment of School-Age Children

School-age children are ages 6–12 years. When caring for these children, nurses will keep in mind that this age group can understand cause and effect and, whenever possible, should be allowed to make decisions. All procedures should be explained to the child. The school-aged child is cooperative and prefers to sit during an exam. When assessing a younger school-aged child, the child may prefer the parent to be present, whereas the older child may prefer privacy.

The nurse will examine the child in a head-to-toe fashion, leaving the genitalia examination for last. The assessment will include general physiological systems, as well as evaluation of the following:

- Nutrition
- Oral health
- Height/weight
- Family system
- Immunizations
- Body mass index

- Vision screening
- Hearing screening
- Behavioral assessment
- Psychosocial assessment
- Developmental surveillance
- Vital signs, including blood pressure

Further education provided includes anticipatory guidance related to environmental safety at home and outdoors, recreational safety, passenger safety, use of media, water safety, violence prevention, fitness, nutrition, cholesterol and hemoglobin screening, school bullying, peer pressure, and academic performance.

Assessment of Adolescents

The adolescent period ranges from 13–17 years of age. The adolescent is autonomous, and before any assessment or examination, the nurse will provide information regarding the plan of care to the client. Matters discussed, such as sexually transmitted infections, contraception, and pregnancy are considered confidential. This age group of clients will be provided health education as well as encouragement to discuss any concerns they may have.

Before the assessment and examination, the nurse will provide information so the client understands what to expect. Although privacy is very important at this stage of development, it is appropriate to offer the client the option for a parent to be present. The examination is carried out the same way as a school-aged child exam, exposing only the areas that need to be examined and examining the genitalia last.

During the examination, it is essential that the nurse communicate with the client using matter-of-fact comments about the normalcy of the developmental findings. The assessment will include general physiological systems as well as evaluation of the following:

- Vision
- Nutrition
- Oral health
- Height/weight
- Family system
- Immunizations
- Body mass index
- Tuberculosis testing
- Cholesterol screening
- Nutrition and exercise
- Behavioral assessment
- Hypertension screening
- Psychosocial assessment
- Growth and development

- Developmental surveillance
- Vital signs, including blood pressure

Additional evaluations include screening for tobacco and substance use or abuse, eating disorders, depression, and sexually transmitted infections.

Further education provided includes anticipatory guidance related to outdoor and recreational safety, media violence, injuries and accidents (specifically MVA and ATVs), possible HIV testing, skin protection, school bullying, peer pressure, academic performance, contraception, STI prevention, intimate partner violence, and exercise.

Assessment of Adult Clients

The adult client ranges from 18 years of age through 64 years. The young adult is fully physically developed by age 20, and before 30, the client is at peak physical functioning. After 30 years of age, there is an unnoticed gradual physical decline for which specific changes can lead to illness and disease. Wellness, prevention, health screenings, and the identification of risk factors are the nurse's primary focus during this stage of life.

Routine physical assessments and screenings are performed at this time, which include the following:

- Vision
- Height
- Weight
- Nutrition
- Skin care
- Vital signs
- Oral health
- Elimination
- Pelvic exam
- Breast exams
- Contraception
- Immunizations
- Sexual activity
- Physical activity
- Testicular exams
- Body mass index
- Sexually transmitted infections

Additional evaluations include screenings for cholesterol, skin cancer, cervical cancer (Pap smear), mental status, emotional status, behavioral disorders, diabetes, blood pressure, cigarette smoking, alcohol or other substance use or abuse, and intimate partner violence.

Further education provided addresses safety issues, such as auto accidents, weapon injuries, violence, infectious diseases, and homicide.

Assessment of Middle Adult Clients

The nursing focus during the assessment of the middle adult is on health promotion. The leading cause of death in this stage of life is related primarily to chronic disease.

Routine physical assessment and health screenings recommended include the following:

- Vision
- Height
- Weight
- Skin care
- Nutrition
- Oral health
- Vital signs
- Elimination
- Pelvic exam
- Breast exams
- Contraception
- Immunizations
- Sexual activity
- Physical activity
- Testicular exams
- Body mass index
- Sexually transmitted infections

Additional evaluations include screenings for cholesterol, skin cancer, cervical cancer (Pap smear), colon cancer (colonoscopy), breast cancer (mammography), mental status, emotional status, behavioral disorders, cardiovascular disease, diabetes, glaucoma, blood pressure, cigarette smoking, alcohol or other substance use or abuse, and intimate partner violence.

Further education is provided addressing safety issues, such as auto accidents.

Assessment of Older Adult Clients

A client age 65 and over is considered to be an older adult. Functional loss is primarily associated with disorders rather than the normal aging process. When conducting a physical examination and providing education to the older adult, modifications are based on the client's cognition, mobility, and range of motion.

Routine physical assessment and health screenings recommended include the following:

- Gait
- Vision
- Height

- Weight
- Balance
- Hearing
- Nutrition
- Mobility
- Nutrition
- Sexuality
- Vital signs
- Oral health
- Muscle tone
- Weight/height
- Immunizations
- Range of motion
- Body mass index
- Bowel and bladder control
- Ability to perform daily tasks and routine self-care

Additional evaluations include screenings for use of tobacco, alcohol, or any other other substance; intimate partner violence or different types of abuse; risk for falls; cognitive, emotional, behavioral, or mental health disorders; sexual activity; cholesterol; skin cancer; cervical cancer (Pap smear); breast cancer (mammography); colon cancer (colonoscopy); diabetes; cardiovascular disease; blood pressure; glaucoma; hearing; and osteoporosis.

Further education is provided addressing safety issues, such as environmental safety and types of prescriptions and dosages.

ANTE/INTRA/POSTPARTUM AND NEWBORN CARE

An essential part of health promotion and maintenance includes caring for the childbearing client and family. The client and family require a great deal of support during the antepartum, intrapartum, and postpartum period, as this is deemed a period of maturational development and a situational crisis. Nursing support includes ongoing psychosocial, spiritual, and physiological assessments. A client's family support system, spiritual beliefs, and cultural practices have an impact on childbearing practices, as well as the client's psychological response and coping mechanisms throughout the pregnancy and into parenthood.

During the antepartum, intrapartum, and postpartum periods of pregnancy, the nurse will provide specialized maternal-fetal assessments to monitor physiological well-being. There are specific maternal physiological adaptations the nurse can expect that are related to maternal hormones and the mechanical pressure the growing uterus places on her body. When a client's pregnancy is confirmed, it is important that the estimated date of delivery is calculated correctly. The nurse can anticipate that each stage of the pregnancy will require specific screenings and tests, which will result in physical maternal/fetal assessment findings appropriate to each stage.

At the beginning of the pregnancy, the client will experience physiological adaptations that are recognized signs and symptoms of pregnancy.

SIGNS AND SYMPTOMS OF PREGNANCY	
Signs	**Symptoms**
Presumptive	These subjective changes reported by the client include symptoms such as amenorrhea, nausea, vomiting, fatigue, and breast changes. These symptoms are not diagnostic of pregnancy because they can be associated with other physiological conditions or changes.
Probable	Probable signs are objective findings by the examiner. These findings include a positive pregnancy test, ballottement, and presence of Chadwick's and Hagar's signs. These findings, when combined with the presumptive signs, strongly suggest a pregnancy.
Positive	Positive signs include objective findings that confirm a pregnancy. These signs include fetal heart tones, visualization of the fetus, and palpation of fetal movement.

When pregnancy is confirmed, it is critical to calculate the estimated date of delivery. A conventional method of calculating the client's estimated date of delivery is the use of **Naegele's rule**. Using the three-step process of Naegele's rule, the first day of the last menstrual period is identified, then three calendar months are counted backward from that date, followed by adding one year and seven days to that date. For example, if the first day of a client's last menstrual period is September 24, 2019, her estimated date of delivery is June 30, 2020. It is important to remember when using Naegele's rule that it is based on a consistent normal menstrual cycle of 28 days.

Routine maternal testing will be performed throughout the pregnancy and is performed based on the weeks of gestation or trimester. The American College of Obstetricians and Gynecologists provides testing recommendations as shown below.

TESTING DURING PREGNANCY	
Stage	**Recommended Tests**
Early in the pregnancy	• Complete blood count (CBC) • Blood type Rh • Urinalysis • Urine culture • Pap test • Rubella • Hepatitis B and hepatitis C • Sexually transmitted infections (STIs) • Human immunodeficiency virus (HIV) • Tuberculosis (TB)
Later in the pregnancy	• A repeat CBC • Rh antibody test • Glucose screening test • Group B streptococci (GBS)

ANTENATAL TESTING PERFORMED BY TRIMESTER	
Trimester	**Recommended Tests**
First trimester	Nuchal translucency screening, ultrasound, maternal serum pregnancy-associated plasma protein A, human chorionic gonadotropin, chorionic villus sampling
Second trimester	Biophysical profile, nonstress test, ultrasound, amniocentesis, maternal triple screen, percutaneous umbilical blood sampling
Third trimester	Biophysical profile, ultrasound, nonstress test, contraction stress test, amniocentesis, vibroacoustic stimulation, amniotic fluid index

Fetal assessment includes the auscultation of the fetal heart rate. The fetal heart rate can be heard with a doppler late in the first trimester and is assessed throughout the pregnancy. The heart rate can be anticipated to be between 110–160 beats per minute. Fetal movement or "quickening" occurs in the second trimester of pregnancy, and client will be instructed to monitor fetal movement or 'kick counts' daily beginning at 28 weeks gestation. Other routine assessments include maternal weight gain, vital signs, measurement of fundal height (after 20 weeks gestation), and urine screening for protein and glucose.

Gestational complications that can occur during the antepartum period include the following:

- Anemia
- Eclampsia
- Endometritis
- Preeclampsia
- Preterm labor
- Placenta previa
- Polyhydramnios
- Isoimmunization
- Oligohydramnios
- Chorioamnionitis
- Ectopic pregnancy
- Abruptio placentae
- Incompetent cervix
- Multiple gestations
- Gestational diabetes
- Hydatidiform mole
- Post-term pregnancy
- Spontaneous abortion
- Substance use and abuse
- Gestational hypertension

- Hyperemesis gravidarum
- Cardiopulmonary disease
- Intrauterine growth restriction
- Sexually transmitted infections
- Premature rupture of membranes
- Disseminated intravascular coagulation
- Urinary tract infections or pyelonephritis
- Preterm premature rupture of membranes
- HELLP Syndrome (Hemolysis, elevated liver enzymes, low platelets)
- Infections: TORCH (toxoplasmosis, other infections, rubella, cytomegalovirus, and herpes)

Throughout the pregnancy, the nurse will provide prenatal education, which includes the following:

- Rest
- Travel
- Nutrition
- Oral health
- Substance use
- Physical activity
- Personal hygiene
- Self-management
- Anticipated discomforts
- Anticipated maternal and fetal changes
- Symptoms to report to the health care provider
- Prescriptions and over-the-counter medications

The nurse's responsibility when caring for laboring clients changes based on the stage of labor. During the admission of the laboring client, it is essential for the nurse to obtain prenatal data to assess the obstetrical history, carefully identifying any conditions that may place the client or the fetus at risk during labor, delivery, or in the postpartum period.

The initial physical evaluation of maternal and fetal well-being includes the following:

- Vital signs
- Leopold's maneuver to determine fetal position
- Auscultation of the fetal heart rate or implementing and interpreting the results of electronic fetal monitoring
- Palpation and monitoring of uterine contractions

- Assessment for rupture of membranes and, if appropriate, fern testing or nitrazine testing

- Vaginal exam (if not contraindicated) to assess cervical dilation, effacement, fetal presentation and position (if possible), and amniotic membranes

- Necessary urine and blood samples

Much of the care, support, and education of the client throughout labor will be based on the current condition of the client as well as birth preferences. Pain management throughout the client's labor and delivery experience is assessed upon admission and remains an ongoing evaluation. Fear, stress, pain, general hygiene, nutritional fluid intake, and elimination are additional factors that are addressed upon admission and throughout the client's labor, delivery, and postpartum care. Throughout this time, the nurse will also provide education and support for the client's partner, as appropriate. The client may experience an event that requires a cesarean section. Throughout this period, the nurse will continue to provide support to the client in addition to implementing necessary procedures and communicating with the health care team to facilitate the delivery of the infant. The health care team members with whom the nurse will most likely collaborate include the health care provider, anesthesiologist, neonatologist, and a neonatal nurse or nurse who will care for the newborn infant immediately after delivery.

From the time the client is admitted in labor throughout the immediate postpartum period, the physiological process is identified by the following four stages.

STAGES OF LABOR	
Stage	Physiological Phase
1	• Latent phase (0–3 cm) • Active phase (4–7 cm) • Transition phase (8–10 cm)
2	• Birth of the baby
3	• Expulsion of the placenta
4	• Immediate postpartum period

During the immediate and general postpartum period, the client and the newborn will be monitored for complications. Throughout this time of transition, the nurse will further assess the client and partner for psychological adaptation and ability to cope with their new role of parenting.

Physiological maternal complications for which the nurse will monitor the client include the following:

- Infection

- Hematoma

- Hemorrhage

- Urinary retention

- Deep vein thrombosis

- Dehiscence of wound repair

Routine postpartum nursing care includes the assessment of vital signs, pain, the need for Rhogam if applicable, and frequently the evaluation of hemoglobin and hematocrit, as well as the following:

- **Heart rate:** normally 120 to 160 beats per minute
- **Breath sounds:** crying is good; assess for weak, irregular, or gasping respiration
- **Breasts:** assess tissue for fullness and nipples for cracks or soreness if breastfeeding
- **Skin:** integrity, temperature, moisture, edema
- **Abdomen:** bowel sounds; if cesarean section, assess dressing or incision
- **Uterus:** fundal height, location, consistency
- **Perineum:** episiotomy, tears, edema, erythema, hematomas
- **Lochia:** amount, odor
- **Bladder:** distension
- **Rectal area:** hemorrhoids
- **Legs:** Homan's sign
- **Incisions:** assess all incisions for redness, edema, exudate, drainage, and approximation

An important part of postpartum care includes providing the client support and education for newborn care (see newborn teaching and care under "Aging Process"). Nursing care of the newborn consists of assisting the client in providing physical care in addition to supporting the emotional and developmental needs of the infant in a safe environment. Throughout the time the client, newborn, and family are receiving nursing care, the nurse will evaluate the ability of the client and partner's ability to provide safe newborn care.

When providing discharge education, the client's self-care instructions include the following:

- Rest
- Nutrition
- Pain relief
- Birth control
- Prescriptions
- Handwashing
- Follow-up care
- Episiotomy care
- Postpartum blues
- Vaginal discharge
- Bowel elimination
- Physical limitations
- Restricted sexual activity
- Cramping or uterine pain

- Breastfeeding: teaching includes nipple care, engorgement, and mastitis

- Nonbreastfeeding: breast support, engorgement, discomfort

- When to notify the health care provider:

  - Symptoms of infection of the uterus (endometritis) incision

  - Urinary tract infection

  - Mastitis

  - Hemorrhage

  - Preeclampsia and eclampsia

  - Cardiovascular and coronary complications

  - Venous thromboembolism

  - Unrelieved pain

  - Mental health conditions, such as postpartum depression

DEVELOPMENTAL STAGES AND TRANSITIONS

The nurse can anticipate providing care and education, as well as evaluating the client based on the client's physical, cognitive, and psychosocial stage of growth and development. It is also essential for the nurse to provide education to other members of the health care team about the expected stages of development throughout the lifespan. Piaget's theory of cognitive development is descriptive of a child's ability to understand concepts based on developmental age. According to Piaget, cognitive development consists of age-related changes that occur in an orderly sequence of stages.

PIAGET'S STAGES OF COGNITIVE DEVELOPMENT	
Stage	Cognitive Development
Sensorimotor Stage (birth to 18–24 months)	The infant learns through movements and sensations (sensorimotor activity). Object permanence occurs when the infant learns that things still exist even when they cannot be seen.
Preoperational Stage (2–7 yrs.)	Symbolic thought emerges. Egocentrism shifts to social awareness, magical thinking, and animism. Playing is essential as a way of understanding the world and working out experiences.
Concrete Operational Stage (7–11 yrs.)	The child understands cause and effect and conservation of matter.
Formal Operational Stage (11 yrs. to adulthood)	The child achieves intellectual thought with abstract thinking and the ability to consider different outcomes.

Erik Erikson's psychosocial stages of development reflect different stages or maturational crisis that, according to Erikson, must be completed to achieve a healthy personality and successful interactions with others.

ERIKSON'S PSYCHOSOCIAL STAGES OF DEVELOPMENT		
Psychosocial Crisis/Conflict	Age	Outcome
Trust vs. Mistrust	Infancy (0–1.5 yrs.)	Infant is completely dependent; caregiver meets infant's basic needs in a sensitive manner
Autonomy vs. Shame	Early childhood (1.5–3 yrs.)	Toddler learns he or she has some basic control of actions and environment
Initiative vs. Guilt	Preschool (3–6 yrs.)	Child becomes purposeful and directive by initiating activities and controlling his or her world through social interaction and play
Industry vs. Inferiority	School age (6–12 yrs.)	Child develops social, physical, and school skills
Identity vs. Role Confusion	Adolescence (12–20 yrs.)	Develops a sense of self
Intimacy vs. Isolation	Early adulthood (20–35 yrs.)	Establishes intimate bonds of love and maintains relationships
Generativity vs. Stagnation	Middle adulthood (35–65 yrs.)	Fulfills life goals that involve family, career, society, and contributing to the development of others
Integrity vs. Despair	Late years (65 yrs.–death)	Reflection on one's life and acceptance of its meaning

The physical development from birth through adolescence is significant. During the first year of life, rapid physical development occurs.

PHYSICAL DEVELOPMENT DURING FIRST YEAR OF LIFE	
Age	Physical Development Milestones
1–3 months	Neck muscles become stronger, turns head side to side when placed on abdomen, strong grasp, brings hands or objects to mouth, looks at hands, listens to sounds, follows and fixes on objects and faces 8–10 inches away, briefly holds rattle or object, socially smiles, coos, babbles.
4–6 months	Rolls from back to side, plays with toes, recognizes familiar faces and objects, displays improved hand-eye coordination, and has clearer vision. By the end of 6 months, the child may be able to sit up; the infant searches for lost objects and begins to fear strangers.
6–9 months	Sits without help for a period of time, picks up larger objects with fingers, tries to crawl or move, picks up and controls an object with both hands, takes objects out of containers, stacks two blocks, can chew or gum finely minced foods.
9–12 months	Stands while holding on, can sit without support, crawls, pulls to stand. By 12 months, the child walks and drinks from a cup.

Throughout the toddler years, physical development slows as the toddler's appetite decreases; however, a diet high in protein is necessary for brain development. By the time an infant is 18 months of age, he or she should be walking alone, may walk up steps, can undress him- or herself, pull a toy when walking, and eat with a spoon. By 2 years of age, the toddler can kick a ball, begin to run, climb up and down furniture without help, throw a ball overhand, and draw straight lines and circles. The 3-year-old child can ride a tricycle, run, and place one foot on a step at a time to climb stairs. The 4-year-old child can hop and stand on one foot for three seconds and catch a bounced ball. The 5-year-old child can jump rope, use scissors, do a summersault, tie his or her shoes, stand on one foot for 10 seconds or longer, climb, and swing. A school-aged child's vision becomes as sharp as that of an adult. The school-aged child can paint, draw, self-groom, and dress independently.

Further physical development includes movement that has become more graceful and motor skills that enable the child to use tools. All of the child's deciduous teeth will be lost. The period toward the middle to end of childhood is considered to be the prepubescence period. Physical development of the adolescent includes a refinement of motor skills and an increase in blood volume and pressure to that of an adult. In addition, puberty occurs, accompanied by growth spurts and sexual maturation with secondary sex characteristics. By the completion of the adolescent period, physical growth will be completed.

Families and children live in diverse arrangements. While some households may fit the model of the traditional nuclear family, a family may also be blended, single-parent, extended, adoptive, multigenerational, childless, or same-gender parents. Family structure, individual roles, and cultural and religious influences all affect an individual's development, health practices, and ability to cope with the changes that occur throughout life. As the client experiences each stage of development, the nurse can anticipate many physical changes that will happen across the client's lifespan. The changes associated with developmental stages include puberty, pregnancy, and the aging process. The nurse will provide education for the client as well as other health care members regarding these anticipated changes that occur in the body throughout the lifespan and will evaluate the client's ability to cope as these changes occur.

Clients will also need further support in coping with the life transitions that may be associated with changes. Examples of transitions in life include attachment to a newborn, parenting, and retirement. Understanding that these are stressors will help the nurse evaluate the client and family's ability to cope with change and provide the necessary support.

HEALTH PROMOTION/DISEASE PREVENTION

Prevention of disease begins with health promotion. The nurse's role includes an understanding of the importance of health promotion and preventative health. The National Center for Chronic Disease Prevention and Health Promotion recommends nurses take the following approaches:

- **Monitor epidemiology and surveillance:** A surveillance system to help prevent or even control diseases is used to plan health promotion and prevent disease. Behavioral, social, and environmental factors can be monitored, and tracking policies may be established that may affect or perpetuate a disease state. Monitoring further allows the nurse to measure the number of people who access preventative care services. The nurse is adept at using health information technology to obtain information that will improve the efficiency of data collection.

- **Improve environments to make it easier for people to make healthy choices:** Healthy environments not only promote healthy behavior, they support the health of the people within the environment. Environments such as schools, child care programs, worksites, and communities are places that can be used to promote health.

- **Health care system interventions:** This allows for the improved use of quality clinical preventive services and the provision of better access to services that can reduce the risk of disease and illness.

- **Community programs linked to services:** Public services provided to populations at risk or to clients who have an active disease process can improve the quality of life, prevent or slow down a disease, avoid complications, and reduce the risk of disease or the need for further health care. Community programs can offer education and treatment to prevent complications for clients with behaviors that are linked to illness.

A client is most likely to participate in preventative health care when general education is provided and access to resources is facilitated. The role of the nurse is to provide screening and general education about wellness for clients who are at risk for illness and disease. All planning is based on several factors, which include age, gender, ethnicity, lifestyle, community, and family history. Cultural, spiritual practices, and language barriers are always considered when promoting the health of any client, family, or community.

Topics of education that focus on prevention include, but are not limited to, the following:

- Exercise

- Oral care

- Nutrition

- Stress/coping

- Sleep hygiene

- Smoking cessation

- Immunization schedule

- Substance use—alcohol, illegal drugs

- Prevention of infection through handwashing, food safety, etc.

- Routine health care provider visits

- Anticipatory health screenings for conditions such as cancer, obesity, or cardiovascular disease

When a client has been identified as being at risk for illness, the client may require the nurse to provide not only assistance in accessing health care, but with monitoring, follow-up care, or the provision of ongoing support. The nurse will also evaluate the effectiveness of any nursing intervention implemented to improve the client's health or prevent illness.

HEALTH SCREENING

The nurse is responsible for understanding the pathophysiology in relation to health screenings based on gender, age, ethnicity, health history, and risk assessments throughout the lifespan. Health screening of clients throughout the lifespan includes the following:

- Injury

- Vision

- Hearing

- Violence

- Diabetes
- Nutrition
- Glaucoma
- Oral health
- Skin health
- Nutritional
- Osteoporosis
- Bone density
- Mammogram
- Mental health
- Immunizations
- Prostate health
- Blood pressure
- Lipid disorders
- Lead poisoning
- Substance abuse
- Testicular cancer
- Colorectal cancer
- Papanicolaou test
- Height and weight
- Coronary heart disease
- Cardiovascular disease
- Sexually transmitted infections
- Rubella serology (women of childbearing age)
- Tobacco use/disease associated with tobacco use

The nurse will utilize the most effective techniques to obtain information from the client. Techniques such as active listening, empathy, validation, reassurance, adaptive questioning, maintaining client privacy, respecting cultural preferences, using open-ended questions, and mindfulness of nonverbal communication will help facilitate a trusting nurse-client relationship.

HIGH-RISK BEHAVIORS

Part of the initial focus of a nursing assessment is to gather data from a client to identify high-risk behaviors. Behaviors may be shaped by actual or potential intrinsic or extrinsic factors that increase the client's risk of injury or physical illness. Intrinsic factors that may contribute to high-risk behaviors include age, sex, past experiences, fatigue, anxiety, or depression. Extrinsic factors include interpersonal influences such as family, peers, or friends, and situational influences, which include work schedules and other outside demands.

Obtaining accurate information about a client's lifestyle practices is important to determine the degree of risk for untoward events or disease. This information gathered from the client can provide the nurse with the opportunity to assist the client in recognizing risk factors. Lifestyle practices such as lack of exercise, poor nutritional choices, frequent substance use, excessive exposure to sun, and smoking are just a few examples of high-risk behaviors that increase the negative impact on the health of the client. When the nurse assists the client in identifying these behaviors, education can be provided about the prevention and treatment of some of the behaviors. Interventions such as smoking cessation, needle exchange, or safe sexual practices can help reduce the client's risk for illness and disease.

LIFESTYLE CHOICES

When assessing a client's lifestyle choices, the nurse's understanding of the social determinants of health is essential. The World Health Organization (WHO) describes the social determinants of health as "the conditions in which people are born, grow, work, live and age, and the wider set of forces and systems shaping the conditions of daily life." Currently, the CDC incorporates social determinants into its Healthy People 2020 program, a national health prevention program that identifies preventable threats to health and provides goals to reduce these health threats.

The five key areas are as follows:

1. **Economic stability:** This domain includes poverty, employment, food security, and housing stability.

2. **Education:** This domain connects education with well-being. Key issues include high school graduation, enrollment in higher education, language, literacy, and early childhood education and development.

3. **Social and community context:** This domain reflects the characteristics within the context for which people learn, play, work, and live and includes civic participation, conditions in the workplace, and general health and well-being.

4. **Health and health care:** This domain reflects the client's understanding of and access to health care services as well as the client's health, health insurance coverage, and health care literacy.

5. **Neighborhood and built environment:** This domain reflects the connection to where a person lives—housing, neighborhood, and environment—and the client's overall health and well-being. Access to transportation, healthy food choices, quality of water and air, as well as exposure to violence and neighborhood crime are all influential to the client's health.

The social determinants of health identify factors that place a client at a higher risk for making unhealthy lifestyle choices. Lifestyle choices such as attitude and perception about sexuality can place a client at increased risk for disease or unplanned pregnancy. An important client assessment includes the need for contraception. The type of contraception chosen is based on the client's age, medical and mental health history, adherence to the selected method, relationship status, and outlook on family planning development. Providing education on issues of sexuality, family planning, safe sexual practice, impotence, and age-related changes such as menopause is included in the nurse's role when addressing the client's lifestyle choices.

Other important assessments include identifying clients who may be environmentally or socially isolated. This isolation may have occurred as a result of residing in a specific geographic location, or it may be due to illness. These clients are at risk for mental health conditions such as depression, and their isolation may further affect their physical health due to their inability to access the necessary resources they need.

Evaluation of the client's use of alternative or homeopathic health care practices is also useful for identifying possible harmful practices to the client's health. The client's acceptance of such practices can be integrated into the plan of care when assisting in making changes to create a healthier lifestyle.

SELF-CARE

Self-care is a process by which individuals and families take an active role in caring for their physical, mental, and emotional health. Before creating a client's plan for self-care, it is important the nurse assesses for the following information:

- Health literacy
- Native language
- Cultural and religious practices
- Home life and family circumstances
- Roles and relationships of family members that will be involved
- Client's understanding and feelings about his or her condition
- Caregiver's understanding of and feelings about the client's condition

Furthermore, the nurse will evaluate a client's ability and or primary caregiver's ability to manage care in the home according to a treatment plan. Integrated into the treatment plan is an assessment of all self-care needs, which will be revised based on the client's condition. The nursing role also includes the provision of assistance, education, and evaluation of the client as well as a caregiver's ability to manage the care to promote wellness and prevent further physical or mental decline. Anticipated client self-care or caregiver responsibilities may include the following:

- **Personal care:** bathing, eating, dressing, toileting
- **Household care:** cooking, cleaning, meal preparation, laundry, shopping
- **Health care:** prescription management and administration, wound treatment, physical therapy, use of medical equipment
- **Emotional care:** companionship, meaningful activities

TECHNIQUES OF PHYSICAL ASSESSMENT

Before performing a physical assessment, the nurse will gather the necessary equipment appropriate for the age of the client. The accuracy of a physical assessment is dependent on the skill and proper order of technique and equipment used throughout. The nurse is responsible for assuring the necessary equipment is available and the information to be included in the client's health history and physical assessment are accurately obtained.

Before the assessment of a client, the nurse will ensure the necessary equipment is available, including the following:

- Scale
- Gloves
- Penlight

- Otoscope
- Stethoscope
- Thermometer
- Tape measure
- Hand sanitizer
- Reflex hammer
- Ophthalmoscope
- Height wall ruler
- Tongue depressor
- Blood pressure cuff
- Watch with a second hand

The nurse is responsible for obtaining information for a complete health history. The components of a health history include the following:

- General assessment
- Chief complaint
- Present health status
- Past health history
- Family history
- Review of systems and physical examination

Basic assessments included in the physical examination are as follows:

- Height, weight
- Vital signs
- Skin, hair, nails
- Neurological examination
- Head, ears, eyes, nose, throat
- Cardiovascular system
- Respiratory system
- Abdomen/gastrointestinal system
- Genitourinary system
- Musculoskeletal system

Techniques used when performing a physical examination include the following:

- **Inspection:** consists of the use of observation with the eyes, ears, and nose.
- **Auscultation:** performed in a quiet room and over bare skin using the appropriate part of the stethoscope.

- **Palpation:** includes light and deep palpation. **Light palpation** is performed with the pads of the fingers depressing 1.5 to .75 inches, which allows for assessment of texture, tenderness, temperature, moisture, pulsations, and masses. **Deep palpation** is performed using the finger pads pressing 1.5 to 2 inches to allow for assessment of the internal organs and masses.

- **Percussion:** used to assess for tenderness or sounds. Sounds include tympany, resonance, hyperresonance, dullness, and flatness. Sounds are elicited by pressing the distal part of the middle finger of the nondominant hand on the body part and using the middle finger of the dominant hand tapping quickly over the point where the other middle finger contacts the client's skin.

SUMMING IT UP

- The nurse's role throughout the **aging process** includes the following:
  - Promotion of client and community wellness through education
  - Assessing health risks
  - Providing care and education
  - Performing comprehensive health assessments and screenings
  - Promoting the prevention of and offering treatment for high-risk health behaviors

- Many physical, psychosocial, and cognitive age-related changes occur throughout a client's lifespan. By providing **anticipatory guidance** to prepare for these changes, the RN helps the client and family identify ways to cope with change, whether it is a **maturational**, **situational**, or **adventitious crisis**.

- **Ante/intra/postpartum and newborn care** includes caring for the childbearing client and family by offering psychosocial, spiritual, and physiological assessments. It also includes providing specialized maternal-fetal assessments to monitor physiological well-being and anticipating the screenings and tests required at each stage of the pregnancy.

- The nurse provides care, education, and evaluates a client based on the client's **physical, cognitive, and psychosocial stage of growth and development**. The nurse also educates other members of the health care team about the expected stages of development throughout a client's lifespan.

- The nurse promotes health to **prevent disease** through the following:
  - Monitoring epidemiology
  - Improving environments to make it easier for clients to make healthy choices
  - Organizing health care system interventions and community programs
  - Providing screening and general education about wellness for clients with risk factors for illness and disease

- The nurse is responsible for understanding the **pathophysiology** in relation to health screenings based on the client's gender, age, ethnicity, health history, and risk assessments. The nurse screens clients for issues involving the following:
  - Injury
  - Vision
  - Hearing
  - Violence
  - Diabetes
  - Nutrition
  - Glaucoma
  - Oral and skin health
  - Osteoporosis

- Bone density
- Various forms of cancer and heart disease
- Substance abuse
- Height and weight
- Sexually transmitted infections
- Numerous other issues

- When performing an assessment, the nurse gathers data to identify **high-risk behaviors** and obtains accurate information about a client's **lifestyle** practices. The nurse then assists the client in identifying those high-risk behaviors and provides education about the prevention and treatment of such behaviors.

- The nurse must understand the **social determinants** of health that place a client at a higher risk for making unhealthy lifestyle choices. This includes examining and identifying the following five key areas:

  1. Economic stability
  2. Education
  3. Social and community context
  4. Health and health care
  5. Neighborhood and built environment

- **Self-care** is a process by which individuals and families take an active role in caring for their own physical, mental, and emotional health. The nurse will also evaluate a client's ability and/or primary caregiver's ability to manage care in the home according to a treatment plan.

- The nurse must gather the necessary **equipment** appropriate for the age of the client before performing a **physical assessment** and is responsible for assuring that the necessary equipment is available and the information to be included in the client's health history and physical assessment are obtained accurately.

- Techniques used when performing a physical examination include **inspection, auscultation, palpation**, and **percussion**.

PRACTICE QUESTIONS: HEALTH PROMOTION AND MAINTENANCE

Practice Questions

> **Directions:** The following are examples of the types of questions you will encounter on the NCLEX-RN exam. Read each question carefully and choose the best answer unless otherwise directed. Check your answers against the answer key and explanations that follow.

1. Which technique should the nurse use to **decrease** the anxiety of a toddler prior to a physical examination?
   1. Encourage the child to ask questions.
   2. Examine with the parent nearby.
   3. Allow the child time to play before the assessment.
   4. Minimize contact with the child throughout the examination.

2. Using Naegele's rule, which is the estimated date of delivery for a client with the first day of the last menstrual period on November 4, 2019?
   1. July 4, 2020
   2. July 27, 2020
   3. August 10, 2020
   4. August 27, 2020

3. The nurse is preparing to provide parental education about the growth and development of an older male child. Which statement will the nurse include in the teaching?
   1. "Your child will finish losing his baby teeth."
   2. "Your child will be able to use abstract thinking."
   3. "Your child's motor skills will be completely refined."
   4. "Your child will begin to develop secondary sexual characteristics."

4. When should the nurse perform Leopold's maneuver on a client admitted to the unit in labor?
   1. During a uterine contraction
   2. Before initiating electronic fetal monitoring
   3. Prior to administering a prescription for pain
   4. After assessing the dilation and effacement of the cervix

5. Which should the nurse take into consideration when preparing to perform a physical assessment on an older adult? **Select all that apply.**
   1. Age
   2. Vision
   3. Mobility
   4. Cognition
   5. Muscle tone
   6. Range of motion

6. For which developmental age group should the nurse begin to provide education about body function?
   1. Toddler
   2. Preschool
   3. Young childhood
   4. Middle childhood

7. Which **initial** assessment question will the nurse ask when evaluating a client for self-care?

   1. "How many family members will be involved in your care?"
   2. "Will your caregivers be able to take some time for respite?"
   3. "Can you tell me what you understand about your condition?"
   4. "What concerns do you have about receiving care in your home?"

8. Which routine blood tests for the newborn should the nurse prepare to discuss with the parents? **Select all that apply.**

   1. Hematocrit
   2. Hemoglobin
   3. Total bilirubin
   4. Metabolic screening
   5. Complete blood count
   6. Blood type and Rh factor

9. The nurse has reviewed the education for a rubella serology test with a pregnant client. Which statement made by the client indicates further teaching is required?

   1. "This test will detect an infection."
   2. "This test will evaluate my immunity."
   3. "If I am immune, I will not need a vaccination."
   4. "If I am nonimmune, I will get a vaccination after I deliver my baby."

10. Which routine vital signs should the nurse be prepared to assess for a preschool child?

    1. Oral temperature, radial pulse, respirations
    2. Rectal temperature, apical pulse, respirations
    3. Tympanic temperature, blood pressure, radial pulse, respirations
    4. Axillary temperature, blood pressure, apical pulse, respirations

Practice Questions

ANSWER KEY AND EXPLANATIONS

1. 3	**3.** 1	**5.** 2, 3, 4, 5, 6	**7.** 3	**9.** 1
2. 3	**4.** 2	**6.** 2	**8.** 4, 6	**10.** 3

1. **The correct answer is 3.** To help decrease anxiety, the toddler should be allowed time to play before the examination. Choice 1 is not an age-appropriate technique because a toddler is not cognitively developed enough to ask questions about the the physical exam. Choice 2 is not the best answer because the examination should be performed with the toddler on the parent's lap, if at all possible. Choice 4 doesn't make sense as the nurse should minimize the contact with the toddler initially to help decrease the anxiety and stress level, not throughout the examination.

2. **The correct answer is 3.** Using Naegele's rule, the first day of the last menstrual period is identified, then three calendar months are counted backward from that date, followed by adding one year and seven days to the date. Keep in mind that 2020 is a leap year. Since the year has one extra day, you need to subtract one day from the end result. The correct answer is August 10, 2020.

3. **The correct answer is 1.** Since an older male child will finish losing his deciduous teeth during childhood, the nurse should include the statement in choice 1 in the teaching. The nurse would include the statements in choices 2, 3, and 4 for an adolescent child.

4. **The correct answer is 2.** Leopold's maneuver is used to assess the position of the fetus and requires four steps of manual palpation of the uterus. This assessment is completed before initiating electronic fetal monitoring, as this method can also be used to identify the best location for which to place the external transducer to obtain a fetal heart rate tracing.

5. **The correct answers are 2, 3, 4, 5, and 6.** Vision, mobility, cognition, muscle tone, and range of motion are evaluated before performing a physical examination. The client's age (choice 1) does not specifically interfere with the nurse's ability to perform a physical exam safely.

6. **The correct answer is 2.** The preschool child, age 3–5 yrs. old, can understand sensory terms and is at a period in cognitive development where the nurse can use simple terms to teach the child about bodily care and function. A toddler (choice 1) is not cognitively developed enough to understand the information. Teaching should begin before young or middle childhood (choices 3 and 4, respectively).

7. **The correct answer is 3.** The initial assessment question stated in choice 3 provides an opportunity to explore the client's understanding of his or her condition. The statement in choice 1 would be appropriate if the client requires assistance from family members so that the nurse can clarify the family members' knowledge of the client's condition before creating a plan of care for self-management. The questions in choices 2 and 4 are better addressed after establishing the client's understanding of his or her condition.

8. **The correct answers are 4 and 6.** Routine newborn blood tests include metabolic screening as well as a blood type and Rh factor. A hematocrit (choice 1), hemoglobin (choice 2), total bilirubin (choice 3), and complete blood count (choice 5) are not a part of routine blood tests, but are assessed based on suspected pathology.

9. **The correct answer is 1.** If the client states that the test will detect an infection, then further teaching is needed because the rubella serology test is used to detect immunity or recent infection; it is not used to identify an active infection. An MMR vaccination for rubella is contraindicated during pregnancy, but is administered to a client that is rubella nonimmune after delivery of the baby.

10. **The correct answer is 3.** The preschool child's vital signs include a tympanic temperature, blood pressure, radial pulse, and respirations. The tympanic temperature is less invasive, faster, and produces accurate results. The axillary temperature (choice 4) has a higher incidence of inaccuracy. The preschool child may be able to follow instructions for an oral temperature (choice 1), but there may be many factors that interfere with an accurate reading, such as drinking fluids before the assessment or mouth breathing. Rectal temperatures (choice 2) are not used for the routine assessment of a preschool child's temperature.

Answers Practice Questions

Psychosocial Integrity

Chapter 5

OVERVIEW

- **Abuse and Neglect**
- **Behavioral Interventions**
- **Coping Mechanisms**
- **Crisis Intervention**
- **Cultural Awareness/Cultural Influences on Health**
- **End-of-Life Care**
- **Family Dynamics**
- **Grief and Loss**
- **Mental Health Concepts**
- **Religious and Spiritual Influences on Health**
- **Sensory/Perceptual Alterations**
- **Stress Management**
- **Substance Use and Other Disorders and Dependencies**
- **Support Systems**
- **Therapeutic Communication**
- **Therapeutic Environment**
- **Summing It Up**
- **Practice Questions: Psychosocial Integrity**
- **Answer Key and Explanations**

The focus of the Psychosocial Integrity Clients Needs category is to assess the nurse's ability to provide and direct the nursing care that supports and promotes the emotional, mental, and social well-being of the client experiencing stressful events, as well as clients with acute or chronic mental illness. The nurse will assess, create a plan of care, provide education, and intervene appropriately for clients experiencing problems that affect psychosocial and physical well-being. Examples of conditions that can affect the physical and mental health of a client include abuse, neglect, grief, loss, and end of life. The client's physical and mental health are also affected by chronic psychological health issues, including addictions, dependencies, depression, dementia, and eating disorders, as well as visual, auditory, or cognitive disorders. It is essential that the nurse recognize nonverbal cues of both physical and psychological stressors.

Using therapeutic communication, the nurse will assess the client's ability to cope with life changes. The nurse also provides support and incorporates behavioral management techniques into client care. The nurse will maintain a safe therapeutic environment when caring for all clients, including those who are experiencing physiological and psychological stressors, those who are at risk for violence, and those clients who are withdrawing from substances or experiencing toxicities. Before creating a care plan for a client experiencing psychological stressors, other factors to consider include the assessment of psychosocial, spiritual, and occupational factors that may affect the care the nurse provides, as well as cultural practices and beliefs and the assessment of family dynamics.

ABUSE AND NEGLECT

The nurse will assess all clients for abuse and identify those who are at an increased risk. A client experiencing abuse may present vague symptoms that can include chronic pain, insomnia, or—if female—gynecological problems. Hypertension and gastrointestinal disturbances may be present as a result of living with chronic stress and high levels of anxiety. Children may appear anxious, clingy, or emotionally withdrawn from their caregiver. In addition, children may display aggressive behavior or angry outbursts, wet the bed, or have nightmares. An older adult may present psychosomatic complaints, fear, anxiety, or nervousness. Before inquiring about abuse, the nurse's priority goal is to establish trust, a rapport, and a safe environment for the client. All assessments for abuse are completed when the client is alone.

Types of abuse for which the nurse will assess include neglect; physical, sexual, emotional, or verbal abuse; bullying; and financial exploitation. Specific subpopulations are at an increased risk of abuse. These subpopulations include women, infants, young children, older adults, and pregnant women, as well as both adults and children who are cognitively impaired, developmentally delayed, physically impaired, or chronically ill.

Child Abuse and Neglect

The CDC has identified a combination of individual, relational, community, and societal factors that contribute to the risk of child abuse and neglect. Individual risk factors include children under 4 years of age and individuals with any special needs that may increase the burden of care.

The nurse can further assess the caregivers for factors associated with an increased risk of abuse. These factors include the following:

- Parental history of child abuse and/or neglect
- Nonbiological, transient caregivers in the home (e.g., mother's male partner)
- Substance abuse or mental health issues, including depression in the family
- Parental thoughts and emotions that tend to support or justify maltreatment behaviors
- Parents' lack of understanding of children's needs, child development, and parenting skills
- Parental characteristics such as young age, poor education, single parenthood, a large number of dependent children, and low income

Family risk factors associated with child abuse include the following:

- Social isolation
- Parenting stress
- Poor parent-child relationships and negative interactions
- Family disorganization, dissolution, and violence, including intimate partner violence

Community risk factors are also considered when assessing risk of abuse. These include the following:

- Community violence
- Concentrated neighborhood disadvantage (e.g., high poverty and residential instability, high unemployment rates, and high density of alcohol outlets)
- Poor social connections

Intimate Partner Violence

The risk for **intimate partner violence (IPV)** is also increased in the presence of certain factors. These factors do not directly cause the abuse but are associated with the risk of harm. It is important to note that some risk factors for intimate partner violence are the same for perpetration, such as a history of childhood physical or sexual victimization.

Similar to child abuse, the CDC has identified a combination of individual, relational, community, and societal factors that contribute to the risk of becoming an IPV perpetrator or victim. These risk factors include the following:

- Young age
- Low income
- Unemployment
- Low self-esteem
- Anger and hostility
- Unplanned pregnancy
- Hostility towards women
- Borderline personality traits
- Heavy alcohol and drug use
- Depression and suicide attempts
- Attitudes accepting or justifying IPV
- Emotional dependence and insecurity
- Poor behavioral control/impulsiveness
- Prior history of being physically abusive
- Low academic achievement/low verbal IQ
- Witnessing IPV between parents as a child
- A desire for power and control in relationships
- Aggressive or delinquent behavior as a youth
- History of experiencing poor parenting as a child
- Lack of nonviolent social problem solving skills
- Antisocial personality traits and conduct problems
- History of experiencing physical discipline as a child

- Having few friends and being isolated from other people
- Belief in strict gender roles (e.g., male dominance and aggression in relationships)
- Being a victim of physical or psychological abuse (consistently one of the strongest predictors of perpetration)

Relationship risk factors for IPV include the following:

- Economic stress
- Social isolation/lack of social support
- Marital instability—divorces or separations
- Parents with less than a high-school education
- Unhealthy family relationships and interactions
- Association with antisocial and aggressive peers
- Marital conflict—fights, tension, and other struggles
- Dominance and control of the relationship by one partner over the other
- Jealousy, possessiveness, and negative emotion within an intimate relationship

Community factors for IPV include the following:

- High alcohol outlet density
- Poor neighborhood support and cohesion
- Poverty and associated factors (e.g., overcrowding, high unemployment rates)
- Low social capital (e.g., lack of institutions, relationships, and norms that shape a community's social interactions)
- Weak community sanctions against IPV (e.g., an unwillingness of neighbors to intervene in situations where they witness violence)

Societal factors for IPV include the following:

- Societal income inequality
- Cultural norms that support aggression toward others
- Weak health, educational, economic, and social policies/laws
- Traditional gender norms and gender inequality (e.g., women should stay at home, not enter the workforce, and be submissive; men support the family and make the decisions)

Elder Abuse

According to the CDC, elder abuse occurs when an act or failure to act causes or creates a risk of harm to an adult age 60 or over and is usually committed by a caregiver or someone the elder person trusts. Frequent types of elder abuse include physical, sexual, emotional, psychological, neglect, and financial exploitation. Many elder abuse cases are unreported because the person is afraid or unable to tell anyone about the abuse. Therefore, it is essential the nurse recognize some of the risk factors of abuse.

Risk factors of abuse include the following:

- Depression
- Lack of social support
- Lack of training in taking care of an older adult
- Use of drugs or alcohol, especially drinking heavily
- High emotional or financial dependence on the older adult
- High levels of stress and low or ineffective coping resources
- Caregivers with inadequately treated mental health disorders
- Caring for older adults who are combative or verbally abusive

Sexual Assault/Abuse

Although anyone is at risk for sexual assault during his or her lifetime, there are various individual, community, relationship, and societal factors associated with an increased likelihood that a child or adult will become a victim of sexual assault. A young child's stage of development and gender contribute to the risk of sexual assault, as do a parent's inability to properly supervise the child and problems occurring within the family.

The most consistently reported factors associated with the sexual abuse of a child include the following:

- Female gender
- History of physical or sexual abuse
    - Ages 12–17 yrs. show a higher incidence of extrafamilial abuse
    - Ages 6–11 yrs. show a higher rate of intrafamilial abuse
- Special needs: physical or cognitive disability, mental health issues, or chronic illness

Identified relationship and family factors associated with child sexual abuse include the following:

- Limited parental supervision
- Parental mental health issues
- Parental use of drugs or alcohol
- Family in which the father is not the child's biological parent

Risk factors associated with the sexual assault of an adult are as follows:

- Female
- Young age
- Depression
- Low income
- Unemployment
- Low self-esteem
- Educational level
- Anger and hostility
- Drug or alcohol use

- Intimate partner violence
- History of sexual assault
- Employment in a sex trade
- Low academic achievement
- Antisocial personality traits
- Borderline personality traits
- History of childhood maltreatment
- Emotional dependence and insecurity
- Perpetrating psychological aggression
- Prior history of being physically abusive
- A desire for power and control in relationships
- Aggressive or delinquent behavior as a youth
- History of experiencing poor parenting as a child
- History of experiencing physical discipline as a child
- Having few friends and being isolated from other people
- Belief in strict gender roles (e.g., male dominance and aggression in relationships)
- Being a victim of physical or psychological abuse (consistently one of the strongest predictors of perpetration)

Relationship factors associated with the sexual assault of an adult are as follows:

- Economic stress
- Multiple sexual partners
- Relationship instability and break-ups
- Unhealthy family relationships and interactions
- Relationship conflicts, fights, tension, and other struggles
- Dominance and control of the relationship by one partner over the other

Community factors associated with the sexual assault of an adult are as follows:

- Gender roles
- Societal factors
- Male sexual entitlement
- Tolerance of sexual assault
- Weak sanctions against sexual abuse
- Weak legal sanctions against sexual assault
- Traditional gender norms (e.g., women should stay at home, not enter the workforce, and be submissive; men support the family and make the decisions)

A primary role of the nurse in caring for clients who have experienced abuse or neglect—or are suspected of such—is to report the abuse as mandated by law. The nurse will further collaborate with the health care team members (health care provider, social worker) to plan interventions that focus on maintaining the safety of the client. Safe interventions may result in the removal of a child from the home environment, placement of a victim of interpersonal violence into a safe shelter, or the transfer of an elderly client to a safer location. A client experiencing interpersonal violence may want to return home. In such cases, the nurse must assess the risk of homicide (especially if there are weapons in the home), as well as ensure a safety plan is in place.

Part of the nursing care for a client suspected of experiencing abuse includes the assessment of the client's level of anxiety and coping responses. The plan also includes an assessment of the client's nonverbal communication. Clients who have experienced violence will exhibit anxiety and possible agitation, rendering them hypervigilant and unable to relax or sleep. The client may also use drugs and alcohol, or possibly be at risk for suicide. Common coping mechanisms of clients who are experiencing abuse include flawed self-beliefs and isolation due to feelings of shame, confusion, despair, and powerlessness.

When creating a plan of care that includes the family, the nurse will assess the family for strengths, stressors, and access to support systems. The nurse can provide support to the client and family by providing education about coping strategies and obtaining the appropriate referrals. Evaluating the client's outcome will allow the nurse to further revise the plan of care to support and promote the safety of the client.

BEHAVIORAL INTERVENTIONS

Maslow's hierarchy of needs is a critical theory that provides a framework for the nurse's care of all clients. This theory is useful in moving the client along a continuum of wellness when focusing on the prioritization of clients. Maslow's hierarchy of needs is based on the theory that the intrinsic need for self-actualization motivates humans. This model is characterized by five levels of needs that must each be successfully met to attain the final level of self-transcendence. These levels need to be met in ranking order, as shown in the following table.

MASLOW'S HIERARCHY OF NEEDS		
Priority	**Hierarchy Level**	**Need**
1	Physiological	Food, water, elimination, rest
2	Safety	Security, protection, stability, structure, order, limits
3	Love and belonging	Affiliation, intimate relationships, friends, love
4	Esteem	Self-esteem related to competency, achievement, and esteem from others
5	Self-actualization	Becoming everything one is capable of becoming

Integrating Maslow's hierarchy of needs will assist the nurse in planning care based on assessment of the client's appearance, mood, and psychomotor behavior, to help the client achieve and maintain behavioral self-control. Before implementing behavioral interventions, the nurse will establish a strong rapport with the client by performing a biopsychosocial assessment in an environment that is safe and conducive to sharing sensitive information. All techniques and tools used during communication and throughout the assessment are based on the client's developmental stage, cognition, current condition, language, and culture.

The data the nurse will gather includes the following:

- Chief complaint
- History of present illness
- Psychiatric history
- History of alcohol and substance abuse
- Medical history
- Family history
- Developmental history
- Social history
- Primary language
- Occupational and educational history
- Cultural preferences
- Spirituality and values
- Coping skills

After gathering information, the nurse will perform a mental status exam before reviewing the physical status and physical assessment of the client. A mental status exam is a structured assessment of the client's behavioral and cognitive functioning. The exam should be modified based on the developmental age or condition of the client.

The components of the exam include the following:

- Mood
- Affect
- Insight
- Judgment
- Behavior
- Cognition
- Appearance
- Thought content
- Thought process/form
- Speech and language

Occasionally a client may require orientation to reality. Reality orientation is used to improve the cognitive and psychomotor function of a client who may be confused or disoriented. Strategies the nurse can use include time, date, the season of the year, frequent use of the client's name, current events, clocks, calendars, signs, labels, photographs, and decorations.

Additional nursing assessments include the identification of risk factors that affect the client and the safety of others. By obtaining the appropriate information and conducting a thorough assessment, the nurse will be better able to understand the client's current problems, identify mutual goals for treatment, and formulate a plan of care comprised of measurable goals. All outcomes will be evaluated, and modifications to the care plan will be made when necessary.

Alterations in a client's behavior require immediate nursing intervention to maintain the safety of the client and others. It is important to determine if the origin of the behavior is due to a physical condition, drug interactions, side effects, or anxiety. The nurse's goal is to use the least restrictive approach when managing a client's behavior and while assisting the client to control his or her behavior.

Unrestrictive nursing client interventions include the following:

- Diversion

- Active listening

- Asking the client to cooperate

- Reducing environmental stimulation

- Offering an "as needed" prescription (PRN)

Environmental safety is always considered when addressing a client's behavior. The nurse should have easy access to leaving the area if needed, and there should be no objects accessible to the client that can be used as weapons or cause injury. Communication with the client is conducted in a calm but respectful nonthreatening manner, while maintaining a safe physical distance between the nurse and the client.

Behavioral modification is a treatment approach based on **operant conditioning**, which replaces undesirable behaviors with more desirable ones through positive and negative reinforcement. Change in behavior can be achieved with the use of strategies such as limit-setting, behavioral contracts, time-outs, and tokens.

All people experience some anxiety at different points throughout their lifespan. Part of the nursing assessment is to assess the level and source of a client's anxiety. Anxiety may result from pathophysiological conditions of the respiratory, cardiovascular, endocrine, neurological, and metabolic systems, or from psychological stressors. Anxiety is also a defense mechanism, related to other mental health disorders or to chronic or situational lifestyle circumstances.

In order to assist the client in developing strategies to reduce anxiety, it is necessary to accurately identify the client's level of anxiety. A client experiencing levels of anxiety that are at a severe or panic level will not be able to problem solve, and behaviors to help relieve the anxiety are unproductive. When developing anxiety reduction strategies for the client, the teaching should include physical signs and symptoms of mild and moderate anxiety to help the client recognize the appropriate time to implement the strategies. The nurse can also recommend the client keep a journal to help identify the triggers of stress.

Strategies that can be offered to the client include the following:

- Yoga

- Music

- Exercise

- Distraction

- Meditation

- Mindfulness

- Biofeedback
- Avoiding smoking
- Adequate sleep
- Deep breathing
- Guided imagery
- Limiting alcohol
- Limiting caffeine

A group setting may be very beneficial to a client experiencing undesirable psychological or behavioral changes as a result of physical or psychosocial conditions. If a group setting is appropriate for the client, advantages include learning new ways to relate to other people; practicing new communication skills; a feeling of cohesiveness; and the knowledge, insights, and experiences of the group leader as well as other members of the group.

COPING MECHANISMS

The assessment of a client's ability to cope, as well as the client's coping style, is essential when a client must adapt to a temporary or permanent role change or a diagnosis of acute or chronic mental illness. Role changes that occur across the lifespan include both situational and maturational changes.

These changes may be temporary or permanent and include such events as a death of a spouse, a spouse newly diagnosed with a chronic illness, death of a parent or child, birth of a child, or loss of a job. When assessing a client's ability to cope with these changes, the nurse will also consider the support system and resources available to the client. Evaluation of the client's acceptance and adaptation to the change will provide the nurse with the opportunity to intervene appropriately if necessary.

A client's coping ability is dependent on the primary and secondary appraisal of the situation. **Primary appraisal** is the extent to which a person perceives an event as benign or threatening and harmful. A **secondary appraisal** is an estimation of whether a person has the resources or abilities necessary to deal with what has already been deemed stressful. If an individual appraises a situation as stressful and has confidence in his or her ability to handle it, the individual can effectively cope with the stressor. In understanding the client's view of a situation, the nurse can assist the client in securing the necessary resources and obtain the necessary referrals that will support the client.

When a client is diagnosed with an acute or chronic mental illness, it may bring up a range of emotions. Before planning care, the nurse will assess the client's reaction to the illness, as well as the coping ability and available support system.

The client with a new diagnosis may experience the following range of emotions:

- Fear
- Guilt
- Hope
- Grief
- Anger
- Relief

- Shock
- Denial
- Shame
- Confusion
- Depression
- Powerlessness

Perceptions of body image affect a client's perception, thoughts, and behaviors about his or her appearance. A client who has experienced an unexpected altered body image requires the nurse's psychosocial support. Body alterations can be a result of disease, violence, or an accident. Other factors across the lifespan that may affect a client's body image perception include puberty, childbirth, and aging. The nurse will assess the client's feelings of acceptance of body changes throughout the lifespan, as well as any unexpected altered body image.

Defense Mechanisms

When adjusting to any situation or change, a client may use defense mechanisms to adapt. Defense mechanisms can help a client cope with emotionally painful feelings, thoughts, and events. The nurse will evaluate whether these mechanisms used by the client will help the client adapt to a situation or become maladaptive.

Defense mechanisms include the following:

- **Compensation:** covering up deficiencies in one area to compensate in another.
- **Conversion:** expression of emotional conflict into a physical symptom
- **Denial:** failure to admit the reality of a situation
- **Displacement:** the transference of emotions associated with a particular person, situation, or object to another nonthreatening person, situation, or object
- **Dissociation:** temporary disruption in thoughts, memory, and sense of identity
- **Identification:** a person patterns him- or herself after others
- **Intellectualization:** processing events analytically without emotion
- **Projection:** placing negative traits or unwanted emotions onto others
- **Rationalization:** self-justification of behavior
- **Reaction formation:** behaving in the exact opposite way a person thinks or feels
- **Regression:** reverting back to an earlier stage of development
- **Splitting:** inability to hold opposing thoughts; actions, beliefs, objects, or persons seen as either positive or negative
- **Sublimation:** substituting a socially acceptable activity for an impulse that is unacceptable
- **Suppression:** denial of a disturbing situation or feeling
- **Undoing:** exhibiting acceptable behavior to make up for negative behavior

CRISIS INTERVENTION

Assessment of a client for potential violence begins with the nurse's awareness of the predictors of violence. A variety of tools exist that can help predict violence; the CDC—in conjunction with The National Institute for Occupational Safety and Health—provides the *Triage Tool*, the *Indicator for Violent Behavior*, and the *Danger Assessment Tool* on its website. During the assessment of a client, the nurse may be able to identify client triggers that may result in violence.

While not all violence can be predicted, some signs and symptoms precede violence. The following signs, symptoms, and factors are associated with acts of violence toward others:

- Threats
- Manic states
- Suicidal risk
- Verbal abuse
- Hyperactivity
- Overcrowding
- Elopement risk
- Unusual silence
- Poor limit setting
- Inexperienced staff
- Anger and irritability
- Loud, aggressive speech
- Agitation and impulsiveness
- Uncharacteristic isolation
- Neurologic abnormalities
- Active paranoid delusions
- Alcohol or drug intoxication
- Provocative or controlling staff
- History of aggression or violence
- Arbitrary revocation of privileges
- Intense or avoidance of eye contact
- Belligerent, hostile, or threatening behavior
- Recent acts of violence, including vandalism
- Physical changes, such as sweating, clenched fists, rapid breathing
- Possession of a weapon or object that can be used as a weapon

Self-violence can be preceded by signs that include the following:

- Isolation
- Loss of love
- Hopelessness
- Rigid thinking
- Physical health
- Gender identity
- Low self-esteem
- Religious beliefs
- Sexual orientation
- Bullying behavior
- Low serotonin levels
- History of depression
- Attitude toward death
- Employment problems
- Feelings of rage or guilt
- Familial history of suicide
- Substance abuse, addiction
- History of psychiatric illness
- History of violence toward others
- Restricted freedom, incarceration
- Difficulty with interpersonal relationships
- Familial history of abuse, neglect, and acts of violence

The nurse's priority is to maintain the safety of staff, the client, and others. The following are techniques used to manage safety:

- Visible security
- Client room search
- Communication with staff
- Identification of triggers
- Provision of a thorough report
- Use of de-escalation techniques
- Visitor limitation or restriction
- Maintaining personal space and presence

- Avoiding secluded areas, remaining near an exit door
- Restricting access to objects that can cause harm
- Ensuring two staff members are present when entering the client's room
- Avoiding clothing or accessories that can be used to cause harm

Identifying a client in crisis is achieved by recognizing certain behaviors. Gerald Caplan categorizes the **behaviors of a crisis** into four phases.

FOUR PHASES OF A CRISIS REACTION	
Phase	**Crisis Reaction**
1	This stage begins with the initial threat to a client's self-concept. The client during this stage responds with defense mechanisms such as rationalization, compensation, and denial and stimulates the use of problem solving techniques to resolve the level of stress and anxiety.
2	If the problem persists and is unable to be resolved, the anxiety continues to increase and functioning begins to become disorganized.
3	During this phase, if the client is unable to resolve the issue and restore balance, the anxiety intensifies to a severe level and then to panic. Automatic relief behaviors such as flight or fight and panic begin to set in.
4	Panic and despair are the hallmark signs of this phase when the client's coping skills are ineffective. The client experiences serious disorganization, confusion, depression, and disorientation; possible violence against self or others may occur.

Before planning client care, the nurse will identify the domain of the crisis and confirm the crisis. The domains include maturational, situational, and adventitious.

Confirmation of the crisis is based on three components: the precipitating event, the perception of the event, and the client's usual coping methods. The goal of the nurse is to return the client to a pre-crisis level using therapeutic communication, decision making, and problem solving. Symptoms identified in the phases of a crisis, as well as the coping mechanisms and defense mechanisms discussed earlier, will assist the nurse in creating a plan of care that is appropriate for the psychopathology of the client. Identification of the proper resources and social supports to help resolve the client's crisis are included in the plan of care.

CULTURAL AWARENESS/CULTURAL INFLUENCES ON HEALTH

The nurse's ability to provide culturally competent care begins with awareness, knowledge, and accurate data collection from all clients. When assessing, planning, and evaluating care for any client, the nurse must consider language barriers, ethnicity, and cultural practices throughout all aspects of care. Considerations also include the client's cultural verbal and nonverbal communication, customs, beliefs, and values. Understanding the cultural concepts of distress identified by the American Psychiatric Association (APA) will assist the nurse in identifying interventions that appropriately meet the client's needs.

The **cultural concepts of distress** include the following:

- **Cultural syndromes:** clusters of symptoms that tend to occur in certain cultural groups, communities, or contexts.

- **Cultural idioms of distress:** ways of communicating emotional suffering that do not refer to specific disorders or symptoms, yet provide a way to talk about personal or social concerns. Frequently, these manifest as physical symptoms (**somatization**).

- **Cultural explanations:** symptom, illness, or distress that is perceived by a culture as having specific local origins or causes.

Furthermore, when the nurse addresses the broad categories of cultural beliefs and attitudes of a client, the nurse is gaining an understanding of the client's cultural beliefs and ability to accept a psychiatric diagnosis.

The following are cultural factors that affect beliefs and attitudes:

- Age
- Pain
- Ethics
- Health
- Gender
- Religion
- Sick role
- Treatments
- Social status
- Disease causation
- Decisions about care
- Geographical location
- Physical location of the disorder

Directly asking the client about specific practices that may enhance the adherence to a treatment plan is appropriate. The nurse will also perform ongoing evaluation of the client's needs to ensure they are met, and, if they are not, the nurse will make the necessary changes. Documenting these findings provides essential communication to other health care team members such as the health care provider, social worker, and any others who are involved in the client's care.

END-OF-LIFE CARE

The nurse will coordinate the appropriate care for a client with a chronic or terminal illness. A client may require palliative care when it is not possible to determine that the life expectancy is less than six months. If the client's life expectancy is less than six months, hospice care will be offered.

One of the primary nursing goals in end-of-life care is to assist and advocate for the client and family in the decision making process. **Advocacy** includes empowering a client to make decisions through providing the education to do so. Topics that are important to include in the discussion are the right to refuse treatment, allowing the client to decide where dying will take place, promoting the use of advance directives, establishing a living will and health care power of attorney, discussing pain management, as well as providing physiological and psychological support throughout the dying process.

Throughout the dying process, the nurse will assess the client and family's anticipatory grieving process and ability to cope and will continue to provide education about the expected physiological and psychological changes that will occur. Throughout the care of the client and family, the nurse will evaluate the understanding of the information by assessing and addressing all barriers to communication. These barriers include language, health literacy, anxiety, inability to cope, and any concerns the client or family may have.

End-of-life client needs include, but are not limited to, the following:

- **Physical comfort:** pain, hydration, nutrition, elimination, respiration, cognitive changes

- **Mental and emotional support:** fear, loss of control, role changes, assessment of coping, end-of-life resolution, anticipatory grief, addressing the developmental tasks of grief

- **Spiritual support:** chaplain, prayer, ritual

- **Resolution of everyday tasks:** financial concerns, employment, pets

The nurse will include multiple domains of the nursing role when providing end-of-life care to a client and family. These domains include the following:

- Management of rapidly changing situations

- Monitoring and ensuring that quality care is provided

- Monitoring diagnostics and physiological functioning

- Administering and monitoring therapeutic interventions

- Organizing collaborative health care team members

- Providing support through listening, advocacy, promoting well-being, ethical decision making

- Teaching through active listening, engagement, and provision of the appropriate treatment information

Support for the family throughout the end-of-life process also requires the nurse to provide education and emotional support. The education encompasses the anticipated physiological and psychological changes in the client that occur as death approaches. Active listening, providing a presence, ongoing assessment of needs, and the provision of respite care are nursing interventions that are essential considerations in meeting the needs of the family. After the death of the client, the nurse will continue to provide an ongoing assessment of the family for complicated grief, which includes chronic, delayed, exaggerated, masked, disenfranchised, or unresolved grief. The nurse will also provide the family members the appropriate resources for support.

FAMILY DYNAMICS

Factors that influence family dynamics and functioning must be taken into consideration when planning care for clients and their families. Factors such as family structure, boundaries, communication, emotional support, socialization, and parenting style all influence the components of a care plan.

It is important to note that dysfunctional families exhibit a variety of patterns. The most common patterns for dysfunctional families include the following:

- Substance abuse

- Parental compulsive behavior

- Threatened or actual violence

- Lack of emotional, physical, or financial support

- Arguing

- Lack of routine

- Fear

- Poor communication

Boundaries are either **diffuse** or **rigid**. A family with diffuse boundaries is overinvolved or enmeshed with each other. Rigid boundaries occur in families who are isolated from one another with minimal communication. Dysfunctional communication includes manipulation, distraction, generalizing, blaming, excessive arguing, criticism, and control. Unhealthy emotional support consists of a dominant pattern of conflict and anger, as well as unmet emotional and physical needs. Socialization is learned through role modeling and requires different types of socialization throughout the developmental process. Families who cannot meet this requirement exhibit a dysfunctional pattern of socialization.

Parenting has a significant effect on family dynamics. Parenting dysfunction is characterized by deficiency; controlling behavior; substance abuse; physical, emotional, or sexual abuse; and neglect. When assessing family dynamics and functioning, parental techniques of discipline should also be included. Stressors and barriers such as the family's current state of housing, finances, employment status, environment, and access to health care are factors that should be assessed in conjunction with family dynamics when planning care. After completing the family assessment, the nurse can evaluate the family's current state and make the appropriate referrals for group or family therapy as appropriate to promote healthy functioning.

The nurse can anticipate the change in family dynamics when a new member is integrated into the family. The adaptation varies based on the nature of family integration; for example, a newborn may evoke feelings of sibling jealousy. Other types of family integration include the assimilation of a blended family, an adopted family, or an older adult into the household. Throughout this process, the nurse will assess the availability of resources, the progression of the family, and the new member's adaptation.

GRIEF AND LOSS

Providing care for a client experiencing loss or grief includes assessing the grief of a client or family. A client or family member who is experiencing anticipatory grief before a loss may be experiencing depression. The nurse may consider using a tool such as the **Anticipatory Grief Scale**, which helps identify clients and family members experiencing anticipatory grief.

Other emotional responses associated with anticipatory grief include denial, sadness, anger, disappointment, as well as other responses. These feelings may be related to the impending loss of life, loss of identity, changes in roles, loss of function, or other events that occur after diagnosis of a severe illness.

When focusing on the client, the nurse will support the client experiencing grief or loss by responding in a meaningful way and incorporating the use of an interdisciplinary team that may include a social worker, therapist, and chaplain. Preparing the client for the anticipatory grief through education and reassuring the client that certain experiences are expected and may become more intense as death nears is a meaningful way to support the client during this process. The nurse will also ensure that the client can discuss somatic concerns and actively participate in the choice of interventions. This discussion is key in providing physical and psychological support and comfort to the client. Assessing previous coping mechanisms, discussing symptom control, and providing updated information about the client's condition will assist the client and family in coping through this time.

MENTAL HEALTH CONCEPTS

Cognitive impairment affects an individual's ability to learn new things, concentrate, or make decisions that affect daily life. Cognitive impairment may occur in relation to dementia, delirium, or other physiological conditions such as injury or illness. All clients will be assessed for medical conditions before the diagnoses of any mental health illness. When assessing a client, one of several tools is used to assist the nurse in screening for cognitive impairment. Tools such as the **Mini-Cog** or **Montreal Cognitive Assessment** can be used to assess cognitive impairment. The **Mental Status Exam (MSE)** can also be used to describe the mental state and behaviors of a client. The MSE can only be used to gather subjective and objective information to assess a client's cognition at that particular point in time, but is still a very useful tool for assessment.

Anticipated findings for a client whose cognition is intact include the following:

- **Appearance:** normal posture, good grooming, good hygiene, appropriate dress, cooperation, facial expression, positive attitude toward health care worker or family

- **Behavior:** eye contact, appropriate psychomotor activity, normal gait, the absence of non-purposeful large and small muscle movements

- **Speech:** appropriate tone, content, volume, and rate

- **Mood:** the euthymic emotional state

- **Affect:**
    - Type—euthymic
    - Range—full
    - Congruency—matches mood
    - Stability—stable

- **Thought process:** connected, flowing, clear, coherent, organized, logical, linear, goal-directed

- **Thought content:** perception, the absence of themes that occupy the client's thoughts

- **Cognition:** appropriate level of consciousness, attention, and concentration; intact short- and long-term memory; ability to use abstraction

- **Insight and judgment:** awareness, ability to anticipate consequences of one's behavior and make decisions

A client with acute or chronic mental illness will exhibit changes in one or more of the categories of the MSE. The changes that occur are related to the type of mental illness and the extent of the disease process the client is experiencing.

Possible abnormal findings in each of the categories associated with mental illness include, but are not limited to, the following:

- **Appearance:** poor posture, under- or overweight, inappropriate dress, disheveled appearance, body odor, and uncooperative behavior

- **Behavior:** poor eye contact or piercing stare, agitation, wringing of hands or psychomotor retardation, tremors, rhythmic or repetitive movements that are predictable but purposeless

- **Speech:** increased (pressured) or decreased (monosyllabic), latency, very articulate or monotone, prosody, slurred, dysarthria, loud, soft, mute, fluent, paucity, talkative, or impoverished

- **Mood:** subjective information obtained from the client

- **Affect:** dysphoric, euphoric, anxious, restricted, blunt, flat, or labile

- **Thought process:** unclear associations, unorganized, incoherent, circumstantial, tangential, loose, a flight of ideas, word salad, clanging, or thought-blocking

- **Thought content:** consists of preoccupations, illusions, ideas of references, audio or visual hallucinations, derealization, depersonalization, delusions, suicidal ideation, homicidal ideation, and paranoia

- **Cognition:** decreased level of consciousness; inability to focus, sustain, or appropriately shift attention; inability to think abstractly

- **Insight and judgment:** unaware of illness or current situation; inability to anticipate consequences of behavior

Understanding acute and chronic mental health disorders and recognizing signs and symptoms associated with the different illnesses is critical in preventing a client's mental health from further deteriorating.

The overall nursing goals for all clients with acute and chronic mental illnesses include the following:

- Reducing or eliminating symptoms

- Confirming symptom control is maintained

- Maximizing the client's quality of life and ability to function

- Promoting and sustaining recovery from the debilitating effects of illness to the maximum extent possible

- Monitoring the client for adverse effects of treatment

- Preventing relapse from occurring

There are more than 200 classified types of mental illness. The major categories are as follows:

- Anxiety disorders

- Mood disorders

- Schizophrenia/psychotic disorders

- Personality disorders

- Dementia

- Eating disorders

- Addiction and dependence

Anxiety Disorders

An anxiety disorder is defined as a persistent sense of apprehension that interferes with personal, occupational, and social functioning. Clients with anxiety may experience chest pain, fear, nightmares, or other somatic discomforts, all of which interfere with day-to-day functioning.

ANXIETY DISORDERS	
Disorder	**Description**
Panic Disorder	Panic disorder is a sudden onset of intense extreme apprehension or fear, usually associated with a fear of impending doom. These attacks are unpredictable and last about ten minutes. Symptoms include heart palpitations, tachycardia, trembling, shortness of breath, nausea, chest pain, dizziness, derealization, paresthesia, or fear of dying.
Obsessive-Compulsive Disorder (OCD)	OCD is an anxiety disorder in which clients have recurring, unwanted thoughts, ideas, or sensations that make them feel driven to do something repetitively. Some of the compulsions a client may experience include handwashing, cleaning, repeating, ordering and arranging things, saying phrases, and checking on things, all of which can interfere with daily activities and social interaction.
Post-Traumatic Stress Disorder (PTSD)	PTSD is a trauma- or stress-related disorder that may develop after exposure to an event in which death or severe physical harm was threatened or occurred. Symptoms of this disorder include flashbacks; jumpiness; difficulty sleeping; hypervigilance; nightmares; loneliness; anger; worry; guilt; and difficulty with relationships, trust, and communication. These symptoms may interfere with a client's daily activities and social interaction.
Phobias	A phobia is an intense, irrational fear of something that poses little or no threat. Phobias include claustrophobia and agoraphobia. Agoraphobia is described as intense fear of or anxiety about being in open or crowded places, leaving home, or being in places from which escape is difficult. Clients with phobias may experience panic, fear, tachycardia, dyspnea, and trembling.
Generalized Anxiety Disorder	Generalized anxiety disorder is characterized by persistent and excessive worry about different things. The client is unable to stop the cycle of worrying.
Separation Anxiety Disorder	Separation anxiety disorder involves developmentally inappropriate levels of significant or intense anxiety when the client is away from a significant other. This anxiety detracts from normal day-to-day activity and may be associated with nightmares, gastrointestinal disturbances, or headaches.

Mood Disorders

Mood disorders are characterized by a serious change in mood that causes a disruption in social, occupational, or other daily activities. Mood disorders include depressive disorders such as **major depressive disorder (MDD)**. It is important to note that the older adult with depression has an increased risk of developing major depression and a disproportional risk for suicide. The psychomotor and cognitive effects of depression in the older adult may be mistaken for a neurocognitive disorder, such as Alzheimer's disease, and is referred to as **pseudodementia**. This can be reversed when the underlying depression is eliminated.

A major depressive disorder is characterized by a persistently depressed mood lasting for a minimum of two or more weeks with the primary symptoms being loss of interest and enjoyment in usual activities and decreased activities overall. At least five of nine symptoms identified in the APA's *Diagnostic and Statistical Manual of Mental Disorders* (*DSM-5*) criteria must be present nearly every day. The client should be assessed for conditions such as substance abuse, medical conditions, other psychiatric disorders, or bereavement before using the diagnostic criteria for major depressive disorder. The severity of a depressive episode may range from mild to severe, and the symptoms may cause significant distress or impairment in social, occupational, or other daily activities.

Recognized symptoms for MDD include the following:

- Depressed mood or irritable most of the day, nearly every day, as indicated by either subjective report (e.g., feels sad or empty) or observation made by others (e.g., appears tearful)

- Decreased interest or pleasure in most activities, most of each day

- Significant weight change (5%) or change in appetite

- Change in sleep—insomnia or hypersomnia

- Change in activity—psychomotor agitation or retardation

- Fatigue or loss of energy

- Guilt/worthlessness—feelings of worthlessness or excessive/inappropriate guilt

- Concentration—diminished ability to think or concentrate, increased indecisiveness

- Suicidality—thoughts of death or suicide or has a suicide plan

Bipolar Disorder

Bipolar disorder is classified as bipolar I or bipolar II disorder. **Bipolar I** disorder is defined as having manic episodes (mania) lasting at least seven days that are severe enough to require hospitalization of the client. Depressive episodes occur with this disorder, lasting for at least two weeks. **Bipolar II** disorder is defined by a pattern of manic and depressive episodes. The manic episodes are not as severe as the symptoms in bipolar I disorder.

Symptoms of mania include the following:

- Reckless behavior

- Excessive irritability, aggressive behavior

- Impulsiveness, poor judgment, distractibility

- Racing speech, racing thoughts, a flight of ideas

- Increased physical and mental activity and energy

- In the most severe cases, delusions and hallucinations

- Decreased need for sleep without experiencing fatigue

- Grandiose delusions, inflated sense of self-importance

- Heightened mood, exaggerated optimism and self-confidence

Symptoms of depression in bipolar disorder include the following:

- Somatic complaints
- Pessimism, indifference
- Feelings of guilt, worthlessness
- Loss of energy, persistent lethargy
- Recurring thoughts of death or suicide
- Inability to concentrate, indecisiveness
- Irritability, anger, worry, agitation, anxiety
- Prolonged sadness or unexplained crying spells
- Significant changes in appetite and sleep patterns
- Inability to take pleasure in former interests, social withdrawal

Schizophrenia

Schizophrenia is characterized by distortions in thinking, perception, emotions, language, sense of self, and behavior. Common experiences for a client with schizophrenia include disorganized thinking and speech; abnormal motor behavior; positive symptoms such as delusions or hallucinations; negative symptoms such as decreased emotional expression, avolition, anhedonia, alogia, and association.

Personality Disorders

Personality disorders are a complex group of mental health disorders. Clients in this group of disorders have difficulty with self-identity, self-direction, and recognizing or acknowledging that they have a disorder. The client may believe that problems originate from outside influences and not from within the self.

The APA has grouped 10 different personality disorders into clusters of similar personality traits and behavior patterns. The clusters and personality disorders are described in the following table.

PERSONALITY DISORDER CLUSTERS	
Cluster/Traits	Personality Disorders/Symptoms
Cluster A: Odd or Eccentric Behavior	• **Schizoid Personality Disorder:** These clients are withdrawn, introverted, non-emotional, distant, and fear closeness or intimacy with others. • **Paranoid Personality Disorder:** The client interprets the actions of others as intentionally threatening or demeaning and displays very guarded or secretive behavior. The client is untrusting and prone to anger or aggressive outbursts due to the perception that others are condescending, unfaithful, or deceitful. • **Schizotypal Personality Disorder:** The client will display odd, eccentric manners of speaking and dressing and will express strange paranoid beliefs. These clients have great difficulty forming relationships or being in social situations. They may talk to themselves and/or react inappropriately or not at all in a conversation.

PERSONALITY DISORDER CLUSTERS	
Cluster/Traits	**Personality Disorders/Symptoms**
Cluster B: Dramatic, Emotional, or Erratic Behavior	• **Antisocial Personality Disorder:** The client ignores the rules of social behavior, acts out conflict, is irresponsible and aggressive, displays no respect for others, and has no remorse for his or her actions. • **Borderline Personality Disorder:** The client demonstrates instability in areas such as mood, self-image, interpersonal relationships, and behavior. The client displays abrupt and extreme mood changes, demonstrates self-destructive actions, fears abandonment, and may self-mutilate or exhibit suicidal gestures to get attention. This type of client is impulsive, views the world in extremes, and may show excessive dependency on another. Generally, this client has very turbulent relationships with others. • **Narcissistic Personality Disorder:** The client has an exaggerated sense of self-importance and seeks constant attention. The client tends to exploit interpersonal relationships, is oversensitive to failure, and often has multiple somatic complaints.
Cluster C: Anxious or Fearful Behavior	• **Avoidant Personality Disorder:** The client is hypersensitive to rejection, timid, and fearful of criticism. The client will avoid social activities that involve interpersonal contact and may have no social contact outside the family. • **Dependent Personality Disorder:** The client demonstrates dependent and submissive behavior, relying on others to make decisions. This client is uncomfortable when alone, is easily hurt by criticism or disapproval, and lacks self-confidence to do things independently. • **Obsessive Compulsive Personality Disorder:** This client has high levels of aspiration and strives for perfection. The client tends to take on more responsibility and is dependable, orderly, and methodical. The client's inflexibility makes him or her incapable of adapting to change. This type of client is also highly cautious and pays attention to every detail, making it difficult to complete tasks. This client feels a sense of isolation and helplessness.

Eating Disorders

Eating disorders occur when a client develops a troubled relationship with food that results in abnormal eating habits and a distorted view of the body. This disorder can be fatal if not addressed and treated properly. The primary eating disorders include anorexia nervosa, bulimia, and binge eating.

A client with **anorexia nervosa** has an intense fear of weight gain, has a distorted body image, and restricts caloric intake in the presence of a significantly low BMI. These clients have a preoccupation with thoughts of food, view themselves as fat even when emaciated, exhibit peculiar handling of food, and will develop a rigorous exercise plan. Their self-worth is based on their weight.

Client behaviors include the following:

- Insomnia
- Flat affect
- Irritability
- Denial of hunger

- Social withdrawal
- Fear of gaining weight
- Avoidance of eating in public
- Preoccupation with food
- Skipping meals or refusing to eat
- Making excuses for not eating
- Developing rigid meal or eating rituals
- Covering up in layers of clothing
- Eating foods low in fat and calories
- Repeatedly weighing or measuring the body
- Dishonesty about how much food has been eaten
- Frequent review of self in the mirror for perceived flaws

A client with **bulimia nervosa** will engage in recurrent episodes of uncontrollable binging, which leads to feelings of loss of control, guilt, and a sense of disgust. The client purges to bring on a sense of relief and to prevent weight gain. Other methods to prevent weight gain include laxative use, vomiting, diuretics, fasting, enemas, and exercise. Client behaviors associated with the disorder include compulsive exercise, eating large amounts of food, and going to the bathroom immediately after meals.

Physical assessment findings for both anorexia and bulimia nervosa include the following:

- Diarrhea
- Petechiae
- Loss of hair
- Ecchymosis
- Constipation
- Tachycardia
- Hypotension
- Hematemesis
- Russell's sign
- Gastric rupture
- Gastric dilation
- Cardiomyopathy
- Mild brain atrophy
- Esophageal rupture
- Cardiac arrhythmias

- Tooth enamel erosion
- Generalized weakness
- Decrease in bone mass
- Electrocardiograph changes
- Swelling of the parotid glands
- Acid base imbalances (alkalosis or acidosis)
- Fluid and electrolyte loss (hypokalemia, hypochloremia)

In addition to the physical assessment findings mentioned above, the following are unique to anorexia nervosa:

- Lanugo
- Cachexia
- Neuropathy
- Amenorrhea
- Bradycardia
- Renal failure
- Muscle wasting
- Hypothyroidism
- Decreased GFR
- Decreased WBC
- Elevated cortisol
- Hypomagnesemia
- Decreased platelets
- Hypophosphatemia
- Hypercholesterolemia
- Cognitive impairment
- Decreased reproductive hormones
- Yellowish discoloration of the skin
- Osteoporosis—increased risk for fracture
- ECG changes—prolonged QT wave, prolonged ST-T wave

A client experiencing a **binge eating disorder** engages in the repeated eating of large amounts of food in a short period of time. Client behavior also includes eating when full, eating until uncomfortably full, eating alone or in secret, and frequently dieting without weight loss. This behavior leaves the client feeling depressed, ashamed, guilty, and disgusted. Binge eating predisposes the client to obesity, which increases the risk of the physiological conditions associated with it.

Addiction and Dependence

According to the APA, **addiction** is defined as a complex condition—a brain disease that manifests by compulsive substance use despite harmful consequences. **Dependence** occurs when the neurons of the brain adapt to repeated exposure to a substance and function normally only when the substance is present. When the substance is not present, a client with a dependency will experience some form of withdrawal. The effect and physiological reaction of the withdrawal is dependent on the substance involved. Over time, clients may develop a tolerance to a substance, leading them to require more of the substance to achieve the same response they initially experienced.

Identifying personalized goals for a client's plan of care is accomplished by providing the client and family with education and by assessing the client's coping ability, support system, and other necessary available resources based on stage of development and cognition. The nurse must also help clients recognize defense mechanisms that may be maladaptive and assist with identifying constructive coping mechanisms. A multi-disciplinary team approach is most often necessary to meet the needs of the client and family. When creating a plan of care, the client and the interdisciplinary health care team will identify interventions to assist the client in managing and coping with the illness and with obtaining the necessary resources to support the client in the appropriate care setting or community.

The nurse can anticipate that management of the disease may include treatments such as physiological stabilization (including the correction of acid-base, electrolyte, and fluid imbalances), cardiac arrhythmias, administration of prescriptions, referrals to therapy (which may include psychotherapy; cognitive behavioral therapy; and family, interpersonal psychodynamic, and group therapies), or integrating desensitization into the client's treatment. Ongoing evaluation for the adherence to treatment is necessary to identify any variances that can be immediately addressed with the client and health care team.

RELIGIOUS AND SPIRITUAL INFLUENCES ON HEALTH

According to NANDA International (NANDA-I), spiritual distress impairs the client's ability to experience and integrate meaning and purpose in life through connectedness with self, others, art, music, nature, or a power greater than oneself. A client experiencing any spiritual distress or a conflict between recommended treatments and religious beliefs requires the support of the nurse to facilitate the interventions necessary to assist the client in resolving any distress. When caring for all clients, the nurse will employ active listening because it conveys presence and empathy, which allows the client to express thoughts, feelings, and concerns. Also, allowing the client to share feelings, concerns, and stories provides the nurse with the client's perspective on the situation. It is essential for the nurse to assesses the client's preferences regarding religious beliefs and practices and to be able to recognize the symptoms of spiritual distress.

Signs and symptoms that are associated with spiritual distress are as follows:

- Difficulty sleeping
- Feeling abandoned by God or other Supreme Being (as defined by the client)
- Feelings of anger or hopelessness
- Feelings of depression and anxiety
- Asking why a situation has occurred
- Questioning the meaning of life or suffering
- Questioning long-held beliefs or the sudden doubt of spiritual or religious beliefs

Nursing interventions are focused on restoring the client's feeling of connectedness and meeting emotional needs; these interventions are constructed based on the client's perception of the distress. The client should be encouraged to participate in choosing the interventions that help to resolve distress or feelings of conflict. Interventions may include supporting the practice of ritual or prayer, or possibly notifying a member of the clergy or a person of the client's choice who is related to the chosen religion or spiritual practice. The nurse will conduct an ongoing evaluation of the client's response to the interventions to ensure the planned outcomes are being met.

Of further concern are the psychological or occupational factors that interfere with the client's ability to adhere to the plan of care. Psychological factors include anxiety, stress, and coping ability. Employment factors may consist of missed work hours, the inability to keep health care appointments due to work hours, loss of wages, and the inability to perform job functions. These areas are assessed on an ongoing basis and, if needed, the care plan is adjusted accordingly. All outcomes are measured and evaluated for the overall effectiveness of the entire plan of care.

SENSORY/PERCEPTUAL ALTERATIONS

All clients are assessed for the presence or risk of sensory perceptual alterations. Sensory alterations place the client at risk for injury, so safety is a priority concern for any client with a sensory perceptional alteration. The different sensory functions that may be altered include taste, smell, vision, hearing, balance, touch (tactile sense), and sensations related to internal organs (visceral sense). Contributing factors to altered sensory function include neurological changes, biochemical factors, psychological stress, chemical alterations, sensory overload, or deprivation. Performing a mental status assessment for clients experiencing altered sensory perception provides valuable information and will help the nurse gain insight into the severity of any existing alterations.

Understanding the factors that can contribute to sensory perceptual alterations will also help prevent them or assist the nurse in identifying the time, place, stimuli, or other factors associated with the alterations. All of this information is necessary to support the nurse in creating a plan of care for the client.

Other factors that place the client at risk for sensory perception alterations include the following:

- Age
- Pain
- Stress
- Discomfort
- Medications
- Invasive tubes
- Proprioception
- Cultural factors
- Social interaction
- Amount of stimuli
- Meaningful stimuli
- Mental health conditions

- Decreased cognitive ability
- Developmental considerations
- Admission to a new environment

Prevention of sensory perceptual alteration is integrated into the plan of care for any client with a risk factor. Preventative measures include the following:

- Managing pain
- Reducing unpleasant odors
- Promoting rest and comfort
- Encouraging physical activity
- Providing stimulation for all of the senses
- Monitoring for mood and behavior changes
- Providing care in a relaxed, unhurried manner
- Assessing for the use of needed sensory aids or prothesis
- Using social activities to stimulate the mind to provide stimuli
- Encouraging family members to participate in activities with client
- Limiting visitors or placing the client in a private room to decrease stimuli

When caring for a client who is experiencing visual impairment, nursing interventions include the following:

- Keeping visual aids accessible
- Maintaining a clutter-free environment
- Speaking in a normal tone of voice
- Using braille and large-print materials
- Providing diversion using the other senses
- Acknowledging your presence in the room
- Keeping the call light within reach of the client
- Orienting the client to the room and furnishings
- Orienting the client to the sounds in the environment
- Providing an explanation before touching the client
- Indicating the conversation is completed before leaving the room
- Walking slightly ahead of the client when assisting with ambulation
- Staying within the client's field of vision (if the client has partial vision)
- Assisting the client with meals by describing the position of plated food using the analogy of time on a clock

When caring for a client who is experiencing hearing impairment, nursing interventions include the following:

- Using a sign language interpreter
- Communicating in writing when appropriate
- Positioning oneself so the light is on the face
- Speaking directly to the client while facing him or her
- Orienting the client to the speaker's presence before speaking
- Ensuring the client's hearing aids are in and working
- Decreasing background noises and distractions before speaking

When caring for a confused client, nursing interventions include the following:

- Wearing a readable name tag
- Addressing the client by name
- Providing a safe environment
- Using closed-ended questions
- Maintaining the client's comfort
- Frequently monitoring the client
- Frequently reintroducing oneself
- Providing reality-based diversions
- Providing frequent client reassurance
- Monitoring the stimuli in the environment
- Managing hallucinations with prescriptions
- Orienting the client to time, place, and person
- Addressing the anticipated needs of the client
- Orienting and reorienting the client to the environment
- Speaking to the client calmly and clearly
- Allowing time for the client to process information and respond
- Using frequent face-to-face contact while maintaining eye contact
- Offering explanations of care using props or aids to facilitate understanding

A client experiencing cognitive or perceptual disturbances may be difficult to engage because the client is distracted, unable to focus, and possibly experiencing memory impairment. The client's inability to process the internal and external environment may result in various misinterpretations that take the form of hallucinations or illusions. An individual with **delirium** is aware that something is wrong and therefore experiences fear and anxiety that may result in psychomotor agitation. The client with cognitive or perceptual disturbances is at risk for injury, self-care deficit, poor nutrition, incontinence, and changes in the sleep/wake cycle. When caring for any client with alterations in sensory perception, the nurse will provide care in a nonthreatening and nonjudgmental manner.

STRESS MANAGEMENT

The nurse will monitor the client for nonverbal cues of physical and psychological stressors with the understanding that different stressors result in different patterns of responses. The client's perception of the degree of stress is most important when providing ongoing monitoring of nonverbal cues of stressors. Perception of stress is based on age, culture, gender, life experience, genetic structure, vulnerability, childhood experiences, and coping strategies. Nonverbal cues of physical and psychological stressors may include increased respiration, heart rate, and blood pressure; muscle tension; nail biting; talkativeness; repetitive behaviors; restlessness; isolation; and an unnatural posture.

Assessing the client's understanding of the stressors or triggers such as environment, fear, noise, uncertainty, change, or lack of knowledge will help the nurse and client identify appropriate measures to include in the plan of care to help alleviate the causative factors. While caring for a client, the nurse can implement measures to provide a therapeutic environment that should help decrease the client's stress. Comfortable lighting and environmental temperature, reduced noise, and privacy are all measures to decrease stress.

Stress management techniques the nurse can suggest to the client include the following:

- Relaxation
- Rest
- Decreased caffeine intake
- Biofeedback
- Meditation
- Deep breathing
- Yoga
- Guided imagery
- Distraction
- Exercise
- Prayer
- Massage
- Journaling
- Hypnosis
- Music therapy
- Cognitive reframing
- Aromatherapy
- Acupuncture
- Humor

By obtaining objective and subjective assessments periodically throughout the client's use of the stress management techniques, the nurse will gather information useful for evaluating the effectiveness of the interventions and ensuring the client meets the outcome of the pre-established goals.

SUBSTANCE USE AND OTHER DISORDERS AND DEPENDENCIES

A client using substances may be at risk for addiction, tolerance, intoxication, or withdrawal. A variety of tools can assist the nurse in screening clients for substance use and dependency. The American Society of Addiction Medicine describes addiction as a "primary chronic disease of the brain reward, motivation, memory, and related circuitry." When a client develops a tolerance, he or she will require a higher amount of the substance in order to obtain the same effect.

Intoxication occurs when the client has taken or used an excessive amount of a substance. The manifestation of physiological symptoms depends on the substance and amount used. Another factor to consider is the route the client is using to take in the substance. Routes for substance use include injecting, inhaling, and swallowing. A client who is injecting or inhaling a substance is at risk for additional physiological injury. Withdrawal occurs when a client stops using a substance. Depending on the substance that is used, the client will exhibit a set of physiological symptoms that can range from mild to life-threatening.

The different categories of psychoactive substances recognized by the APA's *DSM-5* are as follows:

- Opioid
- Alcohol
- Inhalant
- Caffeine
- Tobacco
- Cannabis
- Stimulant
- Hallucinogen
- Sedative, hypnotic, or anxiolytic prescriptions

Other forms of addiction include gambling, compulsive sexual behavior, pornography, shopping, and food. All addictive behavior is associated with the release of dopamine. Providing education to the client about the substance used and including the client in formulating a treatment plan will increase the likelihood of adherence. When caring for a client diagnosed with a substance-related disorder, the nursing priority is to maintain the physiological stability and safety of the client as well as others in contact with the client. The client who is experiencing toxicity or withdrawal is at risk for injury due to an altered perception as well as physiological reactions to the substance. The following information discusses the psychological and physical symptoms of withdrawal for the above-mentioned psychoactive substances, as well as the nursing interventions required to stabilize and maintain client safety.

Opioids

Opioids include drugs like morphine, methadone, heroin, oxycodone, fentanyl, and codeine. Symptoms of intoxication include the following:

- Euphoria
- Confusion
- Weight loss

- Bradycardia
- Hypokinesis
- Constipation
- Hypotension
- Hypothermia
- Altered mood
- Head nodding
- Slurred speech
- Restricted pupils
- Excessive drowsiness
- Respiratory depression
- Psychomotor retardation
- Impaired memory and attention

Symptoms for opioid withdrawal include the following:

- Fever
- Anxiety
- Diarrhea
- Vomiting
- Yawning
- Insomnia
- Tachypnea
- Rhinorrhea
- Lacrimation
- Diaphoresis
- Piloerection
- Tachycardia
- Muscle aches
- Hypertension
- Hyperthermia
- Mood dysphoria
- Pupillary dilation
- Abdominal cramps
- Bone and muscle pain

Withdrawal is based on the administration of an antagonist or the amount of opioid used. Withdrawal from morphine, methadone, and heroin usually begins 6–8 hours after the last dose, reaches intensity during the second or third day, and usually subsides the following week. Treatment initially addresses the client's ability to breathe, as death usually stems from respiratory arrest. The client is also at risk for aspiration during this time. Naloxone is an opioid antagonist that is administered intramuscularly, subcutaneously, or intravenously to reverse the adverse effects of the drug.

Alcohol

Problematic excessive drinking includes binge drinking and heavy drinking. The level of alcohol intoxication is based on the client's blood alcohol level, which is measured in mg/dL. Alcohol withdrawal begins 6–8 hours after the last drink taken when reducing or quitting alcohol consumption after prolonged or heavy use. A mild to moderate withdrawal includes symptoms such as tremulousness, nausea, vomiting, insomnia, agitation, mild perceptual changes, loss of appetite, impaired cognition, depression, headache, fatigue, nightmares, tachycardia, perspiration, mood swings, and weakness. The pulse, blood pressure, and body temperature will increase. The client is at risk for seizures and delirium tremens (DTs), which may occur anytime within the first 72 hours. A client experiencing DTs commonly experiences delusions as well as visual and tactile disturbances. Treatment includes prevention of alcohol withdrawal, symptom relief, correction of fluid and electrolyte imbalances, as well as safety interventions.

Inhalants

Inhalant intoxication levels are based on the amount and type of substance inhaled. High doses of inhalant are associated with fearfulness, illusions, auditory and visual hallucinations, insomnia, muscle weakness, headache, disorientation, convulsions, cardiac arrhythmias, anorexia, coma, blurred vision, nausea, and vomiting. The client may also display apathy, diminished social and occupational functioning, impaired judgment, and impulsive and aggressive behavior. Clients using high doses over a long term are at risk for delirium, dementia, and psychosis. The symptoms may last a few hours or a few weeks. Treatment is based on the pathophysiological findings and psychotic responses.

Caffeine

Caffeine use disorder is not included in the APA's official list of user disorders; however, excessive caffeine use can result in intoxication and withdrawal. Caffeine intoxication is characterized by restlessness, nervousness, rambling speech, excitement, agitation, flushed face, diuresis, gastrointestinal disturbance, tachycardia, and cardiac arrhythmias. Headaches are the most common symptom of withdrawal, but can be accompanied by other symptoms such as fatigue, anxiety, flu-like symptoms, drowsiness, brain fog, irritability, difficulty concentrating, and depressed mood. The symptoms will occur within 12–24 hours of discontinuing its use and can last up to nine days. The symptoms of withdrawal usually occur within the first two days. Gradually reducing the daily consumption of caffeine, combined with adequate hydration, sleep, and exercise, can help the client to adjust to lowered caffeine levels.

Tobacco

Cigarettes, pipes, cigars, and chewing tobacco are the primary methods for using tobacco. Symptoms of withdrawal include irritability, anxiety, depression, difficulty concentrating, restlessness, insomnia, intense craving, headaches, restlessness, sweating, waking at night, increased appetite, abdominal cramping, and constipation. The time frame for withdrawal varies from person to person, but usually the symptoms appear within 24 hours, peaking around day three and lasting several weeks. Treatment focuses on assisting the client to recognize cravings as well as providing nicotine replacement therapies.

Cannabis

A client who is experiencing cannabis intoxication will have a sense of heightened sensations such as depersonalization, derealization, elevated heart rate, dry mouth, increased appetite, unusual fluid accumulation in the eyes, as well as reddened eyes. Symptoms of withdrawal can occur within one week of cessation and may include irritability, anger, aggression, anxiety, nervousness, insomnia, disturbing dreams, weight loss, decreased appetite, depressed mood, restlessness, headaches, fever, chills, sweating, and abdominal pain. Abstinence is the primary treatment, although the client may require hospitalization and a short-term anti-anxiety medication.

Stimulants

Stimulants include cocaine and amphetamines. Symptoms of intoxication include the following:

- Coma
- Anger
- Nausea
- Anxiety
- Seizures
- Vomiting
- Confusion
- Dystonias
- Sensitivity
- Weight loss
- Dyskinesias
- Hypervigilance
- Pupillary dilation
- Muscular weakness
- Cardiac arrhythmias
- Perspiration or chills
- Respiratory depression
- Tachycardia or bradycardia
- Elevated or lowered blood pressure
- Psychomotor retardation or agitation

Symptoms of withdrawal are as follows:

- Fatigue
- Anxiety
- Paranoia

- Irritability

- Depression

- Drug craving

- Increased appetite

- Poor concentration

- Psychomotor retardation

- Hypersomnia (or insomnia)

Treatment for withdrawal depends on the substance used. Antipsychotics may be prescribed if psychosis is present, or diazepam may be administered to treat agitation and hyperactivity. Cocaine withdrawal lasts 1–2 weeks with no physiological disturbances that may require hospitalization. However, clients may experience mood changes, fatigue, depression, and disturbed sleep, as well as an intense craving for the drug.

Hallucinogens

Hallucinogens are intoxicants that produce a disturbance in reality. Hallucinogens include LSD, plants and mushrooms, and dissociative drugs such as phencyclidine (PCP) and ketamine. Symptoms of hallucinogen intoxication include hallucinations, synesthesias, pupillary dilation, tachycardia, sweating, blurred vision, tremors, incoordination, and palpitations. Treatment includes talking with the client to provide reassurance that the symptoms will subside. In severe cases an antipsychotic or benzodiazepine may be prescribed.

Clients experiencing PCP intoxication will display dangerous, violent side effects. Their behavior is unpredictable, impulsive, assaultive, and belligerent. This client is to be considered a medical emergency. Physical symptoms include nystagmus, hypertension, ataxia, dysarthria, hyperacusis, diminished response to pain, hyperthermia, seizures, and coma. Management for PCP intoxication is primarily supportive.

Sedative, hypnotic, or anxiolytic prescriptions include benzodiazepines, carbamates, barbiturates, and hypnotics. Symptoms of intoxication include impaired thinking, slurred speech, incoordination, unsteady gait, nystagmus, mood swings, impaired memory, and decreased blood pressure and pulse. Symptoms associated with withdrawal include rebound hyperactivity, tremors, insomnia, psychomotor agitation, anxiety, and grand mal seizures. The timing of withdrawal is substance-dependent. Treatment consists of the prevention of seizures and a gradual withdrawal of benzodiazepines to prevent seizures.

A client diagnosed with substance use, abuse, or other disorder may experience a wide range of feelings and reactions, such as decreased self-esteem, denial, powerlessness, fear, hopelessness, anger, sadness, and anxiety. The client's ability to participate and adhere to the treatment plan is greatly impacted by the understanding and knowledge of the condition, as well as having adequate coping mechanisms and family support.

Most initial treatments focus on detoxification and medically managed withdrawal, followed by focusing on psychological, social, and behavioral problems associated with use of the substance. During this part of recovery, the treatment plan for most substance use disorders is to focus on prevention of a relapse through the use of treatments that apply to the client's situation. These treatments may include different types of therapy, prescriptions, recovery support groups, psychotherapy, and behavioral therapy through partial hospitalization programs or outpatient treatment. Encouraging the client to participate in support groups will help the client learn new coping skills, obtain peer support, increase accountability, and offer an understanding. The nurse will evaluate the client's response to the treatment plan throughout and will revise the plan using an interdisciplinary approach as needed.

SUPPORT SYSTEMS

Cognitive impairment can be associated with many different diseases or conditions and is not limited to a specific chronological age group. Cognitive impairment can be the result of Alzheimer's disease, stroke, traumatic brain injury, lifestyle, exposure to substances, infection, or developmental disability. Delirium and dementia are two common neurocognitive disorders. Changes in a client's cognition can affect various mental functions such as learning, memory, ability to perceive or identify the relationship of objects in an environment, problem solving, language comprehension, decision making, communication, and the ability to view a situation from different points.

Planning care for a client with impaired cognition is determined by the type of disease and severity of the impairment. A client-centered approach is used when interacting with clients and any family members. If the client is able to participate in care planning cognitively, then most certainly he or she will be included. Caretakers and family should be involved in the plan of care because the client may not be able to recognize further changes in cognition. The amount of support and cooperation from a client who is newly diagnosed with a cognitive condition or disease will vary greatly and is determined by the client's feelings about the diagnosis and potential treatment plan. At the time of diagnosis, the nurse can anticipate providing emotional support and education to the client and family, as well as coordinating care that includes obtaining resources and appropriate referrals.

THERAPEUTIC COMMUNICATION

Clients express their needs through verbal and nonverbal communication. Understanding verbal communication encompasses not only *what* is spoken, but *how* it is spoken. Tone, pitch, volume, scarcity, and speed of the words add additional meaning to what the client is saying. Nonverbal communication includes not only body language but also clothing, appearance, eye contact, body movements, postures, facial expressions, hand gestures, personal space, and the immediate environment.

Both verbal and nonverbal communication from the nurse is vital in establishing a professional therapeutic relationship with the client. Before initiating contact, the nurse will be mindful of factors that interfere with communication. Environmental factors such as background noise and lack of privacy interfere with communication. Personal factors that hinder communication include physical or mental disorders, language barriers, cultural differences, gender-related beliefs, problem solving ability, educational and knowledge level, intellectual developmental disability, and neurocognitive disorders.

When seeking to build a therapeutic relationship with a client, the nurse will use positive attending behaviors, conveying respect for the client's values and beliefs as well as allowing adequate uninterrupted time to communicate with the client. Therapeutic communication focuses on advancing the well-being of the client through the use of several techniques to facilitate communication. The techniques the nurse can use to facilitate therapeutic communication include silence, acceptance, giving recognition, active listening, using touch, an offering of self, and providing broad openings and reassurance.

Clarification techniques used to enhance communication include summarizing, reflecting, and restating. Therapeutic communication creates an environment of trust and comfort that allows the client to verbalize feelings of fear or discomfort safely. A nurse must use effective therapeutic communication techniques during all interactions with the client.

THERAPEUTIC ENVIRONMENT

Many extrinsic factors can interfere with a client's recovery. A client may be worried about finances, limited access to health care, or inadequate family and community support systems. These factors can negatively affect the client's recovery. The nurse will work with members of a multidisciplinary team, such as a social worker or therapist, to assist the client in addressing these stressors.

A standard of care for the psychiatric-mental health registered nurse includes providing a structured, safe, therapeutic, recovery-oriented environment in collaboration with health care consumers, families, and other health care clinicians. Management of a therapeutic environment (also known as a **milieu**) is one of the primary focuses of the mental health nurse. When making room assignments for clients, the nurse will integrate milieu therapy into the decision. Cultivating a therapeutic environment also includes orienting the clients to their rights and responsibilities, providing culturally sensitive care, and maintaining the least restrictive environment that provides a climate for positive change.

SUMMING IT UP

- The purpose of the Psychosocial Integrity category is to assess the nurse's ability to provide and direct nursing care that promotes the client's **emotional, mental, and social well-being**. The nurse is responsible for creating a plan of care, providing education, and intervening appropriately for clients experiencing problems that affect mental and physical well-being.

- The nurse will assess all clients for abuse and identify those who are at an increased risk. The nurse must report any abuse and collaborate with health care team members to plan interventions. Types of abuse for which the RN will assess include the following:

  o Neglect

  o Physical, sexual, emotional, or verbal abuse

  o Bullying

  o Financial exploitation

- According to the CDC, **elder abuse** occurs when an act or failure to act results in risk of harm to an adult age 60 or over. Elder abuse is usually committed by a caregiver or someone the elder person trusts. Many elder abuse cases are unreported because of fear; as such, it is essential the nurse recognize some of the risk factors of abuse.

- A **mental status exam** is a structured assessment of the client's behavioral and cognitive functioning. The assessment is adjusted according to the developmental age or condition of the client. The nurse must perform a mental status exam before reviewing the physical status and physical assessment of the client.

- **Behavioral modification** is a treatment approach based on **operant conditioning** that replaces undesirable behaviors with more desirable ones through positive and negative reinforcement.

- The nurse will assess a client's ability to **cope** whenever that client must adapt to a temporary or permanent role change or a diagnosis of mental illness. Evaluation of the client's ability to accept and/or adapt to change assists the RN in providing the correct intervention, if necessary.

- Being diagnosed with an **acute** or **chronic mental illness** may bring up a range of emotions. Before planning care, the nurse will assess the client's reaction to the illness as well as coping ability and available support system.

- Crisis intervention involves assessing **predictors of violence**. During the assessment, the nurse attempts to identify client triggers that result in violence, as well as any signs, symptoms, and factors associated with acts of violence toward others.

- The nurse must provide **culturally competent care**. The nurse considers language barriers, ethnicity, and cultural practices throughout all aspects of care.

- The nurse will coordinate appropriate care for a client with a **chronic or terminal illness**. Throughout the dying process, the nurse will assess the client and family's anticipatory grieving process and ability to cope and then provide education about physiological and psychological changes that can be expected.

- The nurse must take all factors that influence **family dynamics** and functioning into consideration when planning care for clients and their families.

- When providing care for a client experiencing **grief or loss**, the nurse is responsible for the following:

    ○ Assessing the grief of a client or family

    ○ Responding meaningfully to the client's grief

    ○ Preparing the client for grief through education

    ○ Ensuring the client can discuss somatic concerns and actively participate in the choice of interventions

    ○ Assessing previous coping mechanisms

    ○ Discussing symptom control

    ○ Providing updated information about the client's condition

- The nurse will assess clients for medical conditions before diagnosing any mental health illness. **Major categories of mental illness** include anxiety disorders, mood disorders, psychotic disorders, dementia, eating disorders, addiction, and dependence.

- The nurse must facilitate any interventions necessary to assist a client experiencing **spiritual distress** or a conflict between recommended treatments and religious beliefs.

- The nurse must assess all clients for the presence of or risk for any **sensory perceptual alterations**. When assisting a client with impaired cognition, the nurse may involve family or a caretaker in the plan of care as the client may not be able to recognize further changes in cognition.

- To help manage stress, the nurse will monitor the client for **nonverbal cues of physical and psychological stressors**.

- The nurse must maintain the physiological stability and safety of a client diagnosed with a **substance-related disorder**.

PRACTICE QUESTIONS: PSYCHOSOCIAL INTEGRITY

Directions: The following are examples of the types of questions you will encounter on the NCLEX-RN exam. Read each question carefully and choose the best answer unless otherwise directed. Check your answers against the answer key and explanations that follow.

1. A 9-year-old child tells the nurse that he is home alone for several hours after school before his parent gets home from work. For which type of abuse is the client **most** at risk?

   1. Verbal
   2. Sexual
   3. Physical
   4. Substance

2. A client states to the nurse, "Every time my husband and I argue, I get nauseated." Which defense mechanism should the nurse recognize the client is using?

   1. Projection
   2. Conversion
   3. Displacement
   4. Reaction formation

3. Which client should the nurse anticipate monitoring for suicidal gestures?

   1. An 18-year-old male with antisocial personality disorder
   2. A 28-year-old female with an avoidant personality disorder
   3. A 24-year-old female with a borderline personality disorder
   4. A 32-year-old male client with a schizotypal personality disorder

4. Which physiological finding should the nurse anticipate when assessing a client with bulimia?

   1. Lanugo
   2. Bradycardia
   3. Hypotension
   4. Amenorrhea

5. Which physiological findings should the nurse anticipate for the client experiencing opioid withdrawal? **Select all that apply.**

   1. Rhinorrhea
   2. Piloerection
   3. Hypersomnia
   4. Frequent yawning
   5. Muscular weakness
   6. Pupillary constriction

6. The nurse has provided education for a client experiencing withdrawal from caffeine. Which statement made by the client indicates an understanding of the management of withdrawal?

   1. "I will replace my coffee with herbal tea."
   2. "I should reduce the amount of caffeine daily."
   3. "My headache will be gone within a day or two."
   4. "Drinking fluid will help flush the caffeine from my system."

7. Which question is a nursing **priority** for a client planning to return home where she has experienced interpersonal violence (IPV)?

   1. "Do you have any weapons in the home?"
   2. "Does your partner still live in the home?"
   3. "Would you reconsider going to a safe shelter?"
   4. "Would you consider speaking with a counselor?"

8. Which nursing statement offers an appropriate nursing intervention for a client who appears agitated?

   1. "Would you like to take some medication now?"

   2. "Would you like to speak to your health care provider?"

   3. "Would you like to watch something on television?"

   4. "Would you like to sit in group to help shift your focus?"

9. A client who has active elopement precautions in place is at risk for which of the following?

   1. Agitation

   2. Violence

   3. Impulsivity

   4. Hyperactivity

10. Which statement made by a client will the nurse recognize reflects a family with diffuse boundaries?

    1. "Everyone is always yelling in the house."

    2. "My husband is frequently in and out of jobs."

    3. "The kids do all the cleaning and cooking when we work."

    4. "Whatever my husband wants to do on the weekend, we do."

Practice Questions

ANSWER KEY AND EXPLANATIONS

1. 2	**3.** 3	**5.** 1, 2, 4	**7.** 1	**9.** 2
2. 2	**4.** 3	**6.** 2	**8.** 1	**10.** 3

1. **The correct answer is 2.** Limited parental supervision places the child at the most significant risk for sexual abuse. Perpetrators are usually known, trusted adults who seek out lonely children. There are no factors that put the child at risk for verbal, physical, or substance abuse.

2. **The correct answer is 2.** Conversion is the expression of emotional conflict into a physical symptom. Projection (choice 1) occurs when the client places negative traits or unwanted emotions onto others. Displacement (choice 3) is the transference of emotions associated with a particular person, situation, or object to another nonthreatening person, situation, or object. A reaction formation (choice 4) is behaving in the exact opposite way a person thinks or feels.

3. **The correct answer is 3.** A client with a borderline personality disorder demonstrates self-destructive actions, which can include suicidal gestures to gain attention. The client with an antisocial personality disorder (choice 1) is most at risk for aggressive behavior toward others. The client with an avoidant personality disorder (choice 2) will avoid social situations and is not a threat to self. The client with a schizotypal personality disorder (choice 4) displays odd, eccentric behavior, but is generally not a threat to self.

4. **The correct answer is 3.** A client with bulimia is at risk for hypotension. Lanugo, bradycardia, and amenorrhea are symptoms associated with anorexia nervosa.

5. **The correct answers are 1, 2, and 4.** Symptoms associated with opioid withdrawal include rhinorrhea, piloerection, and frequent yawning. Hypersomnia (choice 3) and muscle weakness (choice 5) are associated with stimulant intoxication.

6. **The correct answer is 2.** The acknowledgment by the client that she should reduce the amount of caffeine daily indicates an understanding of how to manage caffeine withdrawal. The statement in choice 1 indicates the client may not understand that replacing coffee with herbal tea will not lessen the effects of withdrawal. Choice 3 indicates that further education may be required since withdrawal symptoms usually last two days, but may last for up to nine days. The focus of the statement in choice 4 is hydration, not reduction of caffeine intake, which indicates further education may be needed.

7. **The correct answer is 1.** The nurse's priority in this case is to assess the risk for the potential of homicide or committing homicide, which means asking if there are weapons in the home. While asking if a partner who no longer lives with the client is appropriate, choice 2 is not the best answer because the partner may or may not be deterred from committing further acts of violence. Remember, the nurse's first priority is the client. An initial offering and information about a safe shelter (choice 3) is part of the nursing plan of care for a client experiencing IPV. However, the client has a right to refuse, so asking a client if she would reconsider going to a safe shelter may hinder any further communication, as this client may perceive she is being judged. A referral to a counselor (choice 4) is not the priority at this time.

8. **The correct answer is 1.** Offering a PRN medication is the most appropriate intervention for the client experiencing agitation. Choice 2 is not the best intervention technique because contacting the health care provider will not immediately address the client's agitation. While diversional activities

such as watching television can be helpful in certain situations, the stimuli might increase the client's agitation, so choice 3 is not the best intervention either. An agitated client poses a safety threat to others, therefore encouraging the client to sit in a group (choice 4) is not an appropriate intervention.

9. **The correct answer is 2.** A client who is at risk for elopement is at risk for violence toward others. Agitation, impulsivity, and hyperactivity are behaviors associated with violence or other physiological or mental health conditions.

10. **The correct answer is 3.** A household for which the child/parent roles become blurred is reflective of diffuse boundaries. A family who frequently yells at each other (choice 1) is displaying dysfunctional communication. Frequent job changes (choice 2) are stressors and barriers in a family, not a boundary issue. Someone who controls the action of others within a family structure (choice 4) is exhibiting authoritarian behavior, which is a characteristic of a family with rigid boundaries.

Answers Practice Questions

Physiological Integrity

OVERVIEW

- Client Needs for Basic Care and Comfort
- Assistive Devices
- Elimination
- Mobility/Immobility
- Nonpharmacological Comfort Interventions
- Nutrition and Oral Hydration
- Personal Hygiene, Rest, and Sleep
- Client Needs for Pharmacological and Parenteral Therapies
- Contraindications, Interactions, Side Effects, and Adverse Effects
- Dosage Calculation
- Medication Administration
- Total Parenteral Nutrition (TPN)
- Pharmacological Pain Management
- Client Needs for Reduction of Risk Potential
- Monitoring Changes in Client Condition
- Diagnostic Tests and Laboratory Values
- Potential for Alterations in Body Systems
- Potential Complications from Diagnostic Tests, Treatments, and Procedures
- Potential Complications from Surgical Procedures and Health Alterations
- System-Specific Assessments and Therapeutic Procedures
- Client Needs for Physiological Adaptation
- Alterations in Body Systems
- Fluid and Electrolyte Imbalances
- Hemodynamics
- Illness Management
- Pathophysiology and Medical Emergencies
- Summing It Up
- Practice Questions: Physiological Integrity
- Answer Key and Explanations

Chapter 6

The Physiological Integrity Client Needs category of the NCLEX-RN is divided into the following four subcategories:

1. Basic Care and Comfort

2. Pharmacological and Parenteral Therapies

3. Reduction of Risk Potential

4. Physiological Adaptation

The focus of the NCLEX-RN Physiological Integrity category is to assess the nurse's ability to promote physical health and wellness by providing care and comfort, reducing client risk potential, and managing health alterations.

CLIENT NEEDS FOR BASIC CARE AND COMFORT

When addressing basic care and comfort of a client, the nurse will assist the client to compensate for a physical or sensory impairment. Examples include the following:

- Assessing and managing alterations in elimination

- Performing irrigations

- Assessing skin and implementing measures to maintain skin integrity and prevent skin breakdown

- Assisting with the application, maintenance, and removal of orthopedic devices

- Implementing measures to promote circulation

A primary nursing goal for client care and comfort is pain assessment and management. The nurse will assess a client for pain, intervene as appropriate, and provide nonpharmacological comfort measures. A client may choose complementary therapies as part of the treatment. The nurse will provide support for the client's choices, which includes identifying potential contraindications.

The client's nutritional status is monitored and maintained throughout care. Nursing support may include providing the client nutrition through tube feedings, evaluating intake and output, and intervening as necessary.

The nurse will assess the client's ability to perform activities of daily living while promoting a healthy sleep and rest pattern. A client may require postmortem care, and it is the responsibility of the nurse to ensure that this care is performed appropriately according to the agency policy.

ASSISTIVE DEVICES

An interdisciplinary approach is often required when initiating a new assistive device. The nurse may collaborate with other professionals, such as a physical or occupational therapist, prosthetist, speech pathologist, audiologist, or ophthalmologist, when caring for clients who require assistive devices. An **assistive device** is a piece of equipment that will help the client communicate, bathe and perform other general hygiene, dine, dress, ambulate, or transfer. The client may present with existing assistive devices, such as glasses, hearing aids, dentures, a walker, a cane, or prosthetics. The nurse will follow the health care facility's policy and procedures for maintaining the safe use and care of the devices the client brings to the facility.

Many different conditions affect a client's balance, posture, gait, or muscle strength, which place the client at risk for injury, making fall prevention a priority for the nurse. These clients may require the use of crutches, canes, walkers, a wheelchair, a prosthesis, or the use of a gait transfer belt for safe assistance with ambulation or transfer. The nurse is accountable for assessment of the client's needs and evaluation of the correct use of the client's new or existing assistive devices.

The following is a brief review for the proper use of some common physical assistive devices. All of the following devices require that the client have adequate upper body strength.

Crutches

The type of crutches used is based on the length of required use and the type of injury. While the client is standing up straight, all underarm crutches are fitted to allow two inches or three finger-widths between the top of the crutch and the axilla (armpit), and six inches to the side and in front of the client. This space is required so the client does not trip over the crutches.

The hand grips should be even with the top of the hip line, the client's elbow should be flexed 15–30 degrees, and the client's weight should rest on the hands to avoid pressure or damage to the nerve that enters into the axilla. Forearm crutches are designed with a handgrip and metal cuff that partially surrounds the client's arm.

- A **two-point crutch walking pattern** is used by clients who can bear partial weight on either or both lower extremities. The client will move one crutch forward simultaneously with the opposite leg, providing a wide base of support.

- A client with an injury to one leg uses a **three-point crutch walking pattern**. The client begins in a tripod position and initiates a gate pattern when both crutches are placed forward. The client will then swing the legs through, bearing weight on only the uninjured leg.

- The **four-point crutch gait** is the most stable of the crutch gaits and requires bearing partial weight on both extremities. The client will be instructed to move one crutch forward, followed by the opposing leg, and to repeat the pattern by moving the opposite crutch forward, followed by the opposing leg.

The client using crutches is instructed to turn using the stronger leg. When sitting down, the client will back up so that the leg touches the seat, move the weak leg forward, balance on the strong leg, hold the crutches on the weak side, and use the free hand to grip the armrest to slowly sit down. When getting up from a chair, the client will move to the end of the seat with the weak leg forward, holding the crutches on the same side as the weak leg, and use the free hand to help push up from the seat. When going up stairs, the strong leg is always advanced first; when going down stairs, the weak leg is advanced first.

Cane

A cane is either a single-tip or four-pronged device. The cane is held on the unaffected side of the body with the top of the cane level with the hip joint. The client's arm should be comfortably bent when walking. The client is instructed to hold the cane on the stronger side and move the cane forward first, followed by the weaker leg, and then the stronger leg. To turn, the client will use the strong leg. If using a four-pronged cane, it is crucial the client make sure all four prongs are on the ground before placing weight on the cane. When going up stairs, the stronger leg is always used first, followed by the cane, and then the weaker leg. To go down stairs, the client will start with the cane, followed by the weaker leg, and then the stronger leg.

Walker

Walkers may have two wheels, four wheels, or no wheels. If the walker has wheels, it will need to be pushed forward to move, and if the walker has no wheels, it will have to be lifted to move forward. Regardless of what type of walker the client has, all four tips or wheels must be placed on the ground before the client places weight on it. The proper height of the walker is determined when the walker's handle is the same height as the client's hip bone or relaxed wrist when standing up straight. The elbows should be flexed 15–30 degrees when the client is standing inside of the walker with hands on the handgrips.

While looking forward, the client will push or lift the walker forward a few inches—or an arm's length—in front of the body, ensuring all four points or wheels are on the ground before taking a step forward. The client will step forward with the weak leg first then step forward, placing the stronger leg in front of the weaker leg. When standing, the client will lean slightly forward and use the arms to help stand up after all points are on the ground.

The client should be instructed to never pull or tilt the walker to assist with standing up. To stand up straight, the client may need to take a step forward. When going up or down stairs, the walker is placed in front of the client. When going up, the strong leg is used first, placing the weight on the walker; the weaker leg is then brought up the step. When going down, the same process for placing the weight on the walker is used, except the weak leg is placed first, followed by the strong leg.

Wheelchair

General teaching for a client using a wheelchair includes transferring in and out of the chair, maintaining a center of gravity, and positioning the body or chair to desired objects to avoid overreaching and tipping the chair. When a client is being transferred from the bed to a wheelchair, the chair is moved as close to the bed as possible and then locked with the footrests moved out of the way. If the client is not seated, the client is assisted into a seated position.

To get the client into a seated position, the nurse should complete the following steps:

1. Roll the client onto the same side as the wheelchair.

2. Place one arm under the client's shoulders and one behind the client's knees.

3. While bending the knees, swing the client's feet off the edge of the bed and use the momentum created to help the client into a sitting position.

4. Move the client to the edge of the bed and lower the bed so the client's feet are touching the ground.

The next step in the transfer is to complete a pivot turn. The nurse can use a gait belt to help get a grip during the transfer, and during the turn, the client can either hold on to the nurse or reach for the wheelchair.

1. Standing as close as possible to the client, reach around the client's chest and either lock hands behind the client or grab the gait belt.

2. Place the client's outside leg (the one farthest from the wheelchair) between the knees for support.

3. Bending the knees and keeping the back straight, count to three and slowly stand up, using the legs to lift. At the same time, the client places his or her hands by the side of the body and helps push off the bed.

4. Pivot toward the wheelchair and move the feet so the back is aligned with the hips. The client should help support his or her weight on the good leg during the transfer.

5. Once the client's legs are touching the seat of the wheelchair, bend the knees to lower the client into the seat. At the same time, the client reaches for the wheelchair armrest.

If the client starts to fall during the transfer, the nurse should lower the client to the nearest flat surface, bed, chair, or floor.

Client wheelchair safety education to prevent falls or tipping of the chair includes the following:

- Avoid using the wheelchair on uneven surfaces.

- Use available armrests before transferring, if needed.

- Avoid going too fast in the wheelchair or taking sharp corners.

- Avoid forcing the chair up or down staircases, slopes, or inclines.

- Maintain the structure of the wheelchair or motor as recommended.

- Move footrests entirely out of the way when transferring the client.

- Ensure that the client avoids leaning forward, sliding, or positioning too far forward to prevent the client from tipping out of the chair.

- Program the settings for a motorized wheelchair to a speed that is comfortable for the client.

- Avoid placing heavy objects or items on the back of the wheelchair to prevent it tipping backward during a transfer.

- Lock the brakes before assisting the client to get out of or into the wheelchair. The power should be turned off for electric wheelchairs prior to transferring.

- Avoid inclement weather; wheelchairs may lose traction, and the controls of an electric wheelchair should not get wet.

Prosthesis

The physiological nursing priorities for a client with a prosthesis include safety and pain management. Each type of prosthesis will require a unique set of instructions for application. For a client who is a new amputee, an elastic bandage is wrapped around the amputated area when the prosthetic is not used. The client will generally use a prosthetic sock and gel liner before putting on a prosthetic. Personal hygiene is essential to prevent infection and odor. Each day, the client wearing a prosthetic should cleanse the device, examine the residual limb for skin integrity, and cleanse the socket area of the limb with antibacterial soap.

Sensory Considerations

Other factors that place the client at risk for injury include difficulty with speech, vision, hearing, or other sensory perceptual considerations. All clients who have risk factors such as disease processes, or who are receiving prescriptions that place them at risk for impaired communication, speech, vision, or hearing problems, must be assessed by the nurse for changes in sensory conditions.

For a client with risk factors, the nursing assessment is ongoing throughout treatment. Obtaining both subjective and objective information related to sensory risk is integrated into the client's plan of care. Clients who have difficulty with communication, speech, vision, and hearing require the nurse to ensure the environment is safe and adapted to the client's needs.

Nursing interventions for a client with visual challenges are centered on communication, safety, ambulation, self-care, and support. Communication will help the client maintain independence and stay connected to what is occurring. A new environment for a client with visual challenges creates a safety risk due to its unfamiliarity. In order to promote safety, the nurse will ensure the client is oriented to the environment using specific descriptors and avoiding gestures or unclear information. Once the client is adapted to the room, items such as the call light, trash can, chairs, etc., will not be moved without consulting the client.

Safe ambulation for the client includes allowing the client to hold the nurse's arm at the elbow close to the nurse's body so the client can sense direction, as well as providing verbal cues to alert the client when obstacles are in his or her path. The client may use a cane when walking to help detect objects. When entering a client's room, the nurse should always knock on the door, identify him- or herself, and provide the reason for the visit.

Promoting communication and reducing anxiety are nursing priorities when caring for a client who has an auditory sensory impairment. The client is at risk for isolation due to difficulty communicating and the inability to hear. There are many assistive devices available based on the type and extent of hearing loss the client has experienced. For the client who requires a hearing aid, it is essential to ensure that it is working correctly; however, it should be handled only by a person who knows how to care for it properly. A client who is adapting to the use of new hearing aids will require time to adjust and learn how to filter out background noise. Clients who are hearing-impaired may read lips, use sign language, and/or may have been instructed to understand body language. Understanding and incorporating the client's chosen method of communication into the plan of care will help reduce anxiety.

Impaired speech communication may occur as a result of progressive neurological disease, surgical treatment, disfluency, dysarthria, aphasia, or a social communication disorder. For clients with a new speech impairment, the nurse will collaborate with a speech and language pathologist and integrate the speech rehabilitation plan into overall care. The priority nursing goal for a client with speech difficulty is to improve communication and reduce anxiety. There are many devices available that can be used based on the client's condition. Communication boards, high-tech communication technology, and alphabet boards are just a few tools for communication the nurse can implement into the plan of care. The nurse will communicate with the client using his or her preferred method in an effort to increase communication and reduce the client's anxiety.

ELIMINATION

Predisposing and precipitating factors that place a client at an increased risk for altered urinary and bowel elimination include general conditions as well as conditions unique to each gender. Screening for altered elimination, obtaining a comprehensive history, and performing a physical assessment will help the nurse identify the risk factors associated with different types of altered elimination.

The overall treatment and management of a client with altered urinary or bowel elimination is based on the underlying causative factor. Treatments include the following:

- Prescriptive therapy
- Bladder training
- Urinary diversion, such an ostomy pouch or ileal conduit
- Urinary catheterization
- Caffeine reduction
- Reduced fluid intake
- Pelvic floor muscle exercises
- Nutritional therapy
- Vaginal estrogen therapy
- Behavior modification
- Psychotherapy

Some common altered elimination findings include urinary retention, urinary incontinence, and bowel incontinence.

Urinary Retention

Retention of urine in the bladder after voiding contributes to overflow incontinence. Urinary retention may be caused by an infection, mechanical obstruction (e.g., constipation or enlarged prostate), recent surgery, neurological impairment, spinal or peripheral nerve lesions, or the use of specific prescriptions. Noninvasive nursing interventions to promote voiding include the following:

- Providing privacy
- Offering fluids before voiding
- Dipping the client's hands in warm water
- Running warm water over the perineum
- Warming a bedpan if the client has to use one
- Encouraging frequent voiding—at least every four hours
- Allowing the client to listen to the sound of running water
- Encouraging relaxation techniques, such as deep breathing
- Encouraging the client to sit upright on the toilet or bedpan

Urinary Incontinence

Urinary incontinence can be caused by many factors that can be temporary or permanent, including the following:

- Infection
- Pelvic floor laxity
- Neurological impairment
- Dietary intake
- Prescriptions
- Menopause
- Cognitive impairment
- Surgery
- Endocrine issues
- Restricted mobility
- Stool impaction/constipation

Types of incontinence are listed in the following table.

SEVEN TYPES OF URINARY INCONTINENCE	
Type	**Description**
Stress Incontinence	Involuntary leakage of urine caused by intra-abdominal pressure exceeding the intraurethral pressure
Urge Incontinence	A strong urge to void with the inability to make it to the toilet in time
Overflow Incontinence	Involuntary release of urine, often without sensing a urge to urinate; results from incomplete bladder emptying
Mixed Incontinence	A combination of stress and urge incontinence
Functional Incontinence	Inability to get to the bathroom in time, often caused by such factors as dementia, mental illness, or medications or as a result of circumstances that delay getting to the bathroom
Total Incontinence	Continuous, unpredictable loss of urine without distention or awareness of bladder fullness
Transient Incontinence	Temporary loss of bladder control; usually a side effect of another medical issue or a medication

Bowel Incontinence

Bowel incontinence is an involuntary loss of stool that can be caused by the following:

- Infection
- Prescriptions
- Crohn's disease
- Ulcerative colitis
- Paralytic ileus
- Ulcerative colitis
- Neurological impairment
- Weakened or damaged pelvic floor musculature
- Type II diabetes
- Irritable bowel syndrome

Treatment and management are determined by the underlying cause. Treatment may include the following:

- Prescriptions
- Enemas for constipation
- Dietary intervention
- Bowel-training program
- Rectal catheter
- Bowel diversion or a type of ostomy

- Increased physical activity

- Decreased fluid intake

- Monitoring of personal habits

- Pain management

- Management of the client's physical position when defecating

Examples of altered bowel elimination are included in the following table.

BOWEL ELIMINATION DISORDERS	
Disorder	Description
Urge Incontinence	Inability to stop a bowel movement before getting to a toilet
Passive Incontinence	Leakage of fecal matter that occurs without the client realizing
Constipation	Infrequent or difficult bowel movements
Diarrhea	Abnormal frequency and fluidity of bowel evacuation
Fecal Impaction	Presence of hard fecal mass in the rectum that the client is not capable of expelling
Functional Incontinence	Inability to get to the bathroom on time

Regardless of the type of incontinence the client is experiencing, nursing priorities include the prevention of perineal skin breakdown and infection, promotion of privacy, maintenance of the client's dignity, and evaluation of the effectiveness of treatments and interventions. Included in the evaluation are physical assessments and monitoring of intake and output.

Clients with conditions that result in altered elimination are further at risk for emotional and social distress, fear, anxiety, social isolation, loss of self-esteem, and depression. These conditions may interfere with the client's ability to work, attend school or social gatherings, or exercise.

A client who is experiencing incontinence requires meticulous skin care to prevent skin breakdown and infection. Incorporated into the client's care is the frequent washing of the perineal area, taking care to use a cleansing soap that will not dry or further irritate the skin. The health care provider may prescribe the use of moisturizers, barriers, pastes, or sealants to protect the skin. Any skin barrier or moisturizer used to provide added protection will be applied after cleansing and thoroughly drying the skin.

Irrigation may also be prescribed for a client who is experiencing bowel incontinence. Before performing any irrigation, the nurse will identify the client, provide education by explaining the procedure, ensure the client is comfortable and physiologically stable, assemble the equipment, and perform the procedure according to the health care facility's policy and procedures.

MOBILITY/IMMOBILITY

Mobility is assessed through observation of the client's gait and use of ambulatory devices, as well as reviewing the client's history and conducting a physical assessment. The assessment includes gathering data regarding the client's history of falls, substance use, medical history, and current prescriptions. Physical assessment of a client's mobility level includes observation and testing of gait, balance, coordination, muscle strength, tone and symmetry, and active or passive range of joint movement.

Any client with an alteration in the musculoskeletal, nervous, or cardiovascular system is at risk for impaired mobility. Client immobility, whether temporary or permanent, affects various body systems. The impact of immobility on the musculoskeletal system includes weakness, decreased muscle tone, loss of bone and muscle mass, muscle atrophy, contractures, joint stiffness, pain, and an increased risk for falls. When a client is in supine position, the workload of the cardiovascular system is increased and the lungs' ability to expand is decreased, which can result in secretions pooling in the dependent areas of the lungs. Circulatory stasis and weakened calf muscles predispose the client for deep vein thrombosis. These changes contribute to intolerance for completing activities of daily living.

Nutrition alteration includes a reduction of the basal metabolic rate and a breakdown of muscle protein for energy, which causes a negative nitrogen balance if the dietary protein is not adequate. Anorexia may also occur as a result of a decreased appetite. As a result, the immobile client's urinary and bowel functions are altered. Urinary stasis may occur as a result of the client's position, placing the client at risk for urinary tract infections. Excess calcium is also excreted due to the disuse of the bones, putting the client at risk for renal calculi. Decreased appetite and fluid intake result in hypoactive bowels and constipation.

The client's skin integrity is compromised by the edema that may develop from a decrease in circulation and pressure on the bony prominences, which can cause tissue ischemia. Pressure ulcers develop in areas where tissue ischemia occurs as a result of pressure placed on the skin combined with the inactivity of the client.

The psychosocial impact of a client with restricted mobility includes isolation, sensory deprivation, loneliness, anger, depression, anxiety, confusion, altered self-concept, and disruption of sleep and sleep patterns.

Nursing interventions for a client who has restricted mobility are selected to prevent physiological and psychological complications. In order to create an effective and safe nursing plan of care for an immobile client, the nurse must understand the treatment procedures and apply the psychomotor skills necessary to prevent complications. The client's response to all interventions specific to preventing complications from immobility is evaluated throughout the treatment.

The nurse will monitor all areas of the skin—especially the buttocks, coccyx, heels, hips, shoulders, elbows, and ears, as these particular areas are most at risk for breakdown. Assessment of the skin includes the overall observation of color, texture, warmth, and intactness. Any areas of the skin found to be darkened or reddened in tone are of particular concern. To assess the effectiveness of the client's circulation, the temperature, tissue-blanching, and normal reactive hyperemia are evaluated. The **Braden scale** is a standardized skin assessment tool that can be used to help identify clients at risk for compromised skin integrity.

Nursing interventions for the prevention of skin breakdown include the following:

- Assessing the client's skin integrity regularly and during any other opportune time, such as bathing or repositioning

- Keeping the client's skin clean and dry

- Managing the client's incontinence, if present

- Avoiding vigorous rubbing or massaging of the client's skin

- Using an appropriate skin cleanser

- Applying barrier cream or moisturizers, as prescribed

- Transferring or repositioning a client using appropriate equipment, assistive transfer devices, and techniques to reduce skin friction and shear

- Positioning a client on proper support surfaces; utilizing support aides to promote independence

- Monitoring and checking the skin beneath dressings, a prosthesis, or any similar devices when clinically appropriate

- Using equipment, such as siderails, to promote independent mobility

- Repositioning the client every two hours, or reminding the client to reposition his or her body if the client is able to

- Managing the client's pain

- Suspending the client's heels off the bed

- Repositioning facemasks or tubes every two hours, using a barrier dressing if needed

- For clients who are high risk for skin breakdown, limiting the amount of time the client spends sitting in bed with the head elevated

- After repositioning the client, evaluating the position of the bony prominences and the client's heels

- Inspecting all areas of skin that are covered with tape, casts, orthotic devices, cervical collars, pressure stockings, sequential compression devices, IV tubing or boards, or pulse oximeter probes

- Removing excess linens and straightening creases in the bedding

- Offering fluids frequently

- Obtaining a dietary consult as needed for nutritional support

- Implementing the use of pressure-redistributing devices, such as footwear or specialized beds

- Avoiding placing the client in positions in which heat and moisture becomes trapped against the skin

A goal of caring for a client with limited or impaired mobility is to prevent contractures, muscle weakness, and atrophy, as well as to promote circulation to the extremities. This can be achieved through positioning the client to maintain correct body alignment, and/or collaborating with a physical therapist to promote the active and passive ranges of motion. These motions promote circulation to the joints, preventing pressure ulcers, maintaining joint mobility, and reducing stiffness and pain. Contractures are prevented with the use of splints and other supportive devices. As soon as possible, the nurse encourages client mobility to decrease the risk of complications. Movement promotes circulation, and use of the muscles and joints and prevents other physiological complications previously discussed.

Maintaining the correct body alignment for a client is essential in relieving strain, promoting efficient body functioning, preventing complications—such as contractures and pressure ulcers—and promoting comfort. Proper alignment of a client who is in a supine, lateral, or prone position should be the same as if standing. If the client is positioned correctly, an imaginary straight line can be drawn connecting the client's nose, breastbone, sternum, and pubic bone. Many supportive devices may be used to help promote body alignment and comfort, including pillows, blankets, mattress pads, special shoes or boots, or a footboard to maintain foot alignment and prevent foot drop. Orthotic devices such as splints can also be used to restore or improve function, maintain position, and prevent deformity of an extremity. Repositioning an immobilized client involves initially moving the client into proper body alignment; turning the client onto the back, abdomen, or side; and then placing the client's trunk and extremities in the appropriate position. Once attained, the alignment is maintained with supportive devices.

A client with a fracture may require traction. **Traction** involves the use of various weights and pully systems to apply tension on a limb, bone, or muscle that allows for reduction, alignment, immobilization, prevention or correction of deformities, and decreased muscle spasms. Traction is classified as a running or balanced suspension. When the pulling force is in one direction and the client's body acts as counter traction, it is referred to as **running traction**. **Balanced suspension** provides the counter-traction, so the pulling force of the traction is not altered when moving the bed or client.

The client may require **skeletal traction**, which involves surgically inserting screws, pins, wires, or tongs directly into the bone. Alternatively, the client may be placed into **skin traction** using an external fixation device that has pins or wires inserted through the skin and affected bone, which are then connected to a rigid external frame.

Skin traction may be used to apply traction force externally. The traction is connected directly to the client's skin for intermittent or continuous immobilization using an adhesive or nonadhesive traction tape or other devices. The force that is exerted for a client with skin traction is created through the use of weights and pulleys. The nurse may set up traction according to the health care facility's policy and procedure. The basic principles of setting up traction include ensuring all weights hang freely, the prescribed amount of weight is used, and the pulleys are lubricated with a silicone spray.

Based on the type of traction that is prescribed for the client, nursing care will include the following:

- Turning the client every two hours

- Monitoring the client for systemic infection

- Encouraging mobility, as appropriate

- Providing wound care, if applicable

- Teaching the client about safe mobility practices

- Cleaning the fixator, as needed and per policy

- Elevating the client's extremities to prevent swelling

- Assessing pins and traction bars for tightness

- Maintaining the client's alignment in the bed

- Assessing all open wounds for infection and healing

- Encouraging active or providing passive range of motion

- Not lifting or using the halo ring to reposition the client

- Verifying the prescribed weight when assessing equipment

- Assessing affected extremities for pain, pressure, paralysis, paresthesia, pallor, and pulselessness

- Ensuring that the appropriate wrench for the fixation devices is immediately available for the client with a halo

- Evaluating all traction equipment for proper function, including the integrity of the ropes, knots, and pulleys

- Assessing muscle and motor function and skin sensation according to the health care agency's policy and procedures

- Inspecting the skin around the edges of the vest for the client with a halo and change the sheepskin liner when it is soiled or per policy

- Monitoring pin sites for redness, edema, and purulent drainage (which should be reported immediately). Serious drainage may be present around the pin sites.

- Cleaning pins and removing crusts with a sterile applicator. Crust forms from serious drainage and can prevent fluid from draining. If not kept clean, the crust can cause infection.

- Assessing a client with skin traction for allergic reaction to the tape, excoriation of the skin, and pressure sores

A client may require application, maintenance, or removal of other orthopedic devices, which include splints, braces, boots, shoes, and casts. Splints and braces are used to keep joints in functional positions. Boots and shoes called **orthotics** can be used to promote normal foot function, relieve pain, or relieve foot fatigue. Casts are used for a more complex fracture to hold bone fragments in place after a reduction. Casts are primarily made from fiberglass but can be made with plaster. New plaster casts require time to dry and must be handled with the palms of the hand to avoid creating pressure points that result in skin ulceration. The nurse will assess clients with a cast for impaired circulation, peripheral nerve damage, and infection. The overall goal for any client with an orthopedic device is to restore function. Included in the client plan of care is the assessment of skin integrity, pain, the elevation of the extremity to decrease edema, and complications from immobility as discussed previously.

NONPHARMACOLOGICAL COMFORT INTERVENTIONS

Traditional and complementary alternative medicine (TM/CAM) is commonly used in combination with conventional medicine. These nonpharmacological interventions are used alone or in conjunction with pharmacological pain management. A client experiencing mild or moderate pain may benefit from the use of alternative therapy, whereas the client with more severe pain will most benefit from complementary therapy. Various alternative therapies and treatments can be integrated into the client's plan of care. **Biologically based therapy** includes the use of herbs, oils, or special diet. **Mind-body therapies** are used to enhance the mind's ability to affect body function and include guided imagery, meditation, prayer, journaling, and art therapy. When using **manipulative** and **body-based therapies**, pressure or movement of body parts is performed as in chiropractic medicine or massage therapy. **Energy therapies** are used when focusing on electromagnetic fields or biofields of energy. Energy therapy includes acupuncture and reflexology. Nonpharmacological interventions also include practices that have evolved from spiritual tradition, folk medicine, homeopathy, or naturopathy.

When integrating any complementary therapy into a client's treatment, the safety of the combination of treatments must be considered. The therapy may interfere with the effectiveness of conventional treatment for a disease process or may result in unwanted side effects. Some therapies, such as a biologically based therapy, may enhance or minimize the action of the prescriptions used. Several supplements are contraindicated in clients with specific diseases and interfere with medicines. Certain essential oils, such as rosemary, exacerbate epilepsy, high blood pressure, and low blood pressure; are contraindicated in pregnancy; and should be avoided for babies and children. Energy therapy, such as the use of acupuncture, is contraindicated in cases involving lymphedema or edema in limbs and for spinal instability; relative contraindications include epilepsy and hemophilia. Throughout treatment or use of TM/CAM, the nurse will evaluate the outcomes of the therapy.

The most effective physical treatments used to relieve pain include occupational and physical therapy, aqua therapy, and low-impact exercises such as walking or yoga. **Cutaneous skin stimulation** may be used to alleviate pain. Cutaneous skin stimulation includes the application of heat, cold, pressure, vibration, or **transcutaneous electrical nerve stimulation (TENS)**. Adjusting environmental temperature; providing clean, wrinkle-free bedding; or repositioning a client are natural nursing interventions to promote comfort.

Nursing interventions for pain are based on the characteristics and location of the pain. **Acute pain** has a sudden onset, is temporary, and is usually local, whereas **chronic pain** lasts or reoccurs for an indefinite period. Pain is categorized as nociceptive or neuropathic; both types of pain can be acute or chronic. A client experiencing **nociceptive pain** is processing the pain normally. This pain includes **somatic** and **visceral pain**. A client experiencing **neuropathic pain** is demonstrating abnormal pain processing. This type of pain can occur in the absence of tissue damage or inflammation. A client with nociceptive pain will describe the kind of pain he or she is experiencing differently than will a client with neuropathic pain.

DIFFERENT TYPES OF PAIN	
Pain Type	**Location/Characteristics**
Nociceptive somatic pain	When cutaneous or superficial, the pain is described as burning or sharp. When the pain involves deep somatic bone, muscle, blood vessels, or connective tissue, it is usually described as dull, aching, or cramping.
Nociceptive visceral pain	This type of pain is poorly localized, is diffuse, and involves deep cramping. It is usually described as sharp, stabbing, or splitting.
Neuropathic pain	This type of pain is poorly localized and is described as shooting, fiery, shock-like, sharp, or a painful numbness.

Understanding pain will assist the nurse in evaluating the client during a comprehensive pain assessment. Data gathered in the assessment includes identifying the location and intensity of the pain. The method of collecting this data regarding pain will vary and is based on the client's cognitive ability, developmental age, physiological condition, and capacity to communicate.

Many tools can be used to assess pain and it is the nurse's responsibility to choose the correct method. The nurse must evaluate the effectiveness of the tool as well as all planned interventions implemented to prevent or treat a client's discomfort. Other information gathered during a pain assessment includes assessment of the quality, onset, and duration of the pain, as well as any aggravating and relieving factors, the effect the pain has had on the client's function and quality of life, and any comfort interventions used by the client.

A client's culture, past experiences, current treatments, significant medical history, as well as psychosocial history are all considered before creating a plan of care. It is essential for the nurse to understand that many individual factors may affect a client's pain. These factors include age, gender, race, genetics, and culture. After providing education and encouraging the client to identify an acceptable comfort level, the client is encouraged to participate in choosing all nonpharmacological and prescribed treatments.

Palliative, Hospice, and Postmortem Care

Palliative care is offered to clients experiencing chronic or severe illness, with a primary goal of improving the quality of life and providing prevention and relief from pain. Clients offered palliative care may not only receive medical care for their symptoms, but curative treatment as well. Clients with conditions such as heart failure, chronic obstructive pulmonary disease, cancer, and dementia can significantly benefit from palliative care.

Hospice care is offered to clients who have reached the end of life and are no longer receiving curative treatment. The client's symptoms and pain will continue to be managed to provide comfort and support.

Both palliative and hospice care assist the family through the process of the client's illness and death. Assessing a client's need for either palliative or hospice care and providing client and family education are important parts of the nursing role. The nurse will advocate and support a client's decisions regarding the choice to accept palliative or hospice care. Clients receiving palliative or hospice care, as well as the family members, are provided education about the anticipated physiological changes, interventions, and symptom management. The nurse will coordinate the care through collaboration with other health care team members to meet the physiological and psychosocial needs of the client as his or her condition changes. The nurse will also ensure the family is provided resources and emotional support throughout the client's illness and after death. The plan of care will continue to be altered based on the client's desired treatment and evaluation of the client's response to symptom management.

A client who is actively dying requires management determined by the physiological systems in which function is declining. These symptoms may last for weeks, days, or hours before death. The nurse can anticipate providing treatment and comfort measures for the following:

- Pain
- Cough
- Anxiety
- Fatigue
- Dyspnea
- Depression
- Bowel changes
- Anorexia/cachexia
- Nausea and vomiting

As the client transitions from the active phase of dying into the imminent phase of death, the client will begin to withdraw from life. During this period, the client may hallucinate, and interactions with others will decrease. Throughout this transition period, it is important to keep the client as comfortable as possible and minimize the stimuli in the environment.

The following symptoms are associated with a client's transition into the last phase of dying:

- Confusion
- Restlessness
- Increased lethargy
- Cool, clammy skin
- Mottled extremities
- Inability to ambulate
- Rapid or irregular pulse
- Increased respiratory rate
- Decreased or dark urine output
- Inability to move or turn in bed
- Periods of apnea or Cheyne-Stokes breathing
- Inability to clear increased respiratory secretions

Postmortem care begins once death has been determined unless the death has occurred under "unusual circumstances," in which case the care is deferred. If an autopsy is to be performed, devices such as IV lines, nasogastric tubes, tracheostomy appliances, urinary catheters, drainage tubes, or any other invasive device that was present before death must remain in the body. All client and family religious or cultural practices will be integrated into the postmortem care, as the physical care of the body may be dictated based on the specific practices. Postmortem nursing care includes bathing and dressing the client's body and covering the body appropriately. The nurse will adhere to the health care facility's policy and procedures for postmortem care.

Nurses play an essential role in advocating for palliative care and hospice services for individuals and families. This advocacy is accomplished through knowledge and understanding of disease processes and recognition of the benefits both of these services can provide a client and the family. In providing support to the client and family, the nurse can ensure the treatment and plan of care align with the client and family's values.

NUTRITION AND ORAL HYDRATION

Potential or actual problems with chewing or swallowing place the client at risk for aspiration, nutritional deficiency, dehydration, and fluid and electrolyte imbalances. The initial nutritional screening will help the nurse identify a client with a potential chewing or swallowing difficulty. The screening also includes assessing the client's anthropometric measurements, weight history, health history, physical assessment, nutritional history, food and fluid intake, laboratory data, and food-drug interactions, as well as including a psychosocial assessment.

Nutritional deficiencies are reflected in the abnormal findings of a client's hair, nails, eyes, oral cavity, musculoskeletal system, and neurological system. When gathering data, the nurse will ask the client about mouth pain, difficulty chewing, or swallowing difficulty. Specifically included in the initial assessment for a client suspected of altered nutrition or hydration is dentition, ill-fitting dentures, recent changes in appetite or food intake, reported mouth pain, difficulty swallowing, inadequate fluid intake, and body mass index (BMI). The BMI is based on the client's height and weight and reflects the total fat stores in relation to the client's weight. The formula for calculating BMI is as follows:

$$BMI = \frac{Weight\ (lbs.)}{Height\ (inches)^2} \times 703$$

When evaluating the results of a BMI for an adult male or female, the ranges are as follows:

- Underweight: less than 18.5
- Healthy weight: 18.5–24.9
- Overweight: 25–29.9
- Obese: 30–39.9
- Severe obesity: 40 or higher

During the assessment, the nurse will also obtain a prescription history to evaluate potential food and drug interactions that specifically affect the client's nutritional and hydration status. Specific prescriptions can alter appetite, food absorption, and metabolism.

Common substances or medicines that affect a client's overall nutritional status are listed in the following table.

SUBSTANCE EFFECTS ON NUTRITIONAL STATUS	
Symptom	Affected by...
Increased appetite	Alcohol, corticosteroids, antihistamines, psychoactive drugs, sulfonylureas, thyroid hormones, and insulin
Decreased appetite	Antibiotics, glucagon, bulk agents, morphine, and fluoxetine
Reduced absorption of fat	Orlistat
Increased blood glucose levels	Octreotide, opioids, phenothiazines, corticosteroids, thiazide diuretics, and warfarin
Decreased blood glucose levels	ACE inhibitors, aspirin, barbiturates, beta blockers, insulin, monoamine oxidase inhibitors (MAOIs), sulfonamides, and oral hyperglycemic drugs
Decreased blood lipid levels	Aspirin, colchicine, glucagon, niacin, and statins
Increased blood lipid levels	Adrenal corticosteroids, chlorpromazine, growth hormone, estrogen-progesterone oral contraceptives, and vitamin D
Decreased protein metabolism	Tetracycline and chloramphenicol
Affected metabolization of minerals	Diuretics, repeated use of laxatives, oral contraceptives, cortisol, sulfonylureas, certain antibiotics, digoxin, and corticosteroids
Affected absorption and metabolism of vitamins	Alcohol, isoniazid, phenytoin, phenobarbital, anticonvulsants, oral contraceptives, aminosalicylic acid, ethanol, metformin, and proton pump inhibitors

Other methods of evaluating a client's nutritional status include skinfold measurements. The triceps and subscapular folds are typically assessed to estimate the client's body fat. Laboratory assessments will also provide objective information regarding the client's nutritional and hydration status. Relevant laboratory tests include hemoglobin, hematocrit, serum albumin, thyroxine-binding prealbumin, serum transferrin, electrolytes, glucose, BUN, creatinine, complete blood count, serum ferritin, and electrolytes.

A client with dehydration is at risk for falls. The nurse will assess the client for the following physical findings and incorporate a plan for fall prevention as applicable:

- Thirst
- Anuria
- Oliguria
- Headache
- Weight loss
- Tachycardia
- Hypotension
- Constipation

- Dysrhythmias

- Poor skin turgor

- Muscle weakness

- Concentrated urine

- Slow capillary refill

- Postural hypotension

- Altered mental status

- Abnormal electrolytes

- Sunken-appearing eyes

- Weak and thready pulses

- Dry oral mucous membranes

- Elevated BUN and creatinine

- Elevated urine specific gravity

- Low hemoglobin and hematocrit

Fluid replacement is required for a dehydrated client. The method of replacement is determined by the condition of the client. Mild to moderate dehydration is corrected with oral fluids unless the client is experiencing an inability to swallow, nausea, or vomiting. For the client who cannot tolerate oral fluids, IV fluid replacement is initiated. Fluid replacement is based on the client's clinical manifestations and assessment findings. The type of IV fluid prescribed is related to the osmolarity of the blood and on overall cardiovascular status. The health care provider will prescribe the fluid rate based upon the degree of dehydration and the condition of the client's pulmonary, cardiovascular, and renal systems.

All clients receiving fluid replacement will be monitored for overhydration. Symptoms of overhydration include the following:

- Dyspnea

- Headache

- Tachypnea

- Paresthesia

- Tachycardia

- Pale cool skin

- Bounding pulses

- Increased weight

- Visual disturbances

- Distended neck veins

- Elevated blood pressure

- Crackles on auscultation

- Decreased pulse pressure

- Skeletal muscle weakness
- Altered level of consciousness
- Pitting edema in dependent areas

Many conditions require specific food or nutritional requirements. Clients with conditions such as hypertension, diabetes, and cardiovascular disease necessitate dietary modifications. When caring for a client experiencing under- or overnutrition, the nurse can anticipate caloric counts to be included in the plan of care. Additional treatments to improve the nutrition of a client include multivitamins, minerals, and nutritional supplements. Nutritional supplements may consist of scheduled snacks or liquid nutritional shakes.

Common therapeutic diets that may be implemented into a dietary plan are listed in the following table.

THERAPEUTIC DIETS	
Type of Diet	Description
Clear liquid	This type of diet is used for a short period of time due to the limitation of calories and nutrients. Clear liquids include minimum residue fluids that can be seen through. Examples are juices without pulp, broth, and gelatin. This type of diet is generally reserved for clients with gastrointestinal problems, as well as pre- and postoperative clients.
Full liquid	Foods included in this diet may become liquid at room or body temperature and are used for clients who cannot tolerate mechanical soft diets. Full liquids should not be used for extended periods. A full liquid diet consists of liquid dietary supplements, such as ice cream, pudding, strained creamed soups, milk or milk products, yogurt, and juices with and without pulp.
Thickened liquids	In this diet, liquids are thickened by adding a thickening agent. This type of diet is used for those who have difficulty swallowing and are at risk for aspiration.
Pureed	This diet is reserved for clients who cannot safely chew or swallow or have poor dentition. Foods are placed in a blender and blended into the consistency of pulp. This type of food can be passed through a straw and is nutritionally adequate. Nuts, seeds, raw vegetables, and fruits are avoided.
Mechanically altered or soft diet	The consistency of foods in this diet has been modified. This diet is prescribed for those who have difficulty chewing effectively, have poor dentition, or are edentulous. The diet includes chopped or ground meats, fruits, and vegetables.
No concentrated sweets	This type of diet is used for clients with diabetes who have weight and glucose levels under control. Calories are not counted in this diet as they are in the American Diabetes Association (ADA) diet. The client can have foods that do not have sugar.
Diabetic	This type of diet controls the number of calories through carbohydrate, protein, and fat intake to meet the client's nutritional needs and control blood sugars and weight. The **ADA Exchange List** is used for meal planning, and the calorie intake is specific. High-fiber complex carbohydrates from vegetables and fruits are preferred over simple carbohydrates, sugar, and starchy foods. Foods that have a high glycemic index and cause the rapid rise of the body's blood glucose level are avoided.

THERAPEUTIC DIETS	
Type of Diet	**Description**
No added salt	In this diet, the food is seasoned as regular food, but the client is not to add additional salt to the food.
Low sodium	The sodium in this diet is generally restricted to 2 grams/day. The client is instructed to limit salty foods, such as bacon; sausage; chips; crackers; canned vegetables, soups, or meats; and pickled foods. This diet is generally prescribed for clients with heart disease, hypertension, or initial stages of kidney or liver disease.
Low fat/low cholesterol	This diet is used to treat elevated lipid levels and conditions that interfere with how the body uses fats, such as in diseases of the liver, pancreas, or gall bladder. The range of fat intake is limited to no more than 20–30% of the daily caloric intake, and the cholesterol is limited to approximately 250–300 mg/day.
High fiber	This type of diet is prescribed to prevent or treat many gastrointestinal, cardiovascular, and metabolic diseases. Increased fiber should primarily come from legumes, fruits, vegetables, whole wheat bread, and cereals.
Cardiac diet	This type of diet is used to control the intake of foods that contribute to conditions affecting the cardiovascular system. The diet generally consists of maximizing the intake of low-cholesterol and low-sodium foods while minimizing the consumption of animal products, processed foods, canned soups or vegetables, and lunch meats. Clients with hypertension, high cholesterol, atherosclerosis, chronic renal failure, or similar diseases may be placed on some type of cardiac (low-cholesterol, low-sodium) diet.
Renal	This diet plan is individualized for a client who is receiving dialysis; it restricts potassium, sodium, protein, and phosphorus intake. Fresh fruits (except bananas) and vegetables are excellent dietary choices for people on a renal diet. The client's laboratory work will be followed closely on this diet.
Food allergy modification	Foods for which the client has implicated or actual allergies are strictly eliminated. The most common food allergies include milk, eggs, soy, wheat, peanuts, tree nuts, fish, and shellfish. A gluten-free diet has wheat, rye, and barley eliminated, all of which can be replaced with potato, corn, and rice products.
Food intolerance	Lactose is the most common food intolerance. Other intolerances include adverse reactions to products added to foods to enhance taste and color or protect the food from bacterial growth. A client with an intolerance may experience vomiting, diarrhea, abdominal pain, and headaches. Any known food that causes an intolerance is eliminated from the diet.
Tube feedings	All or parts of a client's nutritional needs can be met through enteral tube feedings. A client receiving an enteral tube feeding may receive food by mouth as well if he or she can swallow safely.

Some conditions warrant specialized nutritional support such as **enteral tube feedings**. A client with a functional gastrointestinal tract may require intermittent or continuous enteral tube feedings to meet all nutritional needs. Reasons for enteral feedings include the inability of the client to meet nutritional needs adequately through the oral intake of food, inability to swallow, or refusal to eat. The type of tube and anatomical placement is based on the client's condition and ability to swallow.

Examples of tubes used for enteral feedings include the following:

- **Nasogastric tube:** enters through the nose and terminates in the stomach
- **Nasojejunal tube:** enters through the nose and terminates in the small intestine
- **Nasoduodenal tube:** enters through the nose and extends into the duodenum
- **Jejunostomy tube:** surgically placed through the abdomen into the jejunum of the small intestine
- **Percutaneous endoscopic gastrostomy (PEG) tube:** surgically placed through an incision in the upper left quadrant of the stomach; can terminate directly into the stomach, or can be extended further if necessary

Following insertion of the enteral tube, the client will receive an x-ray to verify correct placement. Monitoring for complications is critical in the care of clients receiving enteral feedings, as they are at risk for aspiration of the contents from the feeding. Factors that increase the client's risk include a high gastric residual volume, high bolus feeding rates, and high feeding volume. Contents of the enteral solution observed in a client's mouth indicate the client is most likely experiencing reflux, placing him or her at risk for aspiration. Any condition that affects the client's esophageal sphincter—such as an endotracheal or tracheostomy tube—also increases the client's chance for aspirating the feeding contents.

Other potential problems associated with enteral feedings include the following:

- Fluid imbalances: dehydration, overhydration
- Electrolyte imbalances: hyponatremia, hypernatremia, hypokalemia, hyperkalemia, hypophosphatemia, hyperphosphatemia
- Glucose abnormalities: hypoglycemia or hyperglycemia
- Gastrointestinal complications: nausea, vomiting, diarrhea or constipation, abdominal distension, pain
- Mechanical complications: tube clogging, tube migration, skin irritation, breakdown from the feeding tube, drainage around the tube

All health care facility policy and procedures should be observed when caring for a client who requires enteral feedings. Nursing interventions to prevent complications and maintain the patency of the enteral tube for a client receiving enteral feedings are as follows:

- Monitoring intake and output
- Assessing the site of the tube
- Providing frequent mouth care
- Cleaning the area around the tube
- Ensuring immediate availability of suction devices at the bedside
- Elevating the head of the client's bed at least 30–45°

- Administering feedings on a pump programmed to the appropriate rate

- Verifying placement of the tube by testing the pH of the gastric contents

- Measuring and recording the residual volumes prior and after each feeding

- Turning off enteral feedings during transport or repositioning of the client

- Logrolling the client into a side-lying position if a semi-Fowler's is contraindicated

- Checking gastric residual volumes before each intermittent feeding, water bolus, or medication administration

- Flushing the tube with 30 mL of water after checking for residual volume, before and after administering an intermittent feeding, or after administering medications

- Assessing the gastric residual volume at least every four hours for all clients receiving a continuous enteral feeding, or as required per the health care facility's policy and procedure

Clients receiving enteral feedings may require the administration of prescriptions. Before administering any medication, the nurse will communicate with the pharmacy about the prescription to be administered and the type and distal location of the enteral tube. Further considerations include the following:

- Obtaining the prescriptions in liquid form rather than a tablet when available

- Using an oral or catheter tip syringe to deliver medications and performing flushes through the current connector

- Monitoring prescriptions administered through a feeding tube, as they might may cause clogging, especially if the prescriptions are crushed

- Administering each medication separately, flushing the tube before, between, and after each medication

- Considering a pharmacy consult for a client who experiences diarrhea while receiving multiple sorbitol-based drugs. For a client with a nasogastric tube who requires a prescription that must be administered on an empty stomach, the feeding may have to be withheld for 1–2 hours before and after administration of the medicine.

Clients who are receiving enteral therapy are at risk for dumping syndrome, and those who have had long-term malnutrition are at risk for refeeding syndrome. **Dumping syndrome** may occur as a result of a rapid infusion of a high-volume feeding that moves too quickly from the stomach to the small intestine and is associated with enteral feeding boluses. To prevent the complication, the formula should be administered at room temperature and the feeding rate increased slowly.

Clients with long-term malnutrition will be monitored for **refeeding syndrome**. This client's body may experience a reaction to digestion after depleted electrolytes shift from the serum to the intracellular space, which can trigger life-threatening arrhythmias and multisystemic dysfunction. The nurse will monitor for intolerance at the onset of enteral feedings by checking heart rate, heart rhythm, and electrolyte levels.

The nurse will assess the client before beginning an enteral feeding and will monitor the client's tolerance of the feeding throughout. The nurse will assess the client's abdomen by auscultating for bowel sounds and palpating for rigidity, distention, and tenderness. Clients who complain of fullness or nausea after a feeding starts may have a higher gastric residual volume. On an ongoing basis, clients will be monitored for gastric distention, nausea, bloating,

> **NOTE**
> Supplements may be ordered for parenteral administration before enteral feedings to reduce the risk of refeeding syndrome in clients with vitamin and mineral deficiencies.

and vomiting. If the client experiences acute abdominal pain, abdominal rigidity, or vomiting, the infusion is stopped and the health care provider notified. A client who has a new onset of pain at or near the insertion site or a nonverbal client with changes in vital signs who is exhibiting agitation and restlessness may have dislodged the feeding tube.

All clients are encouraged to actively participate in choosing dietary foods to help meet their nutritional requirements. Choices are based on cultural preferences, nutritional needs, and the current condition of the client. The nurse will also promote and facilitate the client's independence in eating. The promotion of the client's independence in eating may require special aides to assist the client with feeding him- or herself. Nursing collaboration between health care team members—which may include a language speech pathologist, dietician, occupational therapist, pharmacist, health care provider, respiratory therapist, and dentist—will help establish a plan of care that includes a therapeutic diet to meet the client's nutrition and hydration needs. Clients who are treated for impaired nutrition or hydration require careful ongoing monitoring. Symptoms of improved nutrition are reflected by a change in their current disease state or illness, adequate intake and output, appropriate changes in weight, BMI, trends in laboratory data, physical assessment findings, and subjective information, such as increased energy and a general feeling of well-being.

PERSONAL HYGIENE, REST, AND SLEEP

Hygiene

When assessing a client, the nurse will take into consideration the many factors that may affect the client's ability to perform hygiene. Such factors include culture; religion; available resources; physiological and psychological health; privacy; or lack of required adaptations, such as handrails or shower chairs. During assessment of a client's hygiene practices, it is essential to assess the client's cognitive function, range of motion, skin condition, and overall hygienic practices, as well as to inquire about the client's ability to perform hygiene, frequency of bathing or showering, or changes in the client's ability to perform hygiene.

Physical assessment findings that indicate the client may be having difficulty performing hygiene include an unkempt appearance, body odor, dry skin, rashes, sores, poor cleanliness of hair and nails, and poor oral hygiene. Nursing interventions for the client are based on the client's identified potential or actual hygiene needs. Providing the client and family with education about proper personal hygiene and securing the resources necessary for the client to enhance his or her hygiene are the primary nursing goals.

Rest and Sleep

Rest and sleep have an essential impact on the physiological and psychological health of a client. Rest is needed to conserve and restore energy and helps relieve stress. Sleep is an altered state of consciousness that restores energy, supports physiological well-being, and supports tissue repair and recovery from illness. The psychological effects of a client who does not obtain adequate sleep include diminished mental functioning, decreased ability to concentrate, difficulty making decisions, and irritability, all of which increase the risk for accidents.

Physiological factors that influence the ability to obtain sufficient sleep include the following:

- The reticulating activating system (RAS) and neurotransmitters, which regulate the sleep process
- Acetylcholine and norepinephrine, which influence REM sleep
- Serotonin and gamma-aminobutyric acid (GABA), which affect NREM sleep
- Nerve cells within the hypothalamus, which control the 24-hour circadian rhythms

The circadian rhythms influence biological and behavioral functions, such as body temperature, blood pressure, and hormone and digestive juice production. There are many lifestyles and environmental factors that can affect a client's circadian rhythm, such as work schedules, alarm clocks, prescriptions, pain, substances, food and caloric intake, exercise, fatigue, stress, illness, extraneous noise, and the light-dark cycle of the environment perceived by the retina of the eyes. Melatonin, synthesized in the pineal gland, regulates the circadian phase of sleep and is affected by the light-dark cycle of the natural environment detected by the retinas.

The Sleep Cycle

The normal sleep cycle occurs in five stages and consists of 3–5 cycles of sleep each night. There are two distinct categories of sleep including **nonrapid eye movement (NREM)**, which is further subdivided into four stages. The stages of NREM are characterized by specific brainwave activity, eye movements, and skeletal muscle movements. Throughout NREM, a client's heart rate, respiration, blood pressure, and muscle tone decrease. Sleep energy is conserved, cell division for skin and bone marrow renewal occurs, and epithelial and brain cells are repaired with the release of growth hormone.

Rapid eye movement (REM) is the second category of sleep—a very active stage of sleep characterized by a high degree of cerebral and physiologic activity. This stage of sleep is associated with learning, memory storage, the release of epinephrine, and increased cerebral blood flow. The four stages of sleep are presented below.

THE FOUR STAGES OF SLEEP	
Sleep Stage	**Cerebral and Physiologic Activity**
Stage I NREM Sleep	This is the first stage of sleep, in which the individual is still aware of his or her surroundings. The client is relaxed, drowsy, and thinking is less reality-oriented. This brief stage of sleep lasts up to seven minutes, during which the body's metabolism begins to slow and the temperature and vital signs begin to decrease. Myoclonic body movement may occur at this time.
Stage II NREM Sleep	The client is no longer aware of his or her surroundings. Metabolism and vital signs begin to decrease, and the client is a little harder to awaken.
Stage III NREM Sleep	During this short stage of sleep, the client is much harder to awaken and vital signs, body temperature, and metabolism are decreased. Stage III and IV are considered a slow-wave sleep.
REM Sleep	This is the deepest stage of sleep. During this stage, the client is very difficult to wake, and this is the stage where sleepwalking and bed-wetting occurs. Metabolism is at its lowest point. This stage of sleep decreases with advancing age.

REM sleep is a very active stage of sleep, with a high degree of cerebral and physiologic activity. REM sleep continues to facilitate protein anabolism, but during this same time, there is great fluctuation in autonomic nervous system activity, causing heart rate variability.

When assessing a client's rest and sleep patterns, the nurse will consider the fact that age affects the overall time spent sleeping and the length of each stage of sleep. For example, a newborn requires the most amount of sleep and the older adult requires the least.

Sleep Disorders

Assessing a client with a suspected sleep disorder includes a sleep history, description of sleep patterns, sleep log, consideration of physical illness, life events, lifestyle, stressors, bedtime routines, and sleep environment. Suspected sleep disorders, such as narcolepsy, insomnia, sleep apnea, sleep deprivation, sleep-wake cycle disturbances, and parasomnias can be objectively measured using polysomnography. **Polysomnography** is used to study a client's sleep by recording brain waves, blood oxygen levels, heart rate and rhythm, respiratory rates and patterns, sleep stages, as well as eye, leg, and other body movement or noises made during sleep.

Treatment for sleep disorders is based on the client's diagnosis and may include prescriptions. Nursing interventions designed to help improve rest and sleep focus on incorporating health-promoting principles into the plan of care. These health-promoting principles include the following:

- Promotion of daytime physical activity

- Establishment of bedtime routines and sleep rituals

- Limiting the duration and frequency of daytime naps

- Ensuring a safe, clean, and private sleep environment

- Scheduling client care activities to promote adequate rest

- Identifying prescriptions that may cause wakefulness or decrease REM sleep

- Establishing and adhering to a regular sleep and wake time based on the client's patterns and needs

- Encouraging the client to avoid alcohol, stimulating chemicals such as caffeine, or heavy meals and exercise at least a couple of hours before bedtime

- Promotion of comfort using techniques, such as white noise, dim lighting, pain management, stress reduction techniques, massage, and the elimination of environmental noise

The interventions implemented in a health care setting can also be used at home. While there are some sleep disorders for which there is no cure, such as narcolepsy, it remains essential to implement nonpharmacological measures that promote rest and sleep. Evaluation of the effectiveness of the interventions will allow the nurse and the health care team to modify the treatment plan as needed. Effectiveness of the interventions is reflected in a client acknowledging that he or she feels rested after sleeping.

CLIENT NEEDS FOR PHARMACOLOGICAL AND PARENTERAL THERAPIES

The focus of the NCLEX-RN pharmacological and parenteral therapies subcategory is to assess the nurse's ability to provide care related to the administration of medications and parenteral therapies. Specific areas assessed include the nurse's ability performing the following interventions:

- Safely administer blood products and evaluate the client's response

- Access central venous devices

- Perform calculations necessary for medication administration

- Evaluate the client's response to the medications

Part of the nursing role when administering medications includes providing client education and preparation, as well as observing the "rights" of medication administration. Before administering any medication, the nurse will review pertinent data to ensure it is safe and appropriate for the client. The nurse will participate in medication reconciliation to prevent errors and adverse drug events related to oversights, duplication of medications, or any other discrepancies in the client's medication record. The nurse will titrate dosages of medication based on the client's assessment and parameters prescribed by the health care provider.

Medications will be handled and maintained in a safe, controlled environment, and the client's medications will be evaluated for appropriateness and accuracy. The nurse must be mindful of the potential for client injury when handling or administering high-risk medications. All intravenous infusions and sites will be maintained and monitored by the nurse, and the nurse will adhere to the regulatory guidelines when managing and administering controlled substances. Nursing care also includes the administration and evaluation of the client receiving parenteral nutrition.

CONTRAINDICATIONS, INTERACTIONS, SIDE EFFECTS, AND ADVERSE EFFECTS

Before administering a prescription, the nurse must be knowledgeable about the client's medical and prescription history as well as the client's current condition and any prescribed medical treatments that may interact with the new medication. Prescribed medications may be **contraindicated**, or excluded as a treatment option, based on these factors or other factors such as diet, psychosocial condition, pregnancy, lactation, allergies, and current treatment with alternative or complementary therapies, over-the-counter (OTC) medications, or herbal supplements.

A client may experience a side effect of a prescription. **Side effects** are any effects of a medication that occur in addition to the medication's intended effect. Side effects are predictable and can range from mild and harmless to an actual injury to the client. Client education is essential to provide information about side effects, how to handle them, and when to notify the health care provider. A client who begins a new prescription or has a dosage altered for an existing prescription requires close monitoring for side effects.

Adverse effects are severe, unintended, and often unpredictable effects that occur after taking a prescription. An adverse effect may occur after one dose of the drug or after a period of time. A prescription may result in adverse effects based on the client's gender or race. The client should report all adverse effects to the health care provider, and the client's medication should be immediately discontinued.

Toxic effects occur as a result of an overdose or buildup of the drug in the client's blood. Toxicity is most likely to happen when a client has a history of liver or renal impairment, which renders the organs unable to metabolize and excrete the drug.

Allergic reactions to a prescription occur as a result of a chain reaction that begins with the immune system. An immune response that produces the antibody Immunoglobulin E (IgE) can occur specifically after exposure to a drug, a chemical preservative, or one of the metabolites. These antibodies travel to the cells, which causes the release of chemicals resulting in an immediate allergic reaction. The reaction affects the nose, lungs, throat, sinuses, ears, lining of the stomach, or the skin. This type of reaction occurs within minutes to a few hours of taking the drug. The most common response that occurs is a result of the expansion of the T-cells, which causes a delayed immune response that most often affects the skin, causing rashes that itch. This reaction can occur days to weeks after exposure to the drug.

An **anaphylactic reaction** is a medical emergency. This reaction can occur immediately or several hours after the administration of a prescription and can be fatal. Antibiotics are the most common cause of anaphylaxis, but other drugs can also cause this fatal reaction. A client having an anaphylactic reaction may have varied symptoms such as hives, facial or throat swelling, hypotension, dyspnea, vomiting, or shock. If an anaphylactic reaction is suspected, the nurse will immediately discontinue the drug, administer epinephrine, and—based on the client's condition—administer IV fluids, steroids, and antihistamines while providing respiratory support.

Drug interactions occur when a medication's effect is changed by the presence of another medication or substance. Interactions can delay, increase, or enhance the absorption of either (or both) medication or substance. Many prescriptions, including intravenous fluid, are incompatible with certain medications. Before administering medication with intravenous fluids or mixing any medications in the same syringe, the nurse will consult the pharmacist or a pharmacology resource approved by the health care facility.

Herbal supplements may interact with OTC medications or prescriptions, causing adverse effects. The client may also experience adverse effects when consuming certain foods or drinks that interact with a prescribed medication.

When a client receives a prescription, the nurse will provide education that includes anticipated side effects, adverse effects, potential interaction with other medications, and information as to when to notify the health care provider. Before educating a client, the nurse will perform a medication reconciliation, which includes OTC medications, herbal treatments, allergies, and drug interactions and will report any significant findings to the health care provider.

> **NOTE**
>
> A drug interaction can make a drug less effective. It can also increase the action of a drug or cause unwanted side effects. There are many online tools available to assist consumers in checking for harmful drug interactions.

Client medication education should consist of the following:

- Special storage information

- Indication for the medication

- Safe storage of the medicine away from children

- Name of the medication (generic and brand)

- Dangers of abrupt cessation of the medication

- Signs and symptoms to report to the prescriber

- How to take the medication in relation to meals

- Adverse and side effects specific to the medication

- When and how often the medication should be taken

- Special precautions to follow when taking the medication

- Recordkeeping for medicines, including the reason for taking them

- Information about safe disposal of expired or used medication

- Follow-up testing or visits specifically related to the medication

- Contraindications to taking the medication, including food and drink

- Importance of reporting to any other health care professionals that the client is taking the medication

- Necessity of informing the prescriber if the client is breastfeeding, is pregnant, or has a chance of becoming pregnant while taking the medication

- Review of Consumer Medicine Information (CMI) brochures/leaflets and the need to keep them and written instructions handy for future reference

- Importance of avoiding all other medications, including OTC and complementary drugs without checking with the prescriber first

All side effects, adverse effects, and contraindications of medications and parenteral therapy are reported to the primary health care provider. The nurse will continue to carefully monitor a client who may require an action to counteract a side effect or an adverse effect of a medication. For example, nausea is a common side effect of many drugs and may be treated with another medication. A client prescribed more than one medication that is administered by different routes is carefully monitored for interactions between the medications. The client's response to all medications, any interactions, or attempts to counteract a side effect or adverse effect will be documented in the client's health care record.

Blood and Blood Products

The nurse may be required to administer blood or blood products to replace blood or lost blood components. The nurse must remember that type O (negative) whole blood or red blood cells (RBCs) is a **universal donor** that may be used for any client in an emergency. Clients with type AB (positive) blood are considered a **universal recipient** because they can receive any blood type.

The nurse will conduct a thorough assessment of the client, including pretransfusion baseline vital signs. The nurse will also verify client allergy information (including a possible history of blood transfusion reactions), document the findings, and confirm that informed consent has been obtained. The nurse will ensure the client understands the procedure and rationale and will verify the client has an 18-gauge to 20-gauge intravenous catheter. The nurse will also confirm that the vascular access is patent and the site appears fine. Before the administration of blood or blood products, cross-matching is completed, and laboratory values such as hematocrit, coagulation values, and platelet counts are assessed. The nurse will also assemble all equipment necessary for the administration of blood or blood products and will ensure equipment for managing a reaction is immediately accessible, including intravenous normal saline fluid, oxygen, and suction.

Following the health care facility's policy and procedure, immediately before initiating a blood transfusion the primary nurse and another nurse will verify the following:

- The order for the transfusion
- The client's identification
- The blood group and type for both the client and the product to be administered
- The client's number against the blood product's number
- The expiration date of the blood or blood component
- No unusual clumping, color, or precipitate in the blood, per visual inspection

The blood will be administered using a "Y" filtered tubing and normal saline solution. The nurse will monitor the client for adverse reactions based on the health care facility's policy and procedure. If the client is suspected of having an adverse reaction, the nurse will stop the infusion, keep the intravenous line open with normal saline, intervene as appropriate based on the client's symptoms, notify the blood bank and health care provider, and continue to monitor the client carefully. The nurse can anticipate returning the blood product to the blood bank and obtaining blood or urine samples from the client for laboratory evaluation.

The nurse will monitor the client for complications based on the blood or blood product administered. These products include the following:

- **Packed RBCs:** A packed RBC transfusion is used to treat hemorrhage and improve oxygen delivery to the tissue. One unit of packed RBCs generally increases the hemoglobin by 1 gram per dl and hematocrit by 3 percent.
- **Cryoprecipitate:** This product contains a high concentration of factor VIII and fibrinogen. Cryoprecipitate is administered to clients with hypofibrinogenemia, massive hemorrhage, or consumptive coagulopathy.

- **Plasma:** This includes fresh frozen plasma and thawed plasma. Plasma contains all of the coagulation factors and can be used to reverse anticoagulant effects. Plasma transfusions are recommended in clients with active bleeding or an INR greater than 1.6.

- **Platelets:** A platelet transfusion may be indicated in the prevention or treatment of hemorrhage in clients with platelet function defects or thrombocytopenia.

- **Whole blood:** Transfusion of whole blood is only done in cases of severe hemorrhage. Whole blood contains clotting factors, red blood cells, white blood cells, plasma, platelets, and plasma protein.

- **Albumin:** Albumin is used to help replace circulating blood volume and plasma proteins.

Complications of blood transfusion are based on the type of blood or blood product administered. Complications for which the nurse will monitor the client include the following:

- **Acute hemolytic reactions:** This type of reaction is antibody-mediated. The client's red blood cells are destroyed because of an ABO or Rh incompatibility between the client and the donor's blood. Symptoms of an acute hemolytic reaction include fever, chills, flank pain, changes in vital signs, nausea, headaches, urticaria, dyspnea, chest pain, and shock. Acute hemolytic reactions are life-threatening, placing the client at risk for hypotension, renal failure, and disseminated intravascular coagulation (DIC). Treatment is based on the client's symptoms.

- **Allergic reaction:** An allergic reaction is the most common reaction and occurs due to a hypersensitivity to the plasma proteins in the donor's blood. The reaction can be mild to severe. A mild reaction is characterized by local erythema, hives, itching, and asthmatic wheezing. A more severe reaction includes laryngeal swelling, dyspnea, tachypnea, chest pain, and cardiac arrest. Antihistamines may be administered for a mild reaction, and cardiorespiratory support is included for more severe reactions.

- **Febrile nonhemolytic reaction:** This complication occurs when a client reacts to white blood cells, platelets, or plasma proteins. The client will present with a 2°F or 1°C rise in his or her temperature compared to the pretransfusion reading. Chills, malaise, pruritis, hives, and rashes are common symptoms that occur in a febrile nonhemolytic reaction. Treatment of the symptoms includes the administration of an antipyretic and possibly an antihistamine.

- **Circulatory volume overload:** This usually occurs when whole blood is transfused too quickly or packed RBCs lead to a fluid shift from the interstitial to the vascular space. A client will display signs of fluid volume excess such as dyspnea, headache, tachycardia, hypertension, and distended neck veins. Nursing interventions include stopping the infusion, sitting the client up, and administering oxygen. The overall treatment is aimed at removing the excess fluid.

- **Bacterial contamination:** Bacterial contamination occurs during the donation or preparation of the blood. When this occurs, the infusion is immediately discontinued, and all tubing, filters, and administration sets are removed and saved for cultures while preserving venous access. Treatment is initiated after blood cultures have been obtained and includes administering antibiotics, corticosteroids, and epinephrine as needed. Symptoms of bacterial contamination are abdominal cramping, chills, diarrhea, fever, shock, the onset of renal failure, and vomiting.

All clients will be evaluated for allergic and adverse reactions, and, based on their condition, a therapeutic response to the blood and blood products will be prepared. Client evaluation for a therapeutic response includes physical and laboratory assessment. Documentation of all information is comprehensive and completed promptly per health care agency policy.

Central Venous Access Devices

A client may require venous access for short- or long-term intravenous therapy, hemodynamic monitoring, or difficult venous access. Several types of catheters can be used, including peripheral intravenous devices, a nontunneled central catheter, and a peripheral inserted central catheter (PICC). Dialysis or central venous catheters include the Hickman, Broviac, or Groshong, as well as implanted venous access ports or umbilical venous catheters.

When administering intravenous therapy through a peripheral or central vein, the nurse must consider the purpose and duration of the therapy, as well as the client's age, vascular condition, health history, and diagnosis. The nurse will also use an infusion device to provide accurate administration of fluids and medications. Regardless of the type of infusion of fluids or medications the client requires, the nurse will review with the client the purpose and type of catheter that is required for treatment.

Several different types of catheters are used based on the length and treatment plan of the client.

Central venous catheter (CVC): Also referred to as a central line, a CVC is threaded through the vein until the tip sits in the large vein near the heart (vena cava). Central lines are more difficult to place, but have several advantages over peripheral IVs. Since CVCs extend through shorter internal distances, they are better for clients who have difficulty having a catheter inserted into their veins.

Peripheral intravenous catheter: This type of IV therapy is short-term, intermittent, or used for maintenance of vascular access. The sites most commonly used with peripheral IV therapy include the cephalic, basilic, accessory and upper cephalic, median basilic, median cubital veins of the arms, and the metacarpal veins of the hands. The nurse will select the most distal site to preserve the proximal veins if needed in the future. The size of the peripheral catheter used is based on the length of time access is required, type of medication and fluid being administered, the client's age, and the condition of the veins. The smaller the gauge of the needle, the larger the diameter. Generally, a 16–18 gauge catheter is used for rapid infusion of fluids, trauma, blood, or a client scheduled for surgery. A 20–22 gauge catheter can be used to administer blood and medications. A 24-gauge is used for the older client, children, and general or intermittent infusions. These catheters can typically remain in place for 72 hours but should be removed as soon as possible to prevent infection. An air embolism is a complication of intravenous therapy; therefore, all intravenous tubing is primed and inspected to ensure there is no air.

INTRAVENOUS CATHETERS	
Catheter Type	**Description/Uses/Risks**
Nontunneled CVC	• Has double or triple lumen lines that are inserted into the subclavian vein by the health care provider. • Used for multiple or concurrent venous access and can remain in place for weeks. This access can be used for intravenous therapy, medications, blood administration, or total parenteral nutrition. • Complications associated with insertion include pneumothorax, hemothorax, arterial injury, hemorrhage, infection, air embolism, and thrombosis.
Peripherally inserted central catheter (PICC)	• Has a single- or double-lumen catheter that is inserted via a basilic vein or antecubital space into a central vein, the tip of which terminates in the superior vena cava outside the right atrium. • Used for long-term intravenous therapy. • Does not place the client at risk for pneumothorax, hemothorax, or air embolism and has fewer catheter-related infections.

INTRAVENOUS CATHETERS	
Catheter Type	**Description/Uses/Risks**
Tunneled CVC	• Inserted into the subclavian or jugular vein by the health care provider and tunneled into the subcutaneous tissue of the chest wall before exiting the skin. • Sutured into place and can be used for long-term intravenous therapy. • The client is at risk for the same complications during placement as with the nontunneled CVC.
Implanted ports	• Implanted ports are central venous access devices with a subcutaneous injection port surgically implanted in the chest or an upper extremity. • Used for long-term intravenous therapy.
Hemodialysis catheter	• May be tunneled for long-term needs or nontunneled for short-term needs.
Umbilical vein catheter	• Inserted via the umbilical vein in the umbilical cord with the tip of the catheter positioned at the junction of the inferior vena cava of the right atrium. • Used in neonates.

After initial placement of a CVC, an x-ray must be taken to confirm the placement and position of the tip. Included in the ongoing care is routine assessment of the integrity of all catheters and their insertion sites per health care facility policy. This assessment is also performed prior, during, and after the use of the catheter.

The nurse will assess for the following complications that are specific for the type of catheter used:

- Phlebitis
- Infection
- Embolism
- Hematoma
- Infiltration
- Thrombosis
- Extravasation
- Nerve damage
- Venous spasms
- Catheter rupture
- Lumen occlusion
- Thrombophlebitis
- Catheter migration
- Catheter dislodgment
- Pain, redness, edema, warmth
- Catheter-related bloodstream infection

Care of all intravenous access sites is performed using a sterile technique, and all ports that will be accessed are disinfected before use. Dressing changes for peripheral intravenous sites are completed using aseptic technique, cleansing the site with an approved skin preparation, and then applying a transparent semipermeable dressing. Peripheral capped intravenous sites are flushed with 3–5 mL of 0.9% normal saline.

Nursing care for access and dressing changes of a CVC include the following measures:

- Maintaining hand hygiene at all times during treatment

- Providing maximal barrier precautions, including a sterile drape that covers the client head to toe (with a small opening at the insertion site), head covers, masks, sterile gowns, and gloves for all personnel directly involved in line insertion

- Using a chlorhexidine skin preparation stronger than 0.5% in 70% isopropyl alcohol for antisepsis at the insertion site

- Following removal of the soiled dressing, scrubbing back and forth for 30 seconds and letting the site dry completely. The dressing is not applied until the preparation has dried.

- Monitoring the frequency of dressing changes. Frequency depends on dressing type and integrity. A transparent semipermeable dressing should be used and changed every seven days; a gauze dressing needs changing every 48 hours. If the client is diaphoretic and the site is bleeding or oozing, a gauze dressing may be preferred. All dressings are changed sooner if they are no longer intact, become contaminated or soiled, or there is evidence of inflammation.

- Following the health care facility's recommendation for changing the tubing and caps

- Stabilizing all central catheters to prevent dislodgment, migration, damage, and pistoning (i.e., back-and-forth motion within the vein that can damage the intima and cause phlebitis and infection). Some catheters are sutured into place. In such cases, the sutures are cleaned and all securement devices are replaced during dressing changes.

- Conducting a daily review of the need to continue the central catheter

- Applying an impermeable cover over the dressing before the client takes a shower or bath to protect the site from direct contact with water

- Flushing all catheters with a heparin solution or other type of flush as prescribed to maintain patency, following the health care facility's policy and procedure for flushing capped peripheral IVs. All central catheters are routinely flushed with no less than 10 mL of normal saline, and when withdrawing blood specimens through the catheter, the line will be flushed with at least 20 mL of normal saline. Use the flushing technique that is most appropriate for the type of catheter cap, and clamp the catheter per facility policy.

- Disinfecting the cap and flushing the catheter according to the health care facility's policy and procedures when accessing central venous catheters before and after the treatment or withdrawal of a blood specimen as described above

Expected Actions/Outcomes

Nurses have many resources available to help understand medications with which they are not familiar. Consulting the pharmacist and using approved health care facility resources (such as an electronic resource that provides current evidence-based medication information) or a drug formulary will assist the nurse in finding the information necessary to administer medication to a client safely.

There are several factors the nurse must consider that will impact the anticipated effect and outcome of any medication, including the following:

- Dosage
- Route
- Frequency
- Condition of the client's drug-metabolizing organs (liver and kidneys)
- Age
- Gender
- Weight

Nurses must also be familiar with the pharmacokinetics and pharmacodynamics that affect the action a medication will have on a client. **Pharmacokinetics** includes absorption, distribution, metabolism, and excretion of the drug. **Pharmacodynamics** refers to the half-life of a drug, onset of action, peak plasma levels, and trough.

The **desired action** of a drug is based on the half-life. The **onset of action** of a drug is related to many factors, including the route, drug formulation, and the pharmacokinetic factors previously discussed. Recognizing the onset of action and peak plasma levels is very important when monitoring a client receiving insulin. Peak and trough levels are used to measure and monitor blood levels of certain antibiotics.

A client who is prescribed or receiving an OTC medication, vitamins, herbal supplements, or naturopathic remedies requires education and ongoing monitoring for the effectiveness of the treatment as well as any interactions when more than one medication is taken. The nurse will monitor the client's biochemical response to a drug, which can be systemic or local and is based on the client's response to the medication. Whether taking a medication short-term or for a more extended period, the anticipated results should be therapeutic. Throughout treatment, a client is monitored for side effects, adverse effects, toxicity, and a nontherapeutic response.

DOSAGE CALCULATION

Prior to calculating any dose of a medication or setting up a dosage calculation, the nurse must be able to convert an ordered dose dispensed by the pharmacy and set up the calculation using the same units of measurement.

Common Metric System Equivalents

1 gram (g) = 1,000 milligrams (mg)

1,000 grams = 1 kilogram (kg)

1 mg = 1,000 microgram (mcg)

1 liter (L) = 1,000 milliliters (mL)

1 pint = 2 cups

2 pints = 1 quart

1 gallon = 4 quarts

Common Metric System Equivalents

1 cup = 8 oz.

5 mL = 1 tsp

15 mL = 1 Tbsp

30 mL = 1 oz.

240 mL = 8 oz.

500 mL = 1 pint

1,000 mL = 1 quart

1 kg = 2.2 lbs.

Common conversions the nurse can anticipate when calculating a dosage of medication most commonly occur between units of measure within the metric system and the US standard system of measurement used in the United States.

Common Conversions

lb. = kg × 2.2

kg = lb. ÷ 2.2

mL = L × 1,000

L = mL ÷ 1,000

mg = g × 1,000

g = mg ÷ 1,000

mcg = mg × 1,000

mg = mcg ÷ 1,000

When calculating medication dosages, the nurse must use critical thinking to apply the principles of conversion between different measurement systems and the actual calculation of the prescription. Some high-risk medications require a second nurse to validate the calculation and the safety of the dose. In addition to the clinical decision making used when calculating dosages, the nurse must understand the recommended dosages based on the client's gender, weight, age, and physiological condition.

The following three primary methods can be used to calculate the dosage of medications:

1. Desired Over Have or Formula Method

2. Ratio Proportion Calculations

3. Dimensional Analysis

Examples of these methods, as well as intravenous fluid calculations, follow.

Desired Over Have or Formula Method

$$\text{Dose amount} = \frac{\text{Ordered dose}}{\text{Amount on hand}} \times \text{Quantity}$$

Example

Prescribed: 3 mg IV push

Available: 2 mg/mL

How many mL will the nurse administer?

$$\frac{\text{Ordered dose (3 mg)}}{\text{Amount on hand (2 mg)}} \times \text{Quantity (1 mg)} = \frac{3}{2} = 1.5 \text{ mL}$$

Ratio Proportion Method

Basic Ratio Proportion

$$\frac{\text{Dose on hand}}{\text{Quantity on hand}} = \frac{\text{Desired dose (drug order)}}{\text{Quantity desired } (x)}$$

Example

Prescribed: 1,000 mg

Available: 200 mg tablets

How many 200 mg tablets will the nurse administer?

Solve for x to identify the number of tablets to administer:

$$\frac{\text{Dose on hand (200 mg)}}{\text{Quantity on hand (1 capsule)}} = \frac{\text{Desired dose (1,000 mg)}}{\text{Quantity desired } (x)}$$

$$\frac{200 \text{ mg}}{1 \text{ capsule}} = \frac{1,000 \text{ mg}}{x \text{ tablets}}$$

$$(200 \text{ mg})(x \text{ tablets}) = (1 \text{ capsule})(1,000 \text{ mg})$$

$$x \text{ tablets} = \frac{1 \text{ capsule} \times 1,000 \text{ mg}}{200 \text{ mg}} = \frac{1,000}{200} = 5 \text{ tablets}$$

Calculation of a Medication in a Solution

Example
Prescribed: 2,500 units
Available: 10,000 units/mL
How many mL should the nurse administer?

Set up the ratios between the proportions:

$$\frac{10,000 \text{ units}}{1 \text{ mL}} = \frac{2,500 \text{ units}}{x \text{ mL}}$$

$$10,000 \text{ units} \times x \text{ mL} = 1 \text{ mL} \times 2,500 \text{ units}$$

Solve for x:

$$x \text{ mL} = \frac{1 \text{ mL} \times 2,500 \text{ units}}{10,000 \text{ units}} = \frac{2,500}{10,000} = 0.25 \text{ mL}$$

Dimensional Analysis Method

Example
Prescribed: 650 mg
Available: 325 mg (1 tablet)
How many tablets should the nurse administer?

$$\frac{650 \text{ mg}}{1} \times \frac{1 \text{ tab}}{325 \text{ mg}}$$

Cancel the units:

$$\frac{650 \ \cancel{\text{mg}}}{1} \times \frac{1 \text{ tab}}{325 \ \cancel{\text{mg}}}$$

Multiply across the top and divide across the bottom:

$$\frac{650}{1} \times \frac{1 \text{ tab}}{325} = \frac{650 \text{ tab}}{325} = 2 \text{ tablets}$$

Dimensional Analysis: Conversion

Example
Prescribed: 0.6 mg
Available: 1,000 mcg/mL
How many mL should the nurse administer?

$$\frac{0.6 \text{ mg}}{1} \times \frac{1 \text{ mg}}{1,000 \text{ mcg}} \times \frac{1,000 \text{ mcg}}{1 \text{ mL}}$$

Cancel the units:

$$\frac{0.6 \text{ mg}}{1} \times \frac{1 \text{ mg}}{1,000 \ \cancel{\text{mcg}}} \times \frac{1,000 \ \cancel{\text{mcg}}}{1 \text{ mL}}$$

Multiply across the top and divide across the bottom:

$$\frac{0.6 \text{ mg} \times 1,000}{1,000 \text{ mL}} = 0.6 \text{ mg/mL}$$

Calculating Intravenous Drip Rates

Formula

$$\frac{\text{Volume (mL)}}{\text{Time (min.)}} \times \text{Drop Factor (gtts/mL)} = \text{Flow rate in gtts/min.}$$

Example

Ordered: 250 mL normal saline to infuse over 90 minutes

Infusion set has a drop factor 15 gtts/mL

Calculate the drips per minute

Round to the nearest whole number

$$\frac{250 \text{ mL}}{90 \text{ min.}} \times \frac{15 \text{ (gtts)}}{\text{(mL)}} = \frac{3,750}{90} = 41.66 = 42 \text{ gtts/min.}$$

Formula

$$\frac{\text{Total volume (mL)}}{\text{Infusion time}} = \text{Flow rate (mL/hr.)}$$

Example

Ordered: Infuse 1,000 mL of normal saline over 8 hours

Infusion set drop factor: 15 gtts/mL

Calculate the IV flow rate per minute

Round to the nearest whole number

$$8 \text{ hours} \times 60 \text{ minutes} = 480 \text{ min.}$$

$$\frac{1,000 \text{ mL}}{480 \text{ min.}} \times \frac{15 \text{ (gtts)}}{\text{(mL)}} = \frac{15,000}{480} = 31.25 = 31 \text{ gtts/min.}$$

Formula

$$\frac{\text{Total volume (mL)}}{\text{Flow rate (mL/hr.)}} = \text{Infusion time}$$

Example

Ordered: 750 mL of normal saline is to infuse over 10 hours

For how many mL/hr. will the infusion pump be set?

$$\frac{750 \text{ mL}}{10 \text{ hrs.}} = 75 \text{ mL/hr.}$$

Example

Ordered: Administer 100 mL of an antibiotic over 30 minutes via an infusion pump

For how many mL/hr. will the pump be programed?

$$\frac{100 \text{ mL}}{30 \text{ min.}} \times \frac{60 \text{ min.}}{1 \text{ hr.}} = \frac{6,000}{30} = 200 \text{ mL/hr.}$$

Formula

$$\frac{\text{Flow rate (mL/hr.)}}{\text{Infusion time (hr.)}} = \text{Total Volume (mL)}$$

Example

IV rate is set to deliver 75 mL/hr.

After 6 hours, how many mL of fluid have infused?

$$75 \text{ mL/hr.} \times 6 = 450 \text{ mL}$$

MEDICATION ADMINISTRATION

When providing education about medications for a client, the nurse may have to include additional discussion and demonstration for self-administration of a medication. The client's overall ability to self-administer any medication is evaluated through interview and observation. The interview includes asking a client to describe the steps of administration as well as demonstrating them.

Before any discussion or demonstration regarding self-administration, the nurse will assess the client for the following:

- Knowledge deficits

- Literacy level

- Developmental age

- Financial concerns or fears

- Cultural and religious beliefs that may restrict the type of treatment the client receives

- Functional or cognitive deficits, psychiatric or sensory disorders, level of consciousness, and language barriers

- Health beliefs and expectations of the treatment

This information is essential, as some types of medication require self-administration and are more invasive than others. After establishing that it is acceptable to proceed with the prescribed treatment, providing further information and a demonstration is included in the initial education for self-administration of medications.

Before preparing or administering any prescription, the nurse will evaluate the prescription for appropriateness and accuracy. The health care provider's prescription should include the name of the client, date and time the prescription was written, name of the prescription, dosage strength, form, route of administration, frequency of administration, duration of therapy, indication(s) for use, and the signature of the provider. Based on the indication for the medication, the nurse will also assess the client for allergies, vital signs, current physiological or psychological conditions, laboratory data, current treatments, and prescriptions (to identify potential interactions or contraindications). All medications are prepared and administered in a safe and timely manner.

After verification of the prescription, the nurse will do the following:

- Review the client's condition and allergies.

- Double-check high-risk medications.

- Consult a pharmacist or a facility-approved resource.

- Avoid workarounds, such as borrowing medications.

- Demonstrate familiarity and adherence to the health care facility's medication administration policies.

- Avoid preparing medications in an environment with distractions, such as interruptions, inadequate lighting, or cluttered workspaces.

- Use proper administration devices, such as syringes, needles, infusion tubing, and pumps.

- Check the expiration dates on the medication.

- Avoid overriding safety systems, such as barcoding.

The nurse is responsible for ensuring a client takes his or her medication, or, if necessary, disposing of unused medicine according to the health care facility's policy and procedure. The disposal or "wasting" of some medications—including controlled substances—requires another nurse as a witness as well as detailed documentation. All medications should be securely and appropriately stored until administered. Medications that have been retrieved for administration should not be left unattended or in a client's room.

For client safety, the nurse will remain diligent in following the "rights" of medication administration, which include the following:

- Right client

- Right medication

- Right dose

- Right time

- Right route

- Right client education

- Right documentation

- Right to refuse

- Right client assessment before medicating

- Right client evaluation and monitoring

> **NOTE**
>
> It is imperative that disposal of unused medication is conducted in the presence of a qualified witness and that all documentation is completed. Medication diversion can result in suspension or loss of license, termination of employment, and possible criminal charges.

The nurse may need to mix medications from two vials into one syringe or add a medication to an intravenous solution. Before mixing medications or adding any medication to a solution, the nurse will do the following:

- Check the compatibility of the medications.

- Use aseptic technique throughout the preparation; before drawing up any medication, the tops of the vials will be cleansed according to the health care facility's policy and procedure.

- Use a filter needle or straw for withdrawing medication from ampules.

- Use a needle or blunt tip cannula for withdrawing solutions from vials when possible.

- Use the appropriate syringe and needle.

- Determine the total volume of all medications to be added to a syringe, and whether the volume is appropriate if administering in a specific site, such as intramuscularly.

- Recap all needles using a needle capping device or one-handed technique to avoid contamination of the needle or cap.

- Maintain the sterility of all needles and medications throughout the procedure.

- Avoid contaminating a multidose vial with a second medication, such as insulin.

Before administering any medication, proper handwashing and clean gloves are applied. All health care facility policy and procedures are followed. The client is provided with education and is evaluated, and safety interventions are performed as discussed previously. Medications can be administered using several routes.

Oral Administration

Oral medication comes in different forms, including capsules, tablets, enteric-coated tablets, or liquid. The nurse instructs the client not to chew or disrupt the integrity of capsules or enteric-coated tablets. Liquid medications should be shaken, and many types of medication should not be mixed in beverages such as juice. The nurse consults the pharmacist and pharmaceutical resources if there are any concerns regarding the proper way the client should take the prescription. All **sublingual** medication is placed under the tongue and allowed to dissolve.

Buccal Administration

Buccal medications are placed against the mucous membrane of the cheek. The client is instructed not to chew or swallow either the sublingual or buccal medication.

Ophthalmic Administration

Ophthalmic medications are administered through the eye. A client may require ointments, eyedrops, irrigations, or medicated discs for the treatment of conditions of the eye. **Ointments** are instilled in the lower eyelid from the inner to the outer canthus. When instilling ophthalmic medications, medical asepsis of the applicator must be maintained. The nurse provides the client with tissues to blot any overflow and sits the client up with the head tilted back. The client is instructed to look up and, pulling the lower lid to form a pouch, the nurse instills the drops into the pouch of the lower conjunctival sac. A slight pressure is maintained through the tear ducts to prevent the medication entering systemically through the tear duct.

Before irrigating the eye, the nurse provides the client with a towel and a basin to hold below the face. When irrigating the eye, the nurse fills a sterile irrigation syringe with warm sterile irrigation and, keeping the eye open with the nondominant hand, flushes the eye from the inner to the outer canthus holding the syringe one inch away from the eye.

Medicated discs are placed in the lower eyelid for a prescribed amount of time and removed by lowering the lower eyelid. The exposed medicated disc is removed by pinching it with the gloved thumb and index finger to break the suction.

Otic Administration

Otic medications, such as ear drops or irrigation, may be prescribed to treat infection, soften cerumen, or remove a foreign body. The nurse provides the client with tissues to dry any drainage from the instillation of ear drops. To instill ear drops, the client is positioned so the ear to be treated is in the uppermost position. The auditory canal is straightened in the adult by pulling up and back on the pinna; for a child, the pinna is pulled back and down. The prescribed number of drops are placed in the ear canal, after which the pinna is released. The nurse presses on the tragus to prevent loss of medication and systemic effects, and, if prescribed, cotton will be placed loosely in the auditory canal. When administering medication in both ears, the nurse waits five minutes before applying drops in the second ear.

A client who requires irrigation of the ear will be provided a basin and a towel. The warmed sterile solution is instilled in the ear with a sterile syringe. The nurse straightens the ear canal as described above and flushes the ear until the solution exiting the ear is clear. Loosely placing a piece of cotton in the outer ear canal, the nurse positions the client with the affected side down to help drain fluid. After 10–15 minutes, the nurse removes the cotton and allows fluid to flow outward freely. The nurse stops the procedure if the client indicates he or she is experiencing pain or dizziness.

Inhalation Medication Administration

Medications may be inhaled through a **metered dose inhaler (MDI)** with or without a spacer or a nebulizer. All clients will be assessed before and after treatment. Assessments should include pulse, respiratory rate, breath sounds, pulse oximetry, and peak flow measurement before beginning treatment.

The nurse will perform the following steps for the administration of an MDI:

- Sit the client upright.
- Ensure the canister is in the holder so the client receives the ordered dose, and remove the mouthpiece cover.
- Shake the inhaler.
- Prime the medication if there is a priming button on the bottom.
- Instruct the client to take a deep breath in and exhale completely. Then, place the client's lips around the mouthpiece of the inhaler and position the inhaler in the client's mouth.
- Instruct the client to inhale deeply and slowly while depressing the canister, and—at the peak of the inhalation—to hold his or her breath for 10 seconds or as long as comfortable.
- If another dose is required, instruct the client to wait for 20–30 seconds.
- If another medication is to be inhaled, the client should allow 2–5 minutes between inhalations.
- Allow the client to rinse the mouth with warm water. The inhaler holder and cap should be cleaned with warm running water and allowed to dry.

The nurse will perform the following steps for administration of an MDI with a spacer:

- Insert the MDI into the end of the spacer device.
- Instruct the client to place the spacer mouthpiece in the mouth, close the lips around the mouthpiece, and breathe normally.
- Depress the medication canister to spray one puff into spacer device.
- Instruct the client to breathe in deeply and slowly for about 5 seconds. The client should then hold his or her breath at the end of inspiration for about 10 seconds.
- If another dose is required, instruct the client to wait for 20–30 seconds.
- If another medication is to be inhaled, the client should allow 2–5 minutes between inhalations.
- Allow the client to rinse the mouth with warm water. The inhaler holder and cap should be cleaned with warm running water and allowed to dry.

The nurse performs the following steps for administration of an MDI with a nebulizer:

- Assemble the nebulizer per the manufacturer's instructions or collaborate with a respiratory therapist to set up the equipment.

- Add the medications as prescribed by pouring it into the nebulizer cup. Ensure that the medication is secure and fastened in the device. More than one medication may be mixed if there are no contraindications. Some may require additional dilution with normal saline.

- The client should be positioned at least at a 45° angle.

- The nebulizer is either attached to compressed air (if available) or oxygen.

- Do not cease oxygen if the client is currently receiving; continue through nasal prongs with the nebulizer.

- Turn on the air to the nebulizer and ensure that mist is visibly exiting the chamber. A flow rate of 6–10 L/min. is sufficient.

- Ensure the chamber is connected to a face mask or mouthpiece and the nebulizer tubing is connected to the compressed air or oxygen flowmeter.

- Ensure the client's lips are sealed around the mouthpiece, if used.

- Instruct the client to take slow, deep, inspiratory breaths with a brief 2- to 3-second pause at the end of inspiration, and continue with passive exhalations.

- This breathing pattern will be repeated until the medication is complete and there is no visible misting. This process takes approximately 8–10 minutes.

- After the treatment, turn off the flow meter and disconnect, rinse, and store the nebulizer according to health care facility policy.

- If the inhaled medication included steroids, instruct the client to rinse the mouth and gargle with warm water after treatment.

- After treatment, encourage the client to perform deep breathing and coughing exercises to help expectorate mucus.

Nasogastric Tube Administration

Some oral medications can be administered via nasogastric, gastric, intestinal, and jejunal tubes. Before administration, the placement of the tube is verified. The nurse will take additional precautions to prevent client aspiration or clogging of the tube when administering medications through small-bore feeding tubes. As discussed in the section "Nutrition and Oral Hydration," medication with a special coating cannot be administered through a nasogastric, gastric, intestinal, or jejunal tube, including all enteric-coated, time release, sublingual, and buccal medication.

Topical Prescriptions

Topical prescriptions include creams, pastes, lotions, transdermal patches, or medications applied to the mucous membranes of body cavities, such as the vagina or rectum. Before applying any creams, pastes, or lotions, the nurse must ensure that the area to which the medication will be applied is cleansed. Gloves or another type of applicator may be used to apply the medication. Some areas that are exposed to friction from clothing may require a gauze dressing or other type of dressing over the site. When opening the medication, the nurse will take care to avoid contaminating the opening of the tube or container. The medication is applied using even strokes following the direction of the body's hair growth.

Transdermal Patches

All old transdermal patches are removed before applying a new patch. Ensure the patch is not applied over a site that has hair, a bony prominence, irritated skin, breakdown, a port, or a pacemaker. The backing from the patch is removed, and it is applied to the skin using pressure from the palm of the hand for 10–15 seconds. The nurse avoids massaging the area where the patch is located.

Suppositories

Suppositories are a way to deliver medication to the client when other routes, such as oral, cannot be used. The suppository is designed to dissolve at body temperature, releasing the drug once inside the body.

When inserting a **vaginal suppository**, the nurse will instruct the client to empty her bladder and lie in a dorsal recumbent position; if the position is not tolerated, the nurse will use the Sims' position. The nurse lubricates the applicator or suppository with a water-soluble gel. Separating the labia, the nurse cleanses the vaginal opening and fully inserts the applicator or suppository. The nurse then instructs the client to remain in a side-lying position or with her hips on a pillow for 5–10 minutes.

To insert a **rectal suppository**, the nurse places the client on the left side with the upper knee flexed. Wearing gloves, the nurse lubricates the suppository using a water-based soluble gel. The nurse separates the buttocks and inserts the rounded end of the suppository along the rectal wall (avoiding stool) until the suppository is about 3–4 inches past the internal sphincter. The nurse then cleans the perirectal area and instructs the client to remain in the left lateral position for 5–10 minutes or longer, based on the medication that is prescribed.

Parenteral Medication Administration

Intradermal Layer

An injection into the **intradermal** layer of skin is used for tuberculin or allergy testing. Only a very small volume of medication is injected into the dermis—0.1 mL or less. The client's skin is spread taught, the needle is positioned with the bevel up, and it is inserted at a 10–15° angle. The fluid is administered slowly. After the injection, the needle is withdrawn and sterile gauze is placed over the site. The nurse avoids massaging the site and engages the safety mechanism of the needle and disposes of it properly. If no wheal is observed, then the medication was inadvertently injected into the subcutaneous tissue. Intradermal sites for injection include the anterior aspect of the forearm, upper chest, upper back, and the back of the arm.

Subcutaneous Injection

A **subcutaneous injection** is an injection into the fatty layer under the dermis. This type of injection is used for small volume injections—less than 1 mL—or when the medication is not likely to irritate or damage the subcutaneous tissue. Because the blood supply to this area is less than in muscle tissue, drug absorption is slower. Appropriate needle length and injection technique are dependent on the client's skin and subcutaneous fat thickness.

To avoid a needle stick when raising a skinfold, maintain a distance of greater than an inch between the finger and the thumb. If a raised skin fold is used, the needle should be inserted with the bevel up at a 45° angle. The raised skin should be maintained throughout the injection until the needle is removed. After the injection, gauze is placed over the site, the safety mechanism is engaged over the needle, and the needle is disposed of properly. If the skin is not raised, the needle is inserted at a 90° angle, and the remainder of the procedure is the same as for an injection given at a 45° angle.

The nurse should be mindful of the fact that different injection sites have different absorption rates. For example, injecting insulins in the abdomen has been shown to have the most rapid absorption, while the upper arms are intermediate, and the thigh and buttocks have the slowest absorption. The sites for insulin injection should be rotated within the site to avoid lipodystrophy. The nurse should rotate at least one inch from the previous injection site until the area has been used, then switch to another site until the initial site has healed. Rotating injection sites will help avoid the development of lipodystrophy and maintain a more predictable absorption. Recommended sites for subcutaneous injections include the outer aspect of the upper thigh, outer aspect of the upper arm, and the abdomen, avoiding injections within 1–2 inches around the umbilicus and the upper buttocks.

Intramuscular Injection

Intramuscular injections are typically used to inject less than 3 mL of fluid. The muscle site used depends on the volume of solution to be injected. For example, the deltoid can be used when injecting 1 mL of a solution, whereas the vastus lateralis, ventrogluteal, or dorsogluteal can be used when injecting more fluid. The gluteus maximus and deltoid muscles are used for infants or children who are less than three years old; infants less than 18 months old should not receive an injection of greater than 0.5 mL. When administering intramuscular injections, the landmark is appropriately identified, the skin spread taut, and, with the bevel of the needle up, the needle is injected using a darting motion at a 90° angle. The medication is then injected slowly, the needle is withdrawn, gauze placed firmly over the site, the safety mechanism of the needle engaged, and the needle properly discarded.

Intravenous Medication Injection

Peripheral intravenous fluid may be indicated for many purposes, such as to provide fluids, administer antibiotics or other medications, provide nutrition, replace electrolytes, provide emergency access, or correct a fluid imbalance. When initiating an intravenous medication, the appropriate gauge catheter and the anatomical site will be chosen based on the indication for treatment. The prescribed intravenous fluid is obtained, as is the proper tubing and supplies. All intravenous medications are evaluated for compatibility with the IV solution and any other additives.

Before administering any IV push medications, the flow clamp on the IV tubing is clamped or pinched off above the injection port, the port is cleansed with alcohol, and the prescription is administered according to the recommended rate. After the medication is injected, the clamp is opened and the flow rate is adjusted to the prescribed rate. Before initiating a secondary line or intravenous piggyback, compatibility must be established with the primary IV fluid. The injection port is cleansed with alcohol, and the secondary set is injected into the port using a needleless system or secondary needle set. The primary IV will be lowered so the secondary line can infuse.

After the infusion, the primary IV will continue infusing at the prescribed rate. Keeping both IVs at the same height will allow the primary IV to continue infusing during the infusion of the secondary IV. After the infusion, the secondary line can be removed. Some intravenous medications are prescribed to be titrated. Medications such as insulin, oxytocin, or antihypertensives are titrated according to prescribed parameters that are reflected by the client's condition.

All high-risk medications are handled per the health care facility's policy and procedure. High-alert medications such as blood products, insulin, and anticoagulants are linked to harmful outcomes. Medications identified as a high-alert by the health care facility require double-checking with another nurse to ensure the right client receives the right dose of the right medication. Each nurse will check the medication independently and, if required, will also check the drug calculation, and then compare results.

Medication reconciliation involves obtaining accurate medication history, clarifying that the medication and dosages are appropriate, and conducting reconciliation, which is the documentation of every change in a client's medication. These changes include prescriptions, OTC medications, herbal products, and other home remedies. The health care facility's policy and procedures will define the process and roles of the health care team (including the health care provider, nurse, pharmacist, and other treatment team members) for obtaining, managing, and revising client information for medication reconciliation.

TOTAL PARENTERAL NUTRITION (TPN)

Total parenteral nutrition (TPN) is a form of nutritional support administered through access to central veins, usually through a PICC or subclavian line. The nutritional solution contains proteins, carbohydrates, fats, vitamins, minerals, hyperosmolar glucose, and trace elements. Other additives, insulin, or electrolytes may be mixed into the TPN solution. TPN solutions are prescribed based on the client's age and physiological condition. The purpose of TPN is to restore nutrition, prevent nutritional deficits, or allow the gastrointestinal tract to heal or rest. Before initiating TPN, the nurse will provide education to the client about the need for the TPN in relation to his or her condition. A client receiving TPN requires ongoing monitoring for effectiveness and complications.

The following assessments are included in the plan of the care for a client receiving TPN:

ASSESSMENTS FOR TOTAL PARENTERAL NUTRITION (TPN) CLIENTS	
Assessment	**Description**
Functional Nutritional Assessment	BMI and anthropometric measurements
Skin Integrity	Clients who are adequately nourished and hydrated maintain skin integrity. Any existing wounds should begin to show signs of healing.
Weight	Weight is monitored based on the client's condition.
Vital Signs	Vital signs should remain stable. Any abnormal findings may be related to complications from receiving TPN.
Intake and Output	Intake and output are reflective of the client's cardiovascular and renal condition and should be monitored closely.
Laboratory Evaluation	An initial assessment followed by periodic lab assessments based on the client's condition includes electrolytes, total protein, albumin levels, blood glucose levels, BUN, creatine, CBC, lipid profiles, serum iron levels, urine osmolality, and liver function tests.

The client receiving TPN is at risk for many complications, some of which are shown in the following table.

POSSIBLE COMPLICATIONS OF TPN TREATMENT	
Complication/Disorder	Description
Infection	• TPN is administered in a closed sterile system, and strict aseptic technique is used when setting up and removing TPN tubing. Feedings are to be refrigerated until administered. • Due to the dextrose concentration in the TPN, the client is at an increased risk of infection. • Symptoms of a localized infection at the site of the catheter include redness, tenderness, discharge, fever, chills, and malaise. • Systemic infection or catheter-related bloodstream infection (sepsis) is characterized by tachycardia, hypotension, tachypnea, elevated or decreased temperature, decreased urine output, and an altered level of consciousness.
Hyperglycemia/ Hypoglycemia	• The TPN solution has a high dextrose content, and inadequate insulin coverage will place the client at risk for hyperglycemia. The nurse will monitor the client for symptoms of hyperglycemia, including polydipsia, polyuria, and polyphagia, headache, fatigue, and nausea. • Abrupt TPN rate changes, delayed administration, or a sudden discontinuance of the solution can result in hypoglycemia. Symptoms of hypoglycemia include blurred vision, tachycardia, headache, palpitations, nausea, diaphoresis, irritability, dizziness, unconsciousness, and seizures.
Fluid Overload	• TPN is a hypertonic solution that can create a fluid volume overload through the intravascular shifting of extracellular fluid. • Symptoms of extra fluid volume include shortness of breath, adventitious breath sounds, hypertension, edema, bounding pulses, and distended jugular veins.
Fluid Volume Deficit	• Clients receiving TPN are at risk for dehydration. • Symptoms include dry, poor skin turgor; tachycardia; hypotension; and elevated urine specific gravity.
Essential Fatty Acid Deficiency	• Clients receiving TPN may not receive enough essential fatty acids, which can result in a deficiency. • Symptoms include dry, scaly skin; thrombocytopenia; and poor healing of wounds.

The PICC or central venous lumen line TPN should not be used for any other treatments. When changing or initiating any TPN treatments, the nurse primes all tubing to ensure there is no air in the tubing and instructs the client on how to perform the Valsalva maneuver to avoid an air embolism. TPN is administered using tubing with an inline filter that is changed every 24 hours. The insertion site care and dressing are changed according to the health care facility's policy and procedures. The formula to calculate the TPN flow rate is the same calculation used for intravenous fluid.

Parenteral/Intravenous Therapies

Parenteral and intravenous therapies require the use of different points of venous access. Intermittent parenteral fluid therapy may be necessary for many reasons, such as fluid and electrolyte replacement or administration of medications, anesthetics, diagnostic reagents, blood or blood products, or nutrients and supplements. Provide education for the client as to the indication and anticipated duration of intravenous therapy before initiating treatment.

Intravenous therapy is an invasive procedure that places the client at risk for infection and medication errors if the wrong fluid or rate is infused. Aseptic technique must be maintained throughout all IV therapy, including the preparation of the intravenous fluid for infusion, when spiking the bag and priming the tubing, during the insertion of the IV catheter and initiation of fluid, and when discontinuing the IV system. The expected assessment of a client includes verification of proper placement and patency of the catheter.

> **NOTE**
> Examples of how to calculate intravenous drip rates are located in the section "Dosage Calculation." Parenteral and intravenous therapies require the use of different points of venous access, as discussed in the "Central Venous Access" section.

Throughout the IV therapy, the nurse will monitor the client for complications such as phlebitis, infiltration, extravasation, hemorrhage, hematoma, local site infection, pulmonary edema, air embolism, catheter embolism, and catheter-related bloodstream infection. The length of time the IV catheter remains in place is based on the client's condition and the health care facility's policy and procedures. Peripheral catheters should not be replaced more frequently than every 72–96 hours unless complications occur. All catheters are removed as soon as they are no longer needed or if any complications occur.

Infusing of medications or fluids via an IV pump or client-controlled analgesia device requires the nurse to verify that the right medication is infusing, the programmed dosing is correct, and the equipment alarm systems are audible. The nurse must also ensure that the client is being monitored for the quantity of medication or fluids infused, intake and output, and response to prescribed treatment. Client evaluation is based on the reason for the treatment and may include intake and output, laboratory values, physiological system changes, vital signs, and client comfort.

PHARMACOLOGICAL PAIN MANAGEMENT

The frequency for the assessment and treatment of a client's pain is based on condition, reports of pain, and changes in condition. Generally, **multimodal treatment** is used, which includes the use of two or more classifications of prescriptions to provide ongoing pain relief while avoiding analgesic gaps. This approach also allows for the lowest dose of a drug to be administered, thus decreasing the risk of side effects.

The type of medication and route of administration of a prescription for pain relief is based on the subjective and objective information received during the pain assessment of a client, as well as the origin or source of pain. When administering pain medication, the oral route is the preferred route because it is the least expensive, easiest to administer, and most tolerated. Other considerations include factors that have an effect on the pharmacokinetics of a drug, including the client's condition, age, and if the client is pregnant or lactating. Some medications should be avoided for a young or older client, and the majority of the medications are contraindicated during pregnancy and lactation. Regardless of the type or route of medication administered, the nurse will subjectively and objectively evaluate the client for side effects, adverse effects, allergic response, and therapeutic response to the medication.

> **NOTE**
> Clients may experience **breakthrough pain**, which is an exacerbation of pain in clients whose chronic pain is already subject to long-acting medication.

Commonly Used Analgesics for Pain

Nonopioid analgesics are versatile and have many different agents and formulations that can be administered using different routes. However, nonopioid analgesics are ineffective for neuropathic pain. These agents are used for nociceptive pain, although they are available in combination with opioids. All nonopioid and opioid formulations have a maximum daily dose that should not be exceeded. NSAIDs should be cautiously used and in some cases are contraindicated in client populations, such as older adults, clients with cardiovascular or gastrointestinal risk factors, and clients with bleeding disorders. Acetaminophen should not exceed a daily recommended dose of 4,000 mg/day and is contraindicated in a client with hepatic impairment. Nonopioid analgesics include acetaminophen, aspirin, ibuprofen, NSAIDs, ketorolac, ketoprofen, naproxen, diclofenac, and celecoxib.

Opioid analgesics treat moderate to severe nociceptive pain. Mu-opioid agonists have no dosage ceiling for pain; to prevent tolerance, rotation of opioids can be implemented. The client will develop a tolerance to the side effects (except for constipation) with regular use over several days. Oversedation and respiratory depression can develop in a client, so close monitoring is required for the first 24 hours. Some opioids, such as morphine, produce metabolites that accumulate and result in toxicity. Mu-opioid analgesics include hydromorphone, fentanyl, morphine, hydrocodone, oxycodone, oxymorphone, and methadone.

Adjuvant analgesics have the largest and most diverse group of medications, formulations, and routes of administration. These agents are used to treat neuropathic pain. Due to the varied effects on clients, many agents may have to be trialed to find an effective medication or effective level of mediation. There may be a delayed onset of analgesia because most clients will require titration of a dose over several weeks to evaluate the effectiveness of the drug. Many of the agents have a maximum daily dose, and the side effects can be significant. Over time, the client will develop a tolerance to most of the side effects; the side effects are responsive to a reduction in the dosage of medication. Adjuvant analgesics include drugs from the following classes: anticonvulsants, alpha-2 adrenergic antagonists, muscle relaxants, local anesthetics, and antidepressants.

All controlled substances are administered and the unused portion wasted according to the facility's policy and procedure. The nurse must pay close attention to the policy and procedures as only specific health care workers may witness the waste of a controlled substance. Also, there may be a specified period for the documentation of the waste of the medication. The nurse must have an understanding of the correct way to securely store, handle, transfer, administer, and discard the controlled substance.

CLIENT NEEDS FOR REDUCTION OF RISK POTENTIAL

The focus of the NCLEX-RN Reduction of Risk Potential subcategory is to assess the nurse's ability to reduce the likelihood that clients will develop complications or health problems related to existing conditions, treatments, or procedures. This assessment is accomplished through the nurse's ability to accurately assess and efficiently respond to changes or trends in a client's vital signs, perform diagnostic testing, monitor the results, and intervene appropriately.

During any procedure or diagnostic testing, the nurse will implement the proper precautions to prevent client injury and evaluate the response to procedures and treatments. The nurse will be able to safely obtain blood specimens via venipuncture, a venous access device, or a central line, as well as obtain specimens for other diagnostic tests. The nurse can also expect to perform the insertion, maintenance, and removal of a nasal or oral gastrointestinal tube, urinary catheter, and peripheral intravenous line, as well as maintain a percutaneous feeding tube. A client may require the application of a device to promote venous return. The nurse will apply and monitor the device.

Throughout the period of care, the nurse will continue to monitor the client for trends and changes of condition as well as to implement the appropriate interventions and perform a focused assessment to ensure the client is physiologically stable and responding to treatment. Before any procedure or treatment, and in the perioperative and postoperative periods, the nurse will support the client by providing education. All clients receiving moderate sedation will be monitored by the nurse during and after their procedure.

MONITORING CHANGES IN CLIENT CONDITION

Vital Signs

A client's vital signs are an objective measurement of the physiological functioning. Vital signs include temperature, pulse, respirations, blood pressure, and oxygen saturation. The acceptable parameters of the vital signs are based on the client's age and condition. The frequency of assessment, interpretation, techniques used to obtain a client's vital signs, as well as the nurse's response to changes in vital signs are all based on the client's age, physiological condition, current treatments, and medications. When obtaining vital signs, the nurse must be aware of the anticipated physiology and pathophysiology that affect the client's results.

Temperature, Pulse, and Respiration

A client's internal ability to maintain a temperature within expected ranges is associated with environment, physiological condition, and age. Body temperature is measured in degrees using either the Fahrenheit or Celsius scale. The routes used to measure temperature include oral, axillary, tympanic, rectal, or over the temporal artery on the forehead.

The pulse is reflective of factors such as a client's cardiovascular volume, the electrical conductivity of the heart (which includes rhythm and strength), and the compliance of the arterial system. Anatomical sites used to count beats per minute through the palpation of a pulse include the temporal region, carotid, apical, brachial, radial, femoral, popliteal, posterior tibial, and dorsalis pedis. A **Doppler ultrasound** can also be used to assess pulses that are difficult to detect, and a stethoscope is used to auscultate the apical heart rate. When assessing a pulse through palpation or with a Doppler, the rate, rhythm, and volume are obtained. The rate and rhythm of an apical pulse can be evaluated using a stethoscope.

Adequate respiratory rates and depth are reflective of the functioning of the medulla and pons centers in the brain. Chemoreceptors stimulate these centers throughout the body, and stretch receptors in the lungs, muscles, and joints provide input to the medulla and pons. Therefore, any changes in oxygen, carbon dioxide, or pH levels affect the respiratory centers in the brain. Before assessing a client's respirations, the nurse will consider that many factors, such as age, exercise, cardiovascular or respiratory disease, acid-base balance, medications, pain, and emotions, can all affect the client's respiratory rate. During the assessment, the nurse will observe a client's chest movement and symmetry, respiratory rate, depth, and quality of respirations.

A client's **oxygen saturation (SpO_2)** levels can be measured at a peripheral capillary level through **pulse oximetry**. This measurement reflects the percentage of hemoglobin that combines with oxygen, which is determined by analyzing the amount of light absorbed by oxygenated and deoxygenated blood. Measurement of oxygen saturation is performed noninvasively by clipping a probe to the fingertip, earlobe, or toe of a client, with the fingertip being the primary site used. A client with cold extremities, an injury, nail polish, or who wants to use his or her fingers will require the probe to be placed in an alternate location. Physiological factors that can affect SpO_2 readings include anemia, edema, jaundice, vasoconstriction, lung disease, and hypotension.

Blood Pressure

Blood pressure is determined by the amount of pressure exerted on the walls of the arteries as the blood is pumped out of the left side of the heart and into the arterial circulation. The blood pressure obtained is measured in millimeters of mercury (mmHg) and consists of systolic and diastolic pressure. The **systolic pressure**, which is recorded as the higher number, reflects the peak pressure wave through the arterial system after the left ventricle contracts and forces blood into the arterial system. The **diastolic pressure**, recorded as the lower number, indicates the least amount of pressure on the arterial walls. During this time, the heart is filling with blood and resting between beats.

Blood pressure is regulated by many mechanisms to maintain tissue perfusion. These mechanisms include the autonomic nervous system, renin-angiotensin aldosterone system, antidiuretic hormone, and cardiac output. Factors that affect the blood pressure include age, gender, race, medication, weight, circadian rhythm, fluid volume, food, emotions, pain, and physiological conditions. Blood pressure can be assessed in the upper or lower extremities manually by performing a two-step process, by obtaining a single pressure using a **sphygmomanometer**, or indirectly with a machine.

To avoid inaccurate readings, the blood pressure cuff on a sphygmomanometer or machine must be the correct size and must be positioned correctly. The client's arm should be level with the heart. If the client is sitting, the feet should be flat on the floor. The cuff should not be placed over clothing on the arm, which can be constricting. Additionally, the nurse will avoid taking the blood pressure immediately after the client has exercised or smoked. Blood pressure should not be assessed on an extremity that has an injury, IV, shunt, or arteriovenous fistula, nor should the reading be taken on the side of a mastectomy or nodal removal.

Direct pressure monitoring, referred to as **hemodynamic monitoring**, is an invasive type of monitoring that provides a continuous assessment of a client's cardiovascular system. Common types of hemodynamic monitoring include pulmonary artery pressure monitoring, central venous pressure, and intra-arterial blood pressure monitoring. Specialized equipment is required for the different types of invasive monitoring. A CVP, pulmonary, or arterial catheter will be introduced into the appropriate blood vessel or heart chamber. The catheters require a flush system that includes an IV solution, tubing, stopcocks, and flushing device to provide either manual or continuous flushing. A pressure bag will be applied around the flush solution maintaining a pressure of 300 mmHg to prevent clotting or backflow of blood into the pressure monitoring system. A transducer is required to convert pressures recorded from the arterial system or heart chamber into an electrical signal as well as an amplifier or monitor to increase the size of the electrical signal for display.

Central venous pressure monitoring is obtained by placing the tip of the central venous catheter into the vena cava or right atrium. The placement of the catheter allows for the assessment of right ventricular function and blood return to the right side of the heart. The pressures in the right atrium and ventricle are equal at the end of diastole and range from 1–8 mmHg. Heart failure or hypervolemia will cause pressure to increase. As discussed previously, central venous catheters can also be used to infuse IV fluids and medications and to draw blood specimens.

A **pulmonary artery catheter** typically has four ports, with each port used for a different measurement. The most distal port is used to measure central venous pressure. It is an injectable port used to measure cardiac output. The distal part of the catheter goes into the pulmonary artery and is connected to a pressure line. The pulmonary artery pressure will be consistently visible on the monitor. A balloon port is also present, which is used to determine the pulmonary artery wedge pressure. When the catheter tip is inflated, the catheter advances and wedges in a branch of the pulmonary artery, at which point the tip senses the pressure transmitted from the left atrium, which reflects the **left ventricular end diastolic pressure (LVEDP)**. The pressure that can be measured during the inflation of the balloon is the **pulmonary artery wedge pressure (PAWP)**, which closely reflects the left atrial pressure in clients without left heart or left valvular disease and normal heart rates.

An elevated PAWP pressure may indicate the client is experiencing hypervolemia, mitral regurgitation, or left ventricular failure. A decrease in PAWP occurs with an afterload reduction or hypovolemia. Pulmonary artery pressure parameters are as follows:

- Systolic: 15–26 mmHg

- Diastolic: 5–15 mmHg

- Mean pulmonary artery pressure: 15 mmHg

- Pulmonary arterial wedge pressure (PAWP): 4–12 mmHg

- Cardiac output: 4–7 L/min.

Intra-arterial blood pressure monitoring provides the nurse with continuous monitoring of systemic blood pressure. Clients who are critically ill or have unstable cardiopulmonary systems may benefit from this type of monitoring. The use of arterial lines provides the benefit of being able to obtain blood samples and blood gases from the client. After insertion into the arterial line, the catheter is connected to a flushed and airless tubing and transducer, which is placed at the client's heart level. A waveform reflects the blood pressure, which can be evaluated for accuracy with an ECG waveform or with correlation to manual or indirect blood pressure measurement.

Intracranial Pressure

Cerebral perfusion pressure is the normal amount of pressure required to perfuse the brain, which varies based upon the age of the client. The normal range of cerebral perfusion pressure for an adult is 60–100 mmHg. A client's cerebral perfusion pressure can be calculated by subtracting the intracranial pressure from the mean arterial pressure. An adult client's intracranial pressure range is 5–15 mmHg and is measured using invasive intracranial pressure monitoring. This type of monitoring can be accomplished through the surgical insertion of an intraventricular catheter, subdural screw bolt, or an epidural sensor.

Increased intracranial pressure is the rise in pressure inside the skull that can result from an increase in spinal fluid, blood volume, or brain tissue volume as a result of injury, disease, infection, seizures, stroke, hematoma, aneurysm, or hydrocephalus. Other factors that increase intracranial pressure include anything that increases venous pressure, such as heart failure, suctioning, coughing, the Valsalva maneuver, or laying down after sitting. The nurse will perform a thorough neurological assessment, including the use of the Glasgow coma scale and calculation of the cerebral perfusion pressure, for clients at risk or suspected of increased intracranial pressure.

To prevent complications associated with increased intracranial pressure, the nurse will assess the client for signs and symptoms associated with the condition. Early signs and symptoms related to increased intracranial pressure include the following:

- Headaches

- Emesis

- Change in the level of consciousness

- Irritability

- Sunsetting

- Pupil dysfunction

- Cranial nerve dysfunction seizures

Late symptoms associated with increased intracranial pressure include the following:

- Further decrease in the level of consciousness
- Decreased spontaneous movements
- Posturing
- Papilledema
- Pupil dilation with decreased or no response to light
- Increased blood pressure
- Irregular respirations
- Cushing's triad (a late, ominous sign), widening pulse pressure, irregular and decreased respirations, such as Cheyne-Stokes, and bradycardia

Nursing interventions to help decrease the pressure include positioning the client in bed with the head and neck in midline position and with the head of the bed up at 35–40 degrees to facilitate the venous return. Other interventions include avoiding overhydration and maintaining normal body temperature, oxygen, and carbon dioxide levels. The nurse can also anticipate other treatments to help decrease the pressure, including the administration of an osmotic agent and diuretic to decrease fluid, temporary mechanical hyperventilation to reduce carbon dioxide, careful monitoring of serum sodium, sedation, and muscle relaxation. The treatment goal for the client experiencing increased intracranial pressure is to prevent injury by lowering the pressure.

> **NOTE**
>
> **Cheyne-Stokes respiration** is a specific form of breathing characterized by periods of increasingly deeper (and sometimes faster) respiration followed by a gradual decrease and eventual temporary stop in the client's breathing.

DIAGNOSTIC TESTS AND LABORATORY VALUES

Part of a client's treatment may include diagnostic testing. **Diagnostic testing** requires a client be educated regarding the purpose of testing, preparation for testing, and the implications of the test results, as well as confirming that the client fully understands the information and has provided consent to the testing. To maintain the safety of the client and facilitate the accuracy of testing, the nurse will adhere to the health care facility's policy and procedures—as well as the health care provider's prescriptions—when providing care for a client undergoing diagnostic testing. The client will be identified appropriately, and all specimens labeled and handled according to policy. Documentation is based on the sample obtained during the testing and may include type, quantity, color, odor, and consistency.

Many diagnostic tests, such as laboratory testing, will provide the health care team with a baseline of the client's condition. Throughout treatment, the client may require further testing, and the newer results will be compared to the initial testing results. Periodic testing is referred to as **trending** and allows the health care team to monitor the client for significant changes that may impact his or her health. Common types of diagnostic testing include obtaining oxygen saturation readings; electrocardiograms; glucose monitoring; venous blood sampling; urinalysis; stool analysis; and sputum, throat, or wound cultures.

ECG

The nurse may need to obtain an ECG to monitor and record the electrical activity of a client's heart, which includes the rate and rhythm, evaluation of the effects of cardiac injury resulting from ischemia or disease, evaluation of the effects of medications, or obtaining a baseline reading before a procedure. ECG testing is performed by attaching electrodes to the surface of the client's skin. To obtain an accurate, clear ECG tracing, the leads must be placed and positioned correctly. Before placing the electrodes on the client, the electrodes are attached to the lead cable then placed on the appropriate contact site of the client. Positioning the client will be based on their condition, but the client can be placed supine, semi-recumbent, sitting in a chair, or the tracing can be obtained during ambulation using a telemetry system (battery-operated transmitter). If the client's activity is restricted and the recording is obtained through a hard-wired system, the client will be instructed to remain still and breathe normally. The client's skin should be clean and dry prior to putting the electrodes on, avoiding placement over areas of scar tissue or irritated skin, and clipping the hair if necessary. The electrodes applied should have a pad that has a moist gel to transmit the information.

Blood Glucose Testing

A client may require blood glucose testing at the bedside. This point of care procedure requires obtaining a capillary blood specimen and using a portable glucometer or glucose meter to evaluate the glucose concentration of the specimen. The nurse will obtain a handheld glucose meter with a keypad, display screen, and blood sample port. The client's identification information is programmed into the meter before testing. Some meters include a barcode scanner that can be used to scan the client's ID bracelet, which automatically enters client-specific information into the device.

Aseptic technique is used to obtain a sample of blood from the dermis with a lancet or automated puncture device. The puncture site chosen is highly vascular, but not highly innervated. The preferred puncture sites in children (other than infants) and adults are the lateral aspect of the fingertip or the earlobe. Previous puncture sites; areas of inflammation, bruising, edema, or infection; cyanotic or poorly perfused tissue; or sites with superficial peripheral arteries are avoided in all clients. Puncture site rotation is necessary to allow the tissue to heal. The site will be cleansed using a facility-approved antiseptic and after allowing the site to dry.

After puncturing the area, apply a drop of blood to the blood glucose test strip and insert it into the meter. Based on the test results, the nurse will determine the next course of action to be taken. To avoid errors, the site should be allowed to dry thoroughly before obtaining a sample. The glucose test strips are meter model-specific and cannot be changed between different models of glucometers. The lot number and expiration date of the test strips are checked before use and the lot number programmed or scanned into the meter. The test strips should be stored in a cool, dry location. Prolonged exposure to air, light, or humidity can reduce the accuracy of the blood glucose results. The nurse will ensure that the quality control checks have been performed on the blood glucose meter according to the health care facility's policy and procedure.

Venous Blood Sampling

Many clients require the analysis of blood specimens, which are obtained through **venipuncture**. Considerations when collecting blood specimens include timing, dietary intake, use of the proper blood collection tubes, and labeling and handing the specimen according to the health care facility's policy and procedure.

Steps included in obtaining a blood specimen are as follows:

- Wash hands; use gloves during the blood collection process.
- Identify the appropriate vein for a puncture; the most common site in an adult is the median cubital vein in the antecubital fossa. Choose the correct size needle to avoid hemolyzing the blood.
- Assess the client for allergies or sensitivities to antiseptics, adhesives, or latex.
- Apply the tourniquet 2–4 inches above the site and ask the client to make a fist.

- Prep the site and allow it to dry.

- Firmly pull the skin taut below the puncture site to anchor the vein from rolling, and insert the needle at a 15–30 degree angle with the bevel up.

- After observing a flash of blood, attach the tubes or syringe and remove the tourniquet as the last amount of blood is drawn. Leaving the tourniquet on too long may result in hemoconcentration.

- Remove the needle and press down on the site with gauze.

- Dispose of the needle in an approved container, label the tubes appropriately, place them into transport bags, and deliver the specimens to the lab promptly.

Urinalysis

A **urinalysis** helps provide diagnostic information about the client's renal function, fluid balance, infection, or other disorders. The primary nursing goal when obtaining a urinalysis from a client is to ensure the sample has been collected accurately. Urine testing is performed on a one-time voided sample or a timed collection, such as 24-hour urine. A routine urinalysis requires a simple voided sample, whereas a urine sample needed for a culture requires a clean catch urine collection.

The client submitting a urine sample for evaluation will be instructed to clean the urethral meatus and surrounding areas with approved antiseptic wipes. The client is instructed to void, and, after letting the initial stream of urine pass, place the container under the ongoing stream to obtain a sample. A client who requires a timed urine test will discard the first void and collect all subsequent urine for the remaining prescribed period of time. A client who needs a quick reagent strip testing will provide a midstream sample of urine. When obtaining a urine specimen from an indwelling urinary catheter, the catheter is clamped below the specimen port, and when an adequate sample is present, aseptic technique is used to collect the specimen after which the catheter is unclamped according to the health care facility's policy and procedure.

If a client is menstruating, the nurse will communicate this information to the laboratory. All containers in which timed urine samples are obtained will be stored per the health care facility's policy and procedure to maintain the integrity of the urine. Standard precautions are maintained through the collection and handling of the urine. Urine specimen containers should be labeled with the client's information and transferred in a biohazard bag immediately after collection.

Stool Analysis

A **stool analysis** may be performed to assess for blood, bacteria, viral infection, parasites, and ova. The amount of stool required for analysis is based on the type of testing that is to be performed. When testing for blood, a small amount of stool is placed on a test strip that contains chemically altered filter paper that changes color if the sample contains blood. Stool specimens for obtaining a culture require a small amount of stool, whereas stool to be evaluated for a parasite or ova require a larger sample, preferably obtained from different areas of the stool. The client is provided a stool collection container with a lid. The specimen is obtained from the container using a tongue blade and is placed on the hemoccult testing paper. The remainder of the testing is performed according to the health care agency's policy and procedure. All other specimens for testing will remain in the closed container labeled with the client's identification information, placed in a biohazard bag, and immediately transferred to the laboratory for further testing. The nurse will implement standard precautions throughout the collection and transfer of the specimen.

Sputum Culture

A client may require a **sputum culture** for diagnosis of infection, pneumonia, or tuberculosis. A sputum culture may also be used for the evaluation of cells or of a treatment's effectiveness. The type of container used to transfer a sputum specimen may be specific to the type of testing. Clean gloves should be worn when handling the container, carefully avoiding touching the inside of the sterile container. All specimens should be obtained first thing in the morning after providing oral care. Instruct the client to breathe deeply and cough to expectorate the sputum into the container. If the client has a tracheostomy, he or she will require suctioning with a mucus trap. Obtain 2–10 mL of sputum for accurate results. All specimen containers are labeled with the client's information, placed into a biohazard bag, and transferred immediately to the laboratory for evaluation.

Throat Culture

A **throat culture** is obtained to evaluate the client for bacterial or viral infection and to determine treatment options. Wearing gloves and using a tongue blade and light, the nurse will use the swab end of a sterile culturette, touching only the infected areas of the tonsils or oropharynx. The swab is placed back in the tube and sealed immediately. The container is labeled with the client's information, placed in a biohazard bag, and transported to the laboratory immediately. The nurse will document any redness, swelling, pain, pustules, or discharge. The nurse will use the same technique for a rapid antigen detection test.

Wound Culture

A **wound culture** is obtained when changes in the appearance, amount of drainage, or odor of a wound indicate the wound is infected. An infection places the client at risk for a system infection, poor wound-healing, and tissue destruction. The nurse will adhere to the health care facility's policy and procedure for obtaining a wound culture. Some basic principles include thoroughly irrigating the tissue with normal saline solution, moistening the swab with normal saline solution, swabbing a 1–2 cm area of viable tissue in the wound bed using a Z-stroke or modified swab technique, and collecting the culture before topical or system antibiotics are initiated. Avoid taking a sample from purulent matter or swabbing over eschar tissue. After obtaining the culture, place the swab in an appropriate container (taking care not to touch the sides of the container with the swab), label the container, place the sample in a biohazard bag, and transfer the specimen immediately to the laboratory.

Fetal Heart Rate Monitoring

The normal fetal heart rate (FHR) baseline is 110–160 beats per minute (BPM) and can be monitored intermittently with a Doppler or continuously with an external monitor or internal monitor. The modality of monitoring is based on the clinical situation, which will be discussed further.

Intermittent auscultation is noninvasive and can be utilized to assess the fetus during labor for which there are no existing maternal or fetal complications anticipated. The FHR is auscultated with a Doppler or a **fetoscope** (a specially designed fetal stethoscope), allowing the FHR to be counted. Before listening with a Doppler or a fetoscope, Leopold's maneuver is performed to identify the fetal presentation and position. The Doppler with ultrasonic gel or a fetoscope is placed over the area of maximal intensity. The FHR is auscultated as before, during and after a uterine contraction to assess for the absence or presence of increases or decreases in the FHR baseline. The abdomen is palpated for the presence or absence of a uterine contraction and the FHR counted for 30–60 seconds after the uterine contraction. The frequency of auscultation is based on the phase and stage of labor. Any concerning findings or changes in maternal or fetal condition warrant further auscultation or the implementation of external fetal monitoring.

External fetal monitoring provides continuous fetal and uterine data that is printed out on a fetal heart monitoring strip. An ultrasound transducer is applied to the maternal abdomen after identifying the fetal presentation and position, and a **tocotransducer**—which has a built-in button that is sensitive to pressure—is placed over the fundal portion of the abdomen. The tocotransducer allows for the recording of the uterine contractions' frequency and duration, but does not measure the actual intensity of the contraction. The contractions must be palpated for proper assessment of their intensity.

Fetal electrocardiography can also be obtained using an invasive **fetal scalp electrode**, which attaches to the fetal scalp. This internal electrode transmits the P-R interval of the cardiac cycle and allows for the assessment of beat-to-beat variability. An intrauterine pressure catheter (IUPC) can be placed into the uterine cavity to measure the frequency, duration, and intensity of the uterine contractions. The uterine pressure is recorded in millimeters of mercury (mmHg). The FHR and uterine activity are recorded on a fetal monitor tracing.

Part of the responsibility of the nurse when caring for a client during the antepartum period is to interpret the FHR and uterine contraction pattern. Uterine contractions are quantified as the number of contractions present in a 10-minute window, averaged over 30 minutes. A normal contraction pattern is reflected by five or fewer contractions in 10 minutes and averaged over a 30-minute window. An abnormal pattern termed **tachysystole** is defined as more than five contractions in 10 minutes, averaged over a 30-minute window. The interpretation of a contraction pattern applies to both spontaneous and stimulated labor. Tachysystole should always be qualified as to the presence or absence of associated FHR decelerations.

A reassuring FHR pattern has a FHR baseline of 110–160 BPM with the presence of variability, which is an important indication of fetal oxygenation. Any sustained FHR of below 110 BPM for 10 minutes is considered fetal bradycardia. Any sustained FHR above 160 BPM for 10 minutes is considered fetal tachycardia. The underlying cause of the fetal bradycardia or tachycardia needs to be corrected to return the FHR into a reassuring tracing.

The types of **variability** include **absent**, **minimal**, **moderate**, and **marked**. The FHR baseline and variability is the average heart rate during a 10-minute period that does not include accelerations or deceleration. Variability is quantified by beats per minute and measured from the peak to the trough of a single cardiac cycle. A reassuring FHR pattern will have irregular fluctuation in the baseline and range from 6–25 BPM, which is considered moderate variability. Absent variability is defined as undetected fluctuations in the amplitude of the heartbeat; minimal variability has an amplitude of fewer than 5 BPM.

Conditions that can decrease the FHR variability include fetal sleep cycles, fetal tachycardia, prematurity, medications that cause central nervous system depression, congenital anomalies, fetal hypoxemia, or metabolic acidemia. Marked variability is a FHR that is greater than 25 BPM, and the interpretation is dependent on other factors with which it is associated.

The interpretation of periodic accelerations or decelerations is dependent on the duration and their association with a uterine contraction. **Episodic patterns** are accelerations or decelerations not associated with uterine contractions; **periodic patterns** are accelerations or decelerations associated with uterine contractions. Any increase or decrease of the FHR lasting 30 seconds but less than 2 minutes in duration is referred to as an acceleration or deceleration.

Adequate accelerations for a fetus less than 32 weeks gestational age is ≥ 10 BPM above baseline for ≥ 10 seconds, and for a fetus of greater than 32 weeks gestation, it is ≥ 15 BPM above baseline for ≥ 15 seconds. An increase in heart rate characterizes a prolonged acceleration lasting for 2–10 minutes. The types of decelerations are distinguished based on their waveform. Decelerations are based on their relation to the contraction. Recurrent decelerations include early, late, or variable and occur with ≥ 50% of uterine contractions in any 20-minute segment.

The types of decelerations the nurse will monitor the client for include the following:

- **Early decelerations:** Gradual decrease in the FHR with the onset of the deceleration to the nadir (lowest point), which coincides with the peak of the contraction, is uniform in shape and returns to the baseline at the end of the uterine contraction. The early deceleration is associated with fetal head compression. This type of deceleration is a normal finding with no concern.

- **Late decelerations:** Gradual decrease in FHR with the onset of deceleration to nadir ≥ 30 seconds. The onset of the deceleration occurs after the beginning of the contraction, and the nadir of the contraction occurs after the peak of the contraction. The FHR does not return to baseline until after the contraction is over. This type of nonreassuring deceleration is associated with fetal hypoxia, caused by insufficient oxygenation of the uterus and placenta, such as in the case of maternal hypotension or uterine hypertonicity. Nursing interventions include the following:

  - Placing the client in a side-lying position

  - Discontinuing oxytocin

  - Initiating IV fluid hydration

  - Administering oxygen via a nonrebreather mask

  - Correcting any hypotension

  - Notifying the health care provider

- **Variable decelerations:** Abrupt decrease in FHR of ≥ 15 BPM with the onset of the deceleration to nadir < 30 seconds, lasting less than two minutes. The appearance of variable decelerations is shaped like the letter "U, V, or W." Compression of the umbilical cord vessels (which can occur with or without uterine contractions) results in variable decelerations. Occasional variable decelerations have very little significance; however, if they are persistent, they can cause a repetitive disruption in the fetal oxygen supply. Nursing interventions for the client with variable decelerations include the following:

  - Changing position to wherever the FHR pattern is most improved

  - Discontinuing oxytocin if the FHR tracing is nonreassuring

  - Checking for cord prolapse or imminent delivery by vaginal exam

  - Administering oxygen via a nonrebreather mask

- **Prolonged decelerations:** A decrease in FHR of ≥ 15 BPM measured from the most recently determined baseline rate. The deceleration lasts ≥ 2 minutes, but less than 10 minutes. Nursing interventions include the following:

  - Placing the client in a side-lying position

  - Discontinuing oxytocin

  - Initiating IV fluid hydration

  - Administering oxygen via a nonrebreather mask

  - Correcting any hypotension

  - Notifying the health care provider

When interpreting the FHR, the nurse will document the findings using a three-tiered **fetal heart rate classification system**, with category I reflecting normal findings, category II reflecting indeterminant findings, and category III reflecting abnormal findings. The nurse will monitor for the results of other antenatal testing, which includes a nonstress test, ultrasound, and amniocentesis. The **nonstress test** is used to evaluate the well-being of the fetus. During the test, the FHR and uterine activity are monitored. Two FHR accelerations, lasting 15 seconds and peaking at least 15 beats above the baseline within 20 minutes after 32 weeks gestation is the result of a reactive nonstress test. A nonreactive nonstress test requires further evaluation, which includes additional monitoring time or a biophysical profile.

Ultrasonography

Ultrasonography allows for the evaluation of the maternal reproductive system, fetal growth, age assessment, and fetal and placental anatomy. The ultrasound works through a transducer that sends sound waves through the body that come into contact with tissues, body fluids, and bones. When the sound waves bounce back, they are received by the transducer and turned into images. The images are then viewed as pictures on a video screen.

An ultrasound examination can be performed either abdominally or transvaginally and can be used throughout the pregnancy for different assessments. A transvaginal ultrasound is most likely to be used during the first trimester because a clearer image can be captured. During the first trimester, the uterus is still in the pelvis. The client may have to drink several glasses of water a few hours before the ultrasound to promote visualization of the uterus. During the first trimester, an ultrasound can be used to confirm the pregnancy and viability; assess the fetal heart rate; determine the gestation of the pregnancy; detect multiple gestation; assess the uterus, cervix, ovaries, and placenta; diagnose a pregnancy; provide visualization during a chorionic villus sampling; or identify an ectopic pregnancy.

An ultrasound examination during the second trimester allows for the confirmation of dates, confirms viability, identifies congenital anomalies, assesses the placental location, monitors levels of amniotic fluid volume, measures of the length of the cervix, and provides guidance for testing, such as amniocentesis. During the third trimester, ultrasound examination is used for the previously mentioned evaluations, as well as to detect macrosomia and intrauterine growth restriction. Ultrasound is also used to determine the fetus' position, study Doppler blood flow, evaluate a placenta previa or abruption, establish a biophysical profile, and provide visualization during an amniocentesis or external cephalic version (ECV).

An **amniocentesis** is performed to evaluate the fetal amniotic fluid, which contains fetal cells. Direct ultrasonography is used to minimize complications and help visualize the uterine cavity, after which a needle is inserted through the abdomen and into the uterus to obtain a sample of amniotic fluid. The amniotic fluid is used to evaluate the fetus for congenital disorders or anomalies or to assess for fetal lung maturity. Elevated alpha-fetoprotein levels are associated with neural tube defects. A ratio of lecithin to sphingomyelin of more than 2:1 indicates the fetal lungs are mature and a PG ratio greater than 2 mg/L is associated with a low risk for respiratory distress syndrome. Complications of amniocentesis include amniotic fluid leakage, infection, maternal or fetal hemorrhage, placental abruption, maternal isoimmunization, and amniotic fluid embolism.

Laboratory Values

Chapter 1 reviewed the units of measurements and laboratory values according to the NCLEX-RN Test Plan, with the anticipation that the nurse will be able to identify them.

The defined laboratory values are as follows.

Arterial blood gases

- Arterial blood (pH): 7.35–7.45

- Partial pressure of oxygen (PO_2): 80–100 mmHg

- Partial pressure of carbon dioxide (PCO_2): 35–45 mmHg

- Bicarbonate (HCO_3): 22–26 mEq/L

- Oxygen Saturation (SaO_2): 95%

Electrolytes

- Potassium: 3.5–5 mEq/L

- Sodium: 135–145 mEq/L

Hematology

- Blood urea nitrogen (BUN): 18–21 mg/dL

- Serum Creatinine: 0.8–1.3 mg/dL

- Glucose (Fasting): 65–110 mg/dL

- Glycosylated hemoglobin (HbA1c)

  o Normal HbA1c: < 5.7%

  o Prediabetes HbA1c: 5.7–6.4%

  o Diabetes HbA1c: ≥ 6.5%

Hematocrit

- Hct (Male): 42–52%

- Hct (Female): 35–47%

- Hct (Child): 30–42%

Hemoglobin

- Hgb (Male): 14–18 g/dL

- Hgb (Female): 12–16 g/dL

- Hgb (Child): 10–14 g/dL

- Hgb (Newborn): 15–25 g/dL

International normalized ratio (INR): 0.9–1.2

- Platelets: 150,000–400,000 cells/mm³

- Prothrombin time (PT): 11–14 sec

- Partial thromboplastin time (PTT): 60–70 seconds

- Activated partial thromboplastin time (aPTT): 30–40 sec

- White blood cells (WBC): 5,000–10,000 cells/mm³

Lipids

- Cholesterol (total): < 200 mg/100 mL

Client laboratory values will vary based on age, gender, and the clinical condition of the client. Because laboratory testing can vary, when interpreting laboratory data, the nurse will refer to the laboratory reference ranges identified by the health care facility. Laboratory data provides an initial baseline of a client and may be repeated throughout the treatment to identify changes and trends in the client's condition and to evaluate the effectiveness of treatment. When receiving "critical" laboratory results, the nurse will adhere to the health care facility's policy and procedures, communicating the data to the primary health care provider and implementing interventions to maintain the physiological integrity and safety of the client.

Clients or designated family members are provided education about the purpose of testing, the procedure, the interpretation of the results, and how it will relate to treatment. Clients who have diabetes require frequent glucose monitoring. The frequency of glucose monitoring is based on the client's physiological condition and treatment plan, which includes the administration of insulin and dietary intervention.

> **NOTE**
>
> Information regarding obtaining blood specimens and wound, stool, and urine samples is discussed in the "Central Venous Access Devices" and "Diagnostic Tests" sections of this chapter.

POTENTIAL FOR ALTERATIONS IN BODY SYSTEMS

Airway Aspiration

Maintaining and protecting a client's airway is a priority. The nurse is responsible for recognizing conditions that place the client at risk for **airway aspiration**. Factors correlated with aspiration include the following:

- Dysphagia
- Anesthesia
- Medications
- Advanced age
- Seizure activity
- Impaired swallowing
- Lowered head of the bed
- Neurological disorders
- Delayed gastric emptying
- Increased gastric residual
- Impaired physical mobility
- Drug or alcohol intoxication
- Impaired or absent cough reflex
- Impaired or decreased gag reflex
- Presence of gastrointestinal tubes
- Decreased level of consciousness
- Facial, oral neck surgery, or trauma
- Tracheostomy or endotracheal tube

Skin Breakdown

Assessment of the client includes identifying risk factors associated with skin breakdown. The **Braden Scale for Predicting Pressure Ulcer Risk** or the **Norton Pressure Ulcer Scale** are common tools used to predict the client's risk for the development of a pressure sore.

Risk factors that can result in altered skin integrity include the following:

- Age
- Pain
- Immobility
- Mental status
- Skin moisture
- Poor nutrition
- Support surfaces
- Nutritional status
- Poor blood circulation
- Impaired fluid balance
- Impaired physical activity
- Impaired sensory perception
- Fecal or urinary incontinence
- Skin friction, shearing, or pressure

Ineffective Tissue Perfusion

Tissue is dependent on oxygenated blood flow at the capillary level. Ineffective tissue perfusion can occur in relation to the brain, heart, kidney, gastrointestinal system, and the peripheral systems. Many conditions place the client at risk by interfering with arterial blood flow, including the following:

- Obesity
- Diabetes
- Hypoxemia
- Post-surgery
- Hypertension
- Hypovolemia
- Hypervolemia
- Immobilization of a limb
- Decreased cardiac output
- Interruption of arterial flow
- Interruption of venous flow

- Mismatch of ventilation with blood flow

- Altered affinity of hemoglobin for oxygen

- Decreased hemoglobin concentration in the blood

- Mechanical reduction of venous and/or arterial blood flow

- Impaired transport of oxygen across alveolar and/or capillary membrane

Clients are educated on the prevention of all complications associated with a decreased activity level based on their diagnosed illnesses and disease. The nurse will collaborate with the health care team to implement an individualized plan of care for a client at risk for contractures. The care plan may include exercise, active or passive range of motion, positioning, and splinting.

Diabetic clients require meticulous foot care to prevent infection. A client with diabetes may experience neuropathy and peripheral arterial disease, placing them at risk for foot ulcers, infections, foot deformity, and gangrene, which will result in the loss of the toes or foot. The client requires education on meticulous foot care, which includes daily inspection of the skin integrity of the feet, including between the toes and the bottoms of the feet. Education also includes daily washing, thorough drying, protective shoe wear, promoting blood flow to the feet, trimming the nails carefully and straight across, protecting the feet from extreme temperatures, controlling blood sugar, and avoiding smoking.

When caring for a client, the nurse will obtain baseline data of the client's condition, which includes a physical assessment, current medications, laboratory values, or any other prescribed testing and treatments. Based on these finding, the client will be monitored for changes and response to treatments.

Changes such as the impairment of output related to nasogastric tube drainage, emesis, stool, or urine should be of concern. These changes may be due to a worsening condition, a side effect of a medication or treatment, or an infection and can result in a fluid and electrolyte imbalance.

POTENTIAL COMPLICATIONS FROM DIAGNOSTIC TESTS, TREATMENTS, AND PROCEDURES

Many diagnostic tests, treatments, and procedures place the client at risk for potential complications. For any client, the risk of complications is also dependent on multiple factors, such as the client's clinical condition, presence of comorbidities, age, medications, and the risk factors associated with the procedure or treatment to be performed. The nurse will use the proper precautions to prevent injury and complications that are associated with the prescribed test, treatment, procedure, or diagnosis. The nurse will apply the knowledge of nursing procedures and psychomotor skills to provide care for the client and monitor for complications as well as evaluate responses to procedures and treatments. Cardiac catheterization is an example of a procedure that places the client at risk for complications. Complications the nurse will monitor for in this case would include bleeding, thrombosis, emboli, hematoma, vascular injury, pulmonary edema myocardial infarction, stroke, arrhythmias, and allergic reaction to the medications or contrast.

Bleeding and Shock

Invasive procedures, testing, and treatments place the client at risk for bleeding. Client conditions can also increase the risk of bleeding. Conditions such as traumatic injury, fractures, embolisms, cancer, liver or renal disease, inflammatory bowel disease, genetic bleeding disorders, and medications such as anticoagulants, salicylates, NSAIDs, or chemotherapy drugs, all increase the client's risk for bleeding.

A client may experience external or internal bleeding. External bleeding may be visible from a surgical, arterial, or venipuncture site. Signs and symptoms of internal bleeding are based on the amount of bleeding and the system involved.

A client who is experiencing a significant loss of blood will progress through four adaptive physiological responses to shock. Symptoms associated with the progressive physiological responses to shock include the following:

- Hypotension
- Tachycardia
- Cool, clammy, pale skin
- Light-headedness
- Headache
- Restlessness
- Anxiety
- Vomiting
- Diarrhea
- General weakness
- Vision problems
- Chest pain
- Hematuria
- Oliguria (which can progress to anuria)
- Bruising around the site of the internal hemorrhage
- Laboratory changes such as a decreased hemoglobin and hematocrit
- Metabolic acidosis
- Multiorgan system dysfunction
- Death

Care of the client in shock includes correcting the underlying cause by administering blood, blood products, plasma expanders, crystalloid fluid replacement, oxygen therapy, Trendelenburg positioning, drug therapy, laboratory assessment, arterial blood gases, and possible surgical management. The nurse will determine the client's condition and monitor the effectiveness of treatment frequently until the client is stable.

The client who is in shock will be monitored for the following:

- Cognition
- Vital signs
  - Central venous pressure (CVP)
  - Pulse (rate, regularity, and quality)
- Urine output

- Pulse pressure
- Blood pressure
- Respiratory rate
- Oxygen saturation
- Level of consciousness
- Skin and mucosal color

Positioning

Following a test, treatment, or procedure, the client may require specific positioning to prevent complications. For example, a health care facility's policy and procedures typically require a client who has had a lumbar puncture to remain lying flat on bedrest for a prescribed amount of time. The head of the bed will be elevated for a client who is receiving a tube feeding. Immobilization of a fractured extremity will protect the fracture site and promote healing. Familiarity with the health care facility's policy and procedures, understanding the client's condition, as well as understanding the rationale for the treatment plan, will facilitate healing and prevent client injury.

Nasal or Oral Gastrointestinal Tubes

The nurse may be required to insert, maintain, or remove a nasal or oral gastrointestinal tube. Before the procedure, the nurse will verify the prescription, ensure the client understands the procure, and identify the client using two identifiers.

The nurse will obtain the following supplies necessary for the procedure:

- Prescribed-size NG tube
- Water-soluble lubricant
- 60 mL syringe
- Graduated container
- Tap water or sterile normal saline solution for irrigation
- 1-inch tape or tube fixation device with clamp
- Skin prep and/or skin adhesive
- Emesis basin
- Towels
- Tissues
- Penlight
- Suction equipment
- Pulse oximeter
- Water and straw (if the client is able to swallow)
- Permanent marker
- pH test strips
- Clean gloves and other PPE, as needed

The following describes the steps taken to insert a nasal gastric tube:

- Place the client in a high Fowler's position.

- Assess the client's cough and gag reflex.

- Place a pulse oximeter on the client and assess the vital signs.

- Examine the nostrils for septal deviation.

- Instill 10 mL of viscous lidocaine 2% (for oral use) down the more patent nostril with the client's head tilted backward. Ask the client to sniff and swallow to anesthetize the nasal and oropharyngeal mucosa.

- Measure the length of tube needed for the client by placing the tip of the tube at the tip of the client's nose, extending it to his or her earlobe, and then to his or her xiphoid process. Mark the estimated length with a marker or tape.

- Ask the client to hold the cup of water in one hand and put the straw in the client's mouth.

- Lubricate four inches of the tube tip with a water-soluble lubricant.

- Hyperextend the client's neck and insert the tube down and back.

- When the tube has reached the nasopharynx (back of the throat), have the client tilt the chin forward to rest on the chest.

- Advance the tube while the client is swallowing; provide water to the client (if the client is able to swallow and allowed to drink fluids).

- Encourage the client to breathe through the mouth.

- Advance the tube as gently, quickly, and calmly as possible, rotating the tube if needed and stopping when the tape marking is at the naris.

- Once the tube has been advanced 25–30 cm, stop and listen for air escaping from the tubing. The presence of air indicates the tube might be in the trachea rather than the esophagus. If air is present, withdraw the tube and start again. If there is no air, continue to advance the tube to the distance marker.

- Secure the tube. If using tape, apply a skin prep or adhesive if needed. Gently secure the prepared piece of tape—one end at a time—to the bridge of the nose, forming a sling for the tube.

- Secure the tube away from nasal mucosa by wrapping each of the split ends in opposite directions where it exits the nose.

- Use an approved tube fixation device.

- Place the tube against the client's cheek and use the membrane dressing to anchor it out of the client's line of sight.

- Insert the tube into the clamp of the fixation device and close the clamp. Fasten the end of the tube to the client's gown using a clip or piece of tape.

- Keep the tube clamped until placement of the tube is verified.

- Check the initial tube placement with an x-ray; checking pH may be permitted to confirm correct placement after verification by x-ray.

- Provide oral hygiene.

The tube will require maintenance once the placement is confirmed. The maintenance includes skin care around the tube, oral care, maintenance of tube patency, irrigation of the tube with feedings or medications, monitoring and confirming tube placement, and documenting all output, including the amount, color, and any other characteristics.

The following describes the steps taken to remove a nasogastric tube:

- Place the client in a semi-Fowler's position.

- Place a towel over the client's chest.

- Provide an emesis basin and a cup of water with a drinking straw.

- Disconnect the tube from the pump or the wall suction.

- If the client is receiving a feeding through the tube, stop the feeding, flush the tubing, and then disconnect and clamp the tube.

- Apply clean gloves and remove all tape from the client as well as the tape or clamp that is securing the tube to the client's gown.

- Instruct the client to take a deep breath and hold it.

- While pinching the tube, pull it out smoothly and quickly

- Immediately discard the tubing and the gloves.

Catheterization

A client may require a **urinary catheterization**. This may be via a **straight catheter**, which is a single-lumen device designed for short-term or one-time use. Or, it may be a catheter that is designed to be left in place, such as a **double-lumen indwelling catheter** that continuously drains the bladder, or a **triple-lumen catheter** that remains in place and is used to irrigate the bladder. Follow the health care facility's policy and procedure for single and indwelling catheter insertion. Verify that the supplies you will need for the catheter insertion according to the policy and procedure are available in the urinary catheter kit.

Insertion and Removal

General information required to insert a urinary catheter for a female includes the following:

- Place the client in the dorsal recumbent position.

- Clean the perineal area and dry it thoroughly according to policy.

- Remove gloves and wash hands before proceeding.

- Prepare a sterile field and organize the supplies.

- For the client requiring an indwelling catheter:

  - Remove the cap from the prefilled syringe.

  - Attach the syringe to the injection port and leave it attached.

- Place the sterile drapes under the client and over the perineal area with the perineum exposed.

- Designate the nondominant hand as the clean hand. If right-handed, use the left hand to hold the labia open. If left-handed, use the right hand to keep the labia open and expose the urethral meatus. Do not release the labia.

- Designate the dominant hand as the sterile hand. Use this hand to pick up antiseptic cleaning swabs or the forceps; the forceps will be used to pick up cotton balls soaked in an antiseptic solution.

- Using one cotton ball or swab per wipe, wipe from front to back (i.e., from the anterior end of the labia toward the rectum), using a new cotton ball or swab for each wipe in the following sequence: right labial fold, left the labial fold, then directly over the urinary meatus.

- Discard each cotton ball or swab in the waste receptacle immediately after use.

- Using the sterile hand, pick up the catheter, ensure that the tip is sufficiently covered in lubricant, and coil the distal end of the catheter in the hand.

- Insert the tip of the catheter into the urethral meatus; insertion should be for 2–3 inches or until urine appears. After the urine appears, insert the catheter an additional 1–2 inches. Release the labia.

- If an indwelling catheter was inserted, inflate the balloon and gently tug on the catheter; connect the tubing and secure the catheter with nonallergenic tape or a leg-securing device. Hang the collection drainage bag from the bed frame.

- If a straight catheter was inserted, allow complete drainage or drain 1,000 mL, clamp the tubing, and wait briefly before additional urine is allowed to drain. Remove the catheter after the bladder is emptied.

- Reposition the client for comfort.

- Dispose of catheterization equipment.

General information required to insert a urinary catheter for a male includes the following:

- Position the client in the supine position, with his thighs slightly apart.

- Place the sterile drapes under the client and over the perineal area with the penis exposed.

- Provide perineal care and remove gloves, washing hands before proceeding.

- Follow the facility's policy for the use of lidocaine gel injections.

- Position the penis upright with the nondominant hand, which is designated as the clean hand. (If right-handed, the left hand will be the clean hand; if left-handed, the right hand will be the clean hand.)

- If the client is uncircumcised, use the clean hand to retract the foreskin and hold it in the retracted position.

- If the client is circumcised, use the thumb and index finger of the clean hand to hold the penis below the glans.

- Maintain the position of the penis and foreskin until after the catheter is inserted.

- Wipe from the urethral meatus outward to the base of glans using a new swab or cotton ball for each wipe. Discard cotton balls or swabs, as used, in the appropriate waste receptacle, repeating the process until they are all used.

- Using the dominant hand (designated as the sterile hand) to pick up the catheter, ensure that 5–8 inches of the tip are sufficiently covered with lubricant, and coil the distal end of the catheter in the hand.

- When inserting the catheter, insert the tip of the catheter into the urethral meatus while gently rotating the catheter; insertion should be for 7–9 inches or until urine appears.

- Insert the catheter to the bifurcation ports after urine appears.

- Lower the penis, but keep the catheter secure with the clean hand.

- Replace the foreskin for the uncircumcised male.

- The remaining steps are the same as those for catheter insertion for a female, described above.

Once a catheter is in place, the urinary meatus should be cleaned with soap and water according to the health care facility's policy. When cleansing the penis, retract the foreskin if needed and hold the penis and catheter during the procedure. The urinary bag is kept below the bladder at all times to prevent the urine from back-flowing into the bladder.

To remove the indwelling catheter, empty the urine from the bag, wash hands, and apply clean gloves. Place the syringe in the balloon port on the catheter and wait as the water empties into the syringe. Then gently pull out the catheter, discard the materials, and provide perineal care.

> **NOTE**
>
> Information regarding the selection of catheters and the maintenance of the peripheral intravenous line can be found in the "Central Venous Access" and "Parenteral/Intravenous Therapies" sections of this chapter.

To insert a peripheral intravenous line, prepare the intravenous bag and flush the tubing using aseptic technique. After identifying the site, apply the tourniquet a few inches above the area locating a suitable vein.

- Prepare the site by wiping with an appropriate skin preparation or alcohol swab in a circular motion from the venipuncture site to the surrounding area. Allow the area to dry naturally before proceeding.

- Ask the client to make a fist and anchor the vein by applying manual traction on the skin a few centimeters below the proposed cannulation site to stabilize the vein.

- With the bevel of the cannula facing upward, insert the needle at a 15–30 degree angle into the vein.

- Wait for the first flashback of blood in the flashback chamber of the needle, and as soon as the blood is visible in the cannula, advance the cannula over the needle into the vein.

- Withdraw the needle slightly and the second flashback of blood will be seen along the shaft of the cannula.

- Maintaining skin traction with the nondominant hand, and using the dominant hand, slowly advance the cannula off the needle into the vein.

- Maintaining skin traction with the nondominant hand, and using the dominant hand, lower the angle of the needle catheter and gently advance the cannula off the needle into the vein.

- Release the tourniquet, apply pressure to the vein above the cannula tip, withdraw the needle from cannula, and connect the intravenous tubing to the hub of the catheter.

- Secure the hub of the cannula in place with a semi-occlusive or transparent dressing and a catheter stabilization device.

- Dispose of the needle in the appropriate container and initiate the infusion rate as prescribed.

To remove a peripheral IV catheter, wash hands, apply clean gloves, remove the transparent dressing while stabilizing the catheter, withdraw the catheter slowly, and immediately apply gauze of over the puncture site. Hold pressure until hemostasis is achieved. Assess the catheter tip to ensure it is intact and has been completely removed. Document the removal and appearance of the site.

Tube Care

The many types of invasive tubes require that the nurse monitor and maintain patency of the tube. To maintain the patency of a nasogastric tube, the nurse will flush the tubing before and after each feeding or medication administration. When assessing the patency of a chest tube, the tubing should be checked for kinks and dependent loops. The drainage system should be kept lower than the client's chest. The nurse will ensure the chest tube is securely taped to the connector and that the connector is taped to the tubing that goes into the collection chamber of the chest tube drainage system. A gentle bubbling in the water seal chamber should be present upon the client's exhalation, coughing, or repositioning. Tidaling should be present, the water level in the water seal chamber maintained at the recommended level, and the level in the suction control chamber kept at the prescribed level (unless a dry suction system is used). Following the health care agency's policy, the nurse will document the amount, color, and characteristics of the fluid in the chamber, and then empty the collection chamber or change the system as needed.

Venous Thromboembolism (VTE)

Several conditions place a client at risk for **venous thromboembolism (VTE)**, including medical history, current condition, immobility, and surgery. There are several interventions that are used to prevent VTE interventions by promoting the venous return to the heart, including drug therapy, ambulation, exercises, and the use of specific devices, including **anti-embolism stockings** and **sequential compression devices (SCDs)**.

Before placing compression stockings or SCDs on the client, the nurse will perform a baseline skin and neurovascular assessment of the extremities. When implementing the use of anti-embolism stockings, the nurse will ensure the client has the correct size and they fit correctly. Sizing of the client is done by measuring the length of the client's leg from the gluteal furrow to the base of the heel, the greatest circumference of the calf, and the upper thigh at the gluteal furrow. Assisting the client to apply the stockings will allow the nurse to evaluate how they fit. Stockings that are too loose will not provide enough compression, and stockings that are too tight will inhibit the blood flow to the client's extremities. Instruct the client to wear and remove them according to the health care facility's policy and procedure, and report any pain, numbness, or tingling. Throughout the period the client is wearing the stockings, the nurse will inspect and provide skin care, assess sensation and circulation, and monitor the client's nutritional state.

Venous blood flow can also be enhanced using SCDs, which provide intermittent periods of leg compression. SCDs are generally knee-length unless prescribed otherwise. Antiembolism stockings may also be worn under the SCDs. When choosing the correct size of SCDs, the nurse will adhere to the health care facility's policy and procedures as well as the manufacturer's recommendation. All leg measurements are obtained using a tape measure. The manufacturer's information will also include the proper placement of the SCD sleeve, which generally has a line for the ankle on the sleeve that must line up with the client's ankle and wrap around the client's leg, after which it is secured. The nurse should be able to place two fingers between the SCD sleeves and the client's leg. The tubing from the leg sleeves is then attached to a mechanical pump, at which time the nurse will follow the policy for the proper setting and remain with the client during at least one cycle of compression to ensure the equipment is working correctly. The client will be instructed to keep the SCDs in place and report any pain, numbness, or tingling. The SCDs will be removed according to policy to assess the client's skin, to provide skin care, or during ambulation.

Electroconvulsive Therapy

Electroconvulsive therapy is used in the treatment of clients with conditions such as severe depression, acute mania, and mood disorders with psychotic features. The procedure requires preoperative preparation and postoperative care.

Preoperative assessment includes an electrocardiogram, chest x-ray, urinalysis, CBC, BUN, and electrolyte panel. The client will be required to be NPO, usually for several hours before the procedure. The nurse will ensure the client's hair is clean and dry to allow for electrode contact. All hairpins, bracelets, and body piercings are removed as well as prostheses, dentures, glasses, hearing aids, and contact lenses. The client will also be encouraged to void before the procedure.

During the procedure, an electroencephalogram (EEG) monitors brain waves and an electrocardiogram (ECG) monitors cardiac responses. The client will experience deliberately induced brief seizures (30–60+ seconds) by an electrical current transmitted through electrodes attached to one or both sides of the head. Following the procedure, the nurse will monitor the physiological condition of the client as well as maintain his or her safety. The client will be positioned on the side, and any excessive secretions suctioned as necessary. The nurse will also monitor vital signs and cardiovascular status, assess for muscle soreness and headaches, and reorient the client, as he or she may experience disorientation, confusion, and amnesia.

Complications

Clients receiving specific testing, treatments, or procedures may be at risk for potential circulatory complications, which include embolus, hemorrhage, and shock. The following are the main types of shock the nurse must be able to recognize and assist in managing:

- **Anaphylactic shock:** An extreme allergic reaction that can occur when a client is exposed to a medication such as an antibiotic, contrast medium, or latex. The signs and symptoms include hypotension, constricted airway, hives, flushed skin, confusion, and a swollen tongue and lips. The nurse should prepare to provide oxygen, administer epinephrine, corticosteroids, antihistamines, beta-agonists such as albuterol, and CPR.

- **Cardiogenic shock:** Occurs when the heart muscle's ability to pump is impaired, typically due to a myocardial infarction. A client experiencing cardiogenic shock will display signs and symptoms of decreased cardiac output and mean arterial pressure, including tachycardia, dyspnea, diaphoresis, and decreased urine output. Supportive measures include oxygenation, mechanical ventilation, and oxygen supplementation. The overall client treatment is aimed at improving the function of the heart with interventions such as thrombolytics, inotropic drugs, and procedures such as angioplasty or coronary arterial bypass graft.

- **Hypovolemic shock:** Occurs as a result of a hemorrhage that is unable to be contained. The treatment of hypovolemic shock includes addressing the underlying source of the disorder (hemorrhage) and replacing lost fluids through the administration of intravenous crystalloids, transfusions of blood and blood products, the use of plasma expanders, and the administration of drugs such as dopamine or epinephrine.

> **NOTE**
>
> Hemorrhage and the symptoms leading into hypovolemic shock are covered in the "Potential for Complications of Diagnostic Tests/Treatments/Procedures" section of this chapter.

- **Neurogenic shock:** A type of distributive shock that occurs after damage to the pathways of the central nervous system—particularly the spinal cord—from spinal injury or traumatic brain injury. Vasodilation occurs as a result of a loss of balance between parasympathetic and sympathetic stimulation. The client experiences predominant parasympathetic stimulation, which results in an extended period of vasodilation, which causes a hypovolemic state. Clinical findings include bradycardia; bradypnea; hypotension; warm, dry, flushed skin; and priapism. If the injury is above the third cervical vertebra, the client will experience respiratory arrest; if below the fifth cervical vertebra, the client will demonstrate diaphragmatic breathing. Treatment focuses on supporting the client's airway, breathing, and circulation; restoring sympathetic tone; immobilization; and IV fluids. Pharmacological management incudes vasopressors and atropine.

- **Septic shock:** A type of distributive shock resulting from a system-wide bacterial, viral, or fungal infection, known as **sepsis**. Symptoms of sepsis include decreased urine output, confusion, cyanosis, dizziness, and dyspnea. Abnormal body temperature, pallor, altered level of consciousness, hyperglycemia, thrombocytopenia, increased lactic acid, edema, tachycardia, and tachypnea are also typically present. Treatment focuses on combating the underlying infection and preventing organ damage. In addition, the treatment involves obtaining blood cultures, evaluating liver function, replacing fluid with an IV, and administering oxygen or respiratory support. Administration of antibiotics and vasopressors is also included in the treatment.

- **Obstructive shock:** Caused by the impairment of the heart's ability to pump due to external conditions, such as pulmonary embolus, constrictive pericarditis, tension pneumothorax, cardiac tamponade, pulmonary hypertension, aortic stenosis, or thoracic tumors. In addition to supporting the client's pulmonary and cardiac systems and providing fluid replacement therapy, treatment is based on the underlying problem. For example, if the client is experiencing a pulmonary embolism, the nurse can anticipate the treatment to include intravenous anticoagulants and thrombolytics. A client with cardiac tamponade requires immediate pericardiocentesis with a surgical repair, and the client with a tension pneumothorax requires a needle thoracotomy and chest tube placement. The client's respiratory and cardiac systems require further support.

Treatments and procedures in which medical devices, bandages, restraints, casts, or dressings may be too tight increase the client's risk for neurological complications. Proper application of devices or bandages and monitoring will help prevent injury to a client.

> **NOTE**
>
> Preventing other complications, such as aspiration, is discussed in the "Nutrition and Oral Hydration" section of this chapter. Interventions to prevent contractures, which include foot drop, are discussed in the "Mobility/Immobility" section of this chapter.

When assessing a client at risk for neurological compilations, the nurse will compare findings bilaterally. The assessment includes the evaluation of sensory and motor function as well as peripheral circulation, which includes pain, paralysis, pulses, paresthesia, pallor, capillary refill, and skin temperature. Nursing interventions for any assessment finding that is of concern will focus on restoring circulation and preventing injury. The nurse will follow the health care facility's policy and procedures to monitor the client and manage any abnormal condition, as well as immediately notifying the health care provider of any concern.

POTENTIAL COMPLICATIONS FROM SURGICAL PROCEDURES AND HEALTH ALTERATIONS

The nurse will apply knowledge of pathophysiology when monitoring a client for the potential for post-surgical complications. Complications are not only based on the type of surgical procedure, but also on the client's age, health, comorbidities, current condition, medications, and therapies. The nurse will monitor the client for complications, such as shock, hemorrhage, wound infection, deep vein thrombosis, pulmonary complications, urinary retention, and reaction to anesthesia.

Other complications following surgery include the following:

- Atelectasis

- Pneumonia

- Pulmonary embolism

- Pulmonary edema
- Hypertension
- Hypotension
- Hypovolemic shock
- Dysrhythmias
- Sepsis
- Heart failure
- Pressure ulcers
- Wound dehiscence (splitting open of a wound or incision)
- Wound infection
- Wound evisceration
- Contact allergies
- Skin rashes
- Paralytic ileus
- Gastric ulceration and bleeding
- Hyperthermia
- Hypothermia
- Nerve damage or paralysis
- Contractures
- Urinary tract infection
- Electrolyte imbalances
- Acute kidney injury
- Thrombocytopenia

Postoperative care includes reviewing the results of the laboratory tests performed after surgery to monitor for complications. Tests may include a CBC to evaluate the hemoglobin, hematocrit, platelets, and white blood cell count.

Steps for preventing postoperative complications include the following:

- Initiating preventative measures for VTEs before surgery, such as the use of compression stockings or sequential compression devices to promote venous return
- Promoting mobility and ambulation after surgery
- Preventing aspiration through assessment of the gag reflex and client positioning
- Monitoring intake and output
- Managing pain
- Providing range of motion or muscular strengthening as prescribed

- Turning the client every two hours to prevent skin breakdown

- Ensuring the client receives adequate hydration and nutrition

- Encouraging deep breathing and coughing

- Monitoring dressings, drains, or other implanted devices

- Preventing infection

Thrombocytopenia is a condition characterized by a very low platelet count and the result of many different pathological conditions, such as hemorrhage, aplastic anemia, bone cancer, and infection. General conditions that affect the platelet count resulting in thrombocytopenia include impaired platelet distribution, increased utilization, increased destruction, and decreased production. Medications can cause a drug-induced thrombocytopenia. These medications include heparin, some antibiotics, antimycobacterial agents, vaccines, NSAIDs, antiepileptics, and cardiovascular drugs.

General physical assessment findings associated with thrombocytopenia include petechiae; bleeding from soft tissue, such as the gums; nosebleeds; ecchymosis; oozing from surgical wounds or sites with invasive lines (such as an intravenous catheter); and neurological changes. Treatment varies and is based on the underlying cause, but includes physiological support of the client, assessment of vital signs and for bleeding, replacement of fluids and platelets, monitoring intake and output, evaluation and trending of laboratory results, and protecting the client from injury.

SYSTEM-SPECIFIC ASSESSMENTS AND THERAPEUTIC PROCEDURES

There are procedures that place the client at risk for abnormal circulation distal to the extremities where the procedure was performed. Procedures such as cardiac catheterization, placement of an arterial line, or a cast on a fractured extremity can affect the circulation in the extremity. Regardless of the procedure, the client is at risk for inadequate perfusion to the extremity and requires careful monitoring of the pulses. Pulses can be assessed using palpation or with a Doppler. When assessing a pulse, both extremities are evaluated at the same time to compare the findings.

The rate, rhythm, and amplitude (also known as volume) of the pulse are assessed and recorded using a **pulse volume scale**. The scale grades the strength of a pulse; for example, a score of 0 indicates the pulse is absent. A score of 1+ describes a pulse that is weak and difficult to palpate. A score of 2+ is a normal pulse that is able to be palpated using normal pressure. A score of 4+ indicates a bounding pulse in which the pulsations may be visible to the nurse.

There are many conditions that increase the risk of neurological impairment of a client. A baseline neurological assessment is performed on all clients to detect changes in subsequent assessments. Included in the neurological evaluation is the assessment of the client's history, mental status, and cranial nerves. The Glasgow Coma Scale is used to assess a client's level of consciousness objectively. When assessing the client's motor functions, reflexes, and sensory functions, the nurse will bilaterally compare findings.

Motor function and strength is assessed through observation; bilaterally testing the grip and instructing the client to push, raise, and lower extremities against pressure; assessing deep tendon reflexes; and recording the reflex activity using a scale. The **reflex activity scale** uses a score based on the reflex responses. A score of 0 indicates there is an absence of response, 1+ a hypoactive response that is weaker than normal, 2++ is a normal finding, 3+++ is a reflex that is stronger and more brisk than normal, and a 4++++ is a hyperactive finding. Evaluation of the client's neurological status also includes assessment of sensory functioning through evaluation of the client's bilateral response to pain, changes in temperature, and cerebellar functioning. Cerebellar functioning is evaluated through the assessment of fine motor coordination and equilibrium.

Edema is a result of many conditions, such as heart, liver, or kidney dysfunction; venous obstruction; fluid and electrolyte imbalance; tissue trauma; inflammation; or malnutrition. The consequences of edema include skin breakdown, ulceration, infection, and deep vein thrombosis. When assessing a client's skin, the nurse will include evaluation for edema. Edema usually occurs in the dependent areas of the body, which are based on the client's mobility and activity. Edema is most likely to form in the lower extremities and ankles of a client who sits for long periods in a chair, whereas a client who is confined to a bed will have localized edema in the sacral area. When assessing for edema in the lower extremities, the nurse will evaluate the client for pitting edema using an **edema objective scale**.

EDEMA OBJECTIVE SCALE	
Score	**Description**
1+	A slight indentation of 2 mm; mild indentation returns to normal fairly quickly
2+	A deeper indentation of 4 mm; will last longer
3+	Obvious indentation of 6 mm; lasts for several seconds
4+	Deep indentation of 8 mm; will remain for several minutes

Type I and II diabetic clients are at risk for several complications, including hyperglycemia and hypoglycemia. Type I diabetic clients with severe hypoglycemia are at risk for diabetic ketoacidosis, and a type II diabetic is at risk for hyperglycemic hyperosmolar nonketotic syndrome (HHNS).

Symptoms of **hyperglycemia** include the following:

- Fatigue
- Nausea
- Polyuria
- Vomiting
- Headache
- Confusion
- Polydipsia
- Polyphagia
- Tachycardia
- Poor skin turgor
- Warm, moist skin
- Abdominal cramps
- Orthostatic hypotension

Symptoms of **hypoglycemia** include the following:

- Nausea
- Hunger

- Seizures

- Agitation

- Headache

- Dizziness

- Irritability

- Confusion

- Palpitations

- Tachycardia

- Unconsciousness

- Muscle weakness

- Cool, clammy skin

- Blurred or double vision

Diabetic ketoacidosis results from uncontrolled hyperglycemia, metabolic acidosis, and increased production of ketones. The hyperglycemia and ketone bodies result in metabolic acidosis and may include the following symptoms:

- Coma

- Nausea

- Polyuria

- Lethargy

- Dry skin

- Confusion

- Polydipsia

- Sunken eyes

- Abdominal pain

- Fruity breath odor

- Kussmaul respiration

Hyperglycemic hyperosmolar nonketotic syndrome (HHNS) results from uncontrolled hyperglycemia, which is often triggered by illness or infection. HHNS is characterized by the presence of insulin in a sufficient amount to prevent lipolysis and ketogenesis, but an inadequate amount to facilitate the utilization of glucose. Signs and symptoms of this syndrome include the following:

- Coma

- Fever

- Nausea

- Dry skin

- Seizures

- Lethargy

- Polyuria

- Polydipsia

- Confusion

- Sunken eyes

- Convulsions

- Muscular weakness

When monitoring a client's wound for healing, the nurse will consider factors that can result in delayed or impaired wound healing. These factors include the following:

- Age

- Pain

- Edema

- Trauma

- Anemia

- Necrosis

- Pressure

- Smoking

- Infection

- Hydration

- Body type

- Maceration

- Nutritional status

- Immunosuppression

- Vascular insufficiency

- Impaired physical mobility

- Radiation or chemotherapy

- Chronic disease, such as diabetes, cardiovascular disease, or respiratory disease

- Medications such as steroids, some anti-inflammatories, and antineoplastic medications

The nurse will monitor the client for trends and condition changes based on the assessment data obtained from the client. This data includes subjective and objective information, laboratory values, medications, and prescribed treatments. Care for the client and nursing interventions are based on the health care facility's policy and procedures and standing protocols and must remain within the scope of the nurse's practice. Communication and collaboration with the health care provider and other team members is also implemented based on the client's condition and policy and procedures.

Items included in the client's initial assessment will be evaluated in an ongoing manner and include the following:

- Risk for sensory impairment and falls

- Level mobility

- Evaluation of skin integrity

- Physiological and psychological condition

- Medications, treatments, and procedures

The health care facility's policy and procedures include the identification of the appropriate tools to use during the assessment of the client, which will assist the nurse in gathering both subjective and objective data. Examples of commonly used scales include the **Morse Fall Scale (MFS)**, which is used to identify the client's risk for falls, and the **Braden scale**, which predicts the risk for pressure sores.

A client may require a focused assessment, which is very different from admission or shift assessment. A **focused assessment** is a detailed nursing assessment of a specific body system (or multiple systems) related to the client's current condition. Focused assessments are brief exams that are commonly performed when a client's condition changes or a new complication has developed. As such, the assessments are frequently performed on clients with acute or chronic illnesses.

Therapeutic Procedures

There are different types of anesthesia that may be administered before a test, procedure, or surgery. The type of anesthesia used is based on the client's age, type of procedure, function of the client's organs, medical condition, and comorbidities. Nursing care includes monitoring the client's response and recovery from anesthesia.

General anesthesia provides sedation, reduces anxiety, induces a lack of awareness and amnesia, promotes skeletal relaxation, suppresses undesirable reflexes, and provides analgesia. A client may also receive inhaled gases after administration of an intravenous agent that can be altered by changing the inhalation concentration of the agent. A client receiving general anesthesia will undergo induction to, maintenance of, and recovery from the anesthesia. During the recovery phase, the anesthesia is withdrawn; some agents will require reversal, in which case the client is monitored for the return of consciousness. The client is also monitored for a full recovery of normal physiological function, which includes respiration, acceptable blood pressure, heart rate, reflexes, and no delayed reaction.

Both **local anesthesia** and **regional anesthesia** temporarily disrupt sensory nerve impulse transmission, reducing sensory perception for the body area in which it is administered. Regional anesthesia is used to block the sensation of multiple peripheral nerves, reducing the sensory perception. The different types of regional anesthesia include a field block, nerve block, spinal anesthesia, and epidural anesthesia. The nurse will monitor the client who has had regional anesthesia for a headache, infection, nausea, vomiting, hematoma, decreased urination, and pain at the site of the injection. A local anesthetic is delivered topically in areas, such as the skin or mucous membranes, or by local infiltration, such as into a wound. The nurse will also monitor a client who has received a local anesthetic for edema and inflammation, both of which are early signs of a complication.

Complications of both local or regional anesthesia are primarily related to client sensitivity to the anesthetic agent, incorrect delivery technique, systemic absorption, or overdose. The nurse will observe the client for CNS stimulation followed by cardiac and CNS depression, which indicates the client has had a **systemic toxic reaction** to the anesthesia.

Symptoms such as restlessness, headache, blurred vision, tinnitus, numbness, metallic taste, nausea, tremors, seizures, tachycardia, tachypnea, and hypertension are initial symptoms of toxicity and must be treated. If untreated, they will progress to hypotension, apnea, cardiac arrest, and death. Establishing an airway, administering oxygen, and providing medication are priority measures for managing toxicity. Epinephrine is used to treat sudden unexplained bradycardia.

The nurse is expected to apply knowledge of related psychomotor skills when caring for clients undergoing therapeutic procedures. The health care facility's policy and procedure, procedural training requirements, and standards of care will assist the nurse in meeting this goal.

Throughout the client's treatment, the RN will continue to provide education, which includes home care. The appropriate method for education will be chosen based on the client's health literacy, developmental age, and condition. This education is extended to guardians, parents, spouses, health care surrogates, legal guardians, or any other person the client requests. A client may also require ongoing nursing care in the home, which includes therapy provided by a physical or occupational therapist. A social worker can assist the nurse in providing the client with the resources for the necessary care in the home and community.

> **NOTE**
>
> Client education regarding treatments and procedures begins with informed consent, as discussed in Chapter 3.

When moving or positioning a client with a musculoskeletal injury, the nurse will use precautionary measures to prevent further injury and will promote healing by maintaining proper alignment of the skeleton. Logrolling is used when moving a client who has experienced trauma or a neck or spinal injury. A common use for an abduction pillow is to prevent dislocation of the hip by maintaining alignment and stabilization after replacement.

A client requires monitoring before a procedure in order to establish a physiological baseline assessment. The type of procedure may also necessitate specific types of monitoring, such as ECG or continuous pulse oximetry. The client may require specific drug therapy, laboratory work, and dietary restrictions or may need to remain NPO for a length of time. The health care provider will prescribe treatments before a procedure, and the health care facility's policy and procedures will provide further direction regarding how to carry out the procedure or treatments safely. For example, consider a client who requires monitoring before casting a fracture. The nurse will monitor the client for complications of fractures, including acute compartment syndrome, crush syndrome, hypovolemic shock, fat embolism, venous thromboembolism, and infection.

Following the procedure, the nurse will continue to monitor the client for additional complications such as edema, altered skin integrity, neurovascular impairment, compartment syndrome, and chronic complications such as ischemic necrosis and delayed union. Clients who require therapeutic devices such as chest tubes, drainage tubes, or wound drainage devices, or who require continuous bladder irrigation, require assessment for tube patency. When assessing for patency, the nurse will document measurements of output, appearance, color, odor, and any other assessment parameters associated with the device, drainage, and client condition.

Throughout the preoperative period, the nurse should focus on pre- and postoperative education, safety, and promotion of the psychological and physiological health of the client. All learning principles are based on the client's developmental age and physiological condition. The nurse should anticipate that the client or family member (if applicable) will be able to describe the purpose and expected results of the surgery, ask questions, adhere to the preoperative requirements, verbalize an understanding of the preoperative procedures (such as skin preparation), and demonstrate the correct techniques and exercises to prevent complications after surgery. Common interventions to prevent complications include incentive spirometry, ambulation, splinting the incision, or leg exercises.

The nurse will obtain a history, perform a physical assessment, evaluate laboratory data, prepare the client for any prescribed testing, ensure the informed consent has been obtained, administer any treatments or prescriptions, and remove and secure prosthetics, dentures, eyeglasses, or any other valuables according to the facility's policy and procedure and the health care provider's prescriptions. A facility-approved teaching and preoperative checklist is generally used by the nurse to ensure that all relevant areas are addressed. Any concerning findings are immediately reported to the health care provider.

A client may receive **moderate sedation**, also known as **conscious sedation**, during a procedure. Moderate sedation is administered intravenously and is a sedative, hypnotic, and opioid drug that reduces sensory perception but allows the client to maintain a patent airway. The RN monitors the client's response to the sedation during and after the procedure. Monitoring of the client's airway, level of consciousness, oxygen saturation, capnography, ECG, and vital signs is conducted at minimum per the health care facility's policy and procedure, and more frequently if needed. The client is monitored until awake and oriented and vital signs have returned to the baseline level. Generally, a client's consciousness is evaluated using a sedation scoring system, such as the **Ramsay Sedation Scale** or a scale specified by the health care facility.

CLIENT NEEDS FOR PHYSIOLOGICAL ADAPTATION

The focus of the NCLEX-RN physiological adaptation subcategory is to assess the nurse's ability to manage and provide care for clients with acute, chronic, or life-threatening physical health conditions. The nurse is also expected to be knowledgeable about assisting with invasive procedures, implementing and monitoring a client who requires phototherapy, maintaining the optimal temperature of a client, and monitoring and caring for clients with impaired ventilation or oxygenation who need ventilatory assistance or supplemental oxygen. Additionally, the nurse needs to understand how to monitor and maintain a surgical drain. Other interventions that a client may require include suctioning, wound care or dressing changes, ostomy education and care, pulmonary hygiene, and postoperative care.

The RN will be best able to assist the client toward recovery if the various dimensions of wellness are kept in mind, including physical, emotional, financial, intellectual, career, social, environmental, and spiritual wellness. These dimensions are taken into consideration when planning care for a client recovering from an alteration in body systems. The nurse can address the needs of the client through the use of communication, collaboration, and education. Integrating the client's religious, spiritual, and cultural beliefs into the treatment plan and identifying barriers, such as finances and limited resources, will also assist the client in progressing towards a positive outcome.

Many clients receive dialysis; therefore, it is necessary that the nurse is competent in performing and managing a client receiving peritoneal dialysis, hemodialysis, or continuous renal replacement therapy. The nurse will manage clients with an alteration in hemodynamics, tissue perfusion, or hemostasis, including clients who are hemodynamically unstable or who may require an arterial line, a pacing device to regulate the electrical system of the heart, and telemetry monitoring to assess the pattern of electroconductivity of the heart. Recognizing the pathophysiology related to an acute or chronic condition, providing client education, and evaluating the effectiveness of the treatment plan will help prevent further physiological deterioration of the client.

> **NOTE**
> All clients are at risk for complications. The nurse is responsible for recognizing those risks and the associated physiological changes, intervening in a timely and appropriate manner, and performing emergency care procedures.

ALTERATIONS IN BODY SYSTEMS

A client's ability to cope with alterations to his or her health, including illness and disease, is part of the ongoing nursing assessment. Identifying client attributes of coping, such as health-sustaining habits, life satisfaction, social supports, and effective and healthy response to stress, will assist the nurse in helping the client and family members adapt to the changes in the client's health.

A client's treatment goals are evaluated to determine whether the goals have been met and whether the plan of care should continue, undergo modification, or be terminated. A client's goals can be partially met or unmet due to a change in the client's condition, encountered barriers, or unrealistic goals. A client's care plan is terminated when the goals of treatment have been achieved or when a change in circumstances has occurred.

Prenatal Complications

The signs and symptoms of potential prenatal complications follow.

Anemia

A **physiological anemia** occurs during pregnancy due to the increased plasma volume, which is not pathologic. However, by the second or third trimester of pregnancy, many women lack the iron stores necessary to make hemoglobin, which results in **pathological anemia**.

Iron-deficiency anemia is the most common anemia in pregnancy; when severe enough, it is associated with low birth weight infants and preterm labor. When related to other complications, such as preeclampsia, the cardiac workload is increased to compensate for the reduction of the oxygen-carrying capacity of the blood, placing the client at risk for congestive heart failure. **Folic acid deficiency anemia** is a form of anemia that is corrected through dietary intake and folic acid supplementation. Other anemic conditions include **sickle cell hemoglobinopathy** and **thalassemia**.

Preeclampsia

Preeclampsia is hypertension with proteinuria that develops after 20 weeks gestation in a client who does not have hypertension. In the absence of proteinuria, preeclampsia may be defined as hypertension along with either thrombocytopenia, impaired liver function, new-onset renal insufficiency, pulmonary edema, or new-onset cerebral or visual disturbances. Preeclampsia can cause damage to other organs—specifically the liver and kidneys—and may result in seizures. It is associated with abruptio placentae and HELLP syndrome.

Preterm labor is characterized by regular contractions that occur on or after the 20th week and before the 37th week of gestation. Preterm labor is associated with a change in cervical effacement, dilation, or both or with a clinical presentation of regular uterine contractions and cervical dilation of at least 2 cm.

Eclampsia

Eclampsia is a condition associated with preeclampsia. Eclamptic seizures are usually preceded by signs and symptoms of a headache, blurred vision, photophobia, epigastric pain, and altered mental status. The seizures are characterized by a tonic contraction of all body muscles followed by tonic-clonic convulsions. Immediate maternal seizure-induced complications may include tongue biting, head trauma, aspiration, fractures, and placental abruption. Fetal risk factors include preterm birth or death as a result of placental abruption.

Endometritis

Endometritis is an infection of the uterus that usually begins as a localized infection at the placental site in the postpartum period. Symptoms include fever, lethargy, chills, tachycardia, uterine tenderness, and foul-smelling lochia.

Hypertension

Chronic hypertension is either present before pregnancy or is initially diagnosed during pregnancy and persists longer than 12 weeks postpartum. Clients who have chronic hypertension are at risk for superimposed preeclampsia.

Gestational Hypertension

Gestational hypertension is the onset of elevated blood pressure or other systemic findings, such as proteinuria, after 20 weeks of pregnancy and usually resolves within the first week postpartum. A client with gestational hypertension is at risk for preeclampsia.

Placenta Previa

Placenta previa is a condition in which the placenta partially or totally covers the mother's cervix—the outlet for the uterus. The placenta may be close enough to the cervix to cause painless bleeding when the lower segment of the uterus effaces or the cervix dilates. The location of the placenta places the client at risk for hemorrhage, placental abruption, or preterm delivery, while the fetus is at risk for anemia, Rh isoimmunization, IUGR, low birth weight, decreased oxygenation, and fetal death.

Oligohydramnios

Oligohydramnios occurs when the amount of amniotic fluid is lower than expected for the fetus' gestational age. It is sometimes defined as an amniotic fluid index of less than 5 cm. However, because that value is adjusted according to gestational age, it can vary. Causes of oligohydramnios include congenital anomalies, twin-to-twin transfusion, some medications, post-term pregnancy, ruptured membranes, and fetal demise. Maternal and fetal risk factors include cord compression, IUGR, preterm birth, fetal pulmonary hyperplasia, and aspiration of meconium-stained fluid.

Polyhydramnios

Polyhydramnios is a condition during pregnancy in which an excess of amniotic fluid is present. It is usually diagnosed when the amniotic fluid index is greater than 24 cm. Polyhydramnios is associated with maternal diabetes, fetal malformations, genetic conditions, multiple pregnancies, fetal anemia, and viral infections. Maternal symptoms associated with polyhydramnios include preterm labor, shortness of breath, fetal malpresentation, and edema. Complications related to the condition include premature birth, premature rupture of membranes, placental abruption, cord prolapse, stillbirth, postpartum hemorrhage, and cesarean delivery.

Isoimmunization

Rh incompatibility occurs when the client's blood is Rh-negative, the fetus is Rh-positive, and the fetal blood cells are transferred into the maternal circulation. The transfer accidentally occurs as a result of abdominal trauma, amniocentesis, or after the delivery of the placenta. This transfer of fetal blood cells into the maternal circulation results in the stimulation of maternal antibody production. If this sensitization to Rh antigens occurs during labor, there is no effect on the baby. However, if the sensitization occurs earlier in the pregnancy or the client has a subsequent pregnancy with an Rh-positive fetus, the previously formed maternal antibodies to Rh-positive blood cells can enter the fetal circulation where they will attack and destroy fetal erythrocytes. When the fetal erythrocytes are damaged, this will result in progressive fetal hemolysis, anemia, and fetal erythroblastosis.

Hemolytic disease can also occur when the maternal antigens differ from the fetus. This hemolytic condition is usually less severe than the Rh incompatibility but can cause fetal hydrops.

Chorioamnionitis

Chorioamnionitis is caused by a bacterial infection of the amniotic cavity and is characterized by maternal fever, tachycardia, uterine tenderness, and purulent amniotic fluid. This condition most commonly occurs after rupture of the membranes or during prolonged rupture of the membranes. Maternal risk factors include bacteremia and dysfunctional labor. Fetal complications include bacteremia, pneumonia, and meningitis.

HELLP Syndrome

HELLP is an acronym for hemolysis, elevated liver enzymes, and low platelets. **HELLP syndrome** is a life-threatening condition associated with preeclampsia. Vasospasms occur, resulting in the micro vessels destroying red blood cells and platelets causing hepatocellular necrosis and edema. Risk factors associated with HELLP syndrome include liver infarction, rupture or hemorrhage, acute renal failure, abruptio placentae, eclampsia, pulmonary edema, disseminated intravascular coagulation, adult respiratory distress syndrome, and death. Fetal complications include intrauterine growth restriction (IUGR), respiratory distress syndrome, preterm birth, and death.

Ectopic Pregnancy

Ectopic pregnancy occurs when the fertilized ovum is implanted outside of the uterine cavity; the condition is classified according to the site of implantation. The majority of ectopic pregnancies occur in the fallopian tube, placing the client at high risk for hemorrhage. The signs and symptoms of an ectopic pregnancy include abdominal pain, delayed menses, and abnormal vaginal bleeding. The client is at risk for hemorrhage and death as a result of a fallopian tube rupture, which is characterized by unilateral abdominal pain, referred shoulder pain, signs of shock, and Cullen's sign.

> **NOTE**
> **Cullen's sign** is a bruising and edema that appears in the fatty tissue around the umbilicus.

Abruptio Placentae

Abruptio placentae is the detachment of part or all of the placenta from the uterine wall after 20 weeks gestation. Clinical manifestations are based on the degree of placental separation. Symptoms of abruptio placentae include vaginal bleeding; uterine contractions; abdominal tenderness; and abdominal pain, which may be localized or diffuse over the uterus, with a board-like abdomen. Maternal complications are based on the degree of separation but can include hemorrhage, thrombocytopenia, and hypofibrinogenemia. Fetal complications include oligohydramnios, IUGR, preterm birth, hypoxemia, and stillbirth.

Incompetent Cervix

An **incompetent cervix** is a painless cervical dilation without contractions that can result in the delivery of the fetus *before* 20 weeks gestation (considered a miscarriage) or *after* 20 weeks gestation (a viable fetus). Signs and symptoms include pink-tinged vaginal discharge, rupture of membranes, increased pelvic pressure, and cervical dilation. Maternal and fetal complications include a preterm delivery, with a fetal outcome based on the gestational age at birth.

Multiple Gestations

A client with more than one fetus is at risk for preterm labor and birth, preeclampsia, gestational diabetes, anemia, miscarriage, twin-twin transfusion syndrome, abnormal amniotic fluid index, fetal cord entanglement (monozygotic twins), cesarean delivery, and postpartum hemorrhage. Fetal risk factors include preterm birth, congenital birth defects, complications from maternal anemia and preeclampsia (as previously discussed), low birth weight, IUGR, and fetal demise.

Diabetes

Complications from diabetes are based on glycemic control. Maternal and fetal surveillance is frequently performed throughout the pregnancy to monitor the well-being of the mother and fetus. Maternal risk factors include miscarriage, the development of preeclampsia, polyhydramnios, infection, ketoacidosis, and hypo- or hyperglycemia. Fetal risk factors include congenital malformations, respiratory distress syndrome, IUGR, large for gestational age (SGA), fetal macrosomia, hypoglycemia after birth, birth injuries, and stillbirth.

Gestational Diabetes

Gestational diabetes is diagnosed earlier in the pregnancy based on abnormal fasting blood glucose levels. Gestational diabetes can be controlled through diet, exercise, glucose monitoring, and pharmacological therapy, if necessary. Fetal surveillance is performed to monitor fetal growth and well-being. Fetal risks include fetal macrosomia, perinatal death, birth injuries, and neonatal hypoglycemia.

Hydatidiform Mole

A **molar pregnancy** is a rare condition in which the trophoblast cells that normally develop into the placenta instead grow into an abnormal mass within the uterus. A hydatidiform mole is classified as either partial (both the placenta and embryo are abnormal) or full (involves an abnormal placenta with no embryo). Signs and symptoms are based on the classification and include uterine growth that does not correlate with gestational age, dark brown or bright red vaginal bleeding, hyperemesis gravidarium, abdominal cramping, preeclampsia, and hyperthyroidism. A full hydatidiform molar pregnancy places the client at risk for choriocarcinoma.

Post-Term Pregnancy

A **post-term pregnancy** is a pregnancy that is longer than 42 0/7 weeks gestation. Maternal symptoms include fatigue, physical discomfort, maternal weight loss, frustration, depression, and anxiety. Maternal risks include labor dystocia, perineal injuries, chorioamnionitis, endometritis, postpartum hemorrhage, oligohydramnios, meconium-stained fluid, and increased risk of assisted or operative delivery. Fetal risks include abnormal fetal growth, small for gestational age, fetal macrosomia, cord compression related to oligohydramnios resulting in fetal hypoxia, meconium aspiration, shoulder dystocia, fetal injury, and stillbirth.

Spontaneous Abortion

A pregnancy that ends before 20 weeks gestation is referred to as a **miscarriage** or **spontaneous abortion**, placing the client at risk for bleeding and infection.

Substance Use and Abuse

Maternal and fetal effects from substance use and abuse are based on many factors, such as the type of substance, amount, and duration of abuse. Maternal complications related to substance abuse may include bacterial infections or neurological, cardiovascular, pulmonary, renal, liver, and gastrointestinal problems, such as hypertension, endocarditis, seizures, and cerebrovascular accident. The client is also at risk for sexually transmitted infections such as HIV, hepatitis, malnutrition, vitamin deficiencies, and psychiatric

> **NOTE**
> Physiological and psychological symptoms associated with specific substances are discussed in the "Substance Use Disorders and Dependencies" section in Chapter 5.

comorbidities. Effects specifically associated with the pregnancy include placenta previa, abruptio placentae, premature rupture of membranes, spontaneous abortion, IUGR, preterm delivery, maternal and fetal withdrawal, birth defects, long- and short-term neonatal developmental effects, and maternal and fetal death.

Hyperemesis Gravidarum

Hyperemesis gravidarum is characterized by excessive vomiting during pregnancy that causes weight loss, electrolyte imbalance, nutritional deficiencies, metabolic imbalance, renal and gastric impairment, and ketonuria. The client is at risk for fluid and electrolyte imbalance and altered nutrition. Effects on the fetus include IUGR and low birth weight.

Cardiovascular Disease

When the mother enters the pregnancy with a pre-existing cardiac issue, the maternal and fetal outcomes are based on the risk factors of **maternal cardiac disease**, including treatment, prognosis, and whether the cardiovascular disorder is acute or chronic. The addition of the cardiovascular demands associated with pregnancy to the existing cardiac disorder results in an increased level of risk. The client is monitored for signs and symptoms associated with cardiac decompensation or heart failure, such as arrhythmias, heart palpitations, generalized edema, neck vein distension, inadequate tissue perfusion, dyspnea, frequent moist cough, symptoms of thromboembolism (including pain), redness, tenderness or swelling in the extremities, chest pain, sudden weight gain, and activity intolerance. Fetal complications include preterm birth and IUGR.

Sexually Transmitted Infections

Prenatal symptoms and complications related to sexually transmitted infections are associated with the specific disease. Maternal complications range from immunosuppression, preterm labor, preterm rupture of membranes, chorioamnionitis, and endometritis. Fetal complications are based on the type of sexually transmitted infection and the outcome of the pregnancy.

Preterm Premature Rupture of Membranes

Preterm premature rupture of membranes occurs any time before 37 0/7 weeks gestation. Chorioamnionitis is the most common complication. Other complications include retained placenta, placentae abruption, hemorrhage, sepsis, and death. Fetal complications include intrauterine infection, cord prolapse, oligohydramnios, umbilical cord compression, and pulmonary hypoplasia if the rupture of membranes occurs before 20 weeks gestation.

Other Obstetrical Complications

An obstetrical client can experience unexpected complications. The laboring client with preeclampsia is at risk for experiencing many complications, including eclampsia. Nursing interventions for the client experiencing eclampsia are the same as managing a seizure with a nonpregnant client. The nurse will remain at the bedside and will protect the client from injury with the following interventions:

- Raising and padding the siderails of the bed
- Maintaining airway patency by turning the client's head to one side or placing the client in a lateral position
- Calling for assistance
- Initiating emergency medical measures as indicated by the client's status during the seizure

The client who labors and delivers in less than three hours after the onset of contractions has experienced **precipitous labor**. The client is at risk for complications such as uterine rupture; lacerations of the cervix, vagina, vulva, or perineum; amniotic fluid embolus; and postpartum hemorrhage. Fetal risk factors include head trauma and hypoxia.

Nursing interventions for the client experiencing precipitous labor include providing emotional support, encouraging the client to pant between contractions, remaining with the client, and notifying other staff for assistance. If the infant's head is crowning and delivery is imminent, the nurse will tear the amniotic sac if it is still intact, and apply gentle pressure to the fetal head (pressing toward the vagina) to prevent fetal head trauma and lacerations to the perineum and vagina. After the emergence of the baby's head, the nurse will assess the neck to see if the umbilical cord is wrapped around it. If it is, the nurse will try to gently slip the cord over the baby's head or pull it gently to get some slack so it can be slipped over the shoulders. Using a gentle downward pressure, the nurse delivers the anterior shoulder from under the symphysis pubis and applies a gentle pressure upward to deliver the posterior shoulder. The rest of the baby may deliver quickly. After delivering the baby, the nurse will use a bulb syringe (if needed) to remove mucous first from the infant's mouth and then the nose. Placing the newborn on the mother's abdomen, the nurse dries the newborn quickly to prevent heat loss and to ensure the warmth of the newborn is maintained.

An obstetrical client may have risk factors predisposing her to hemorrhage. The treatment for **postpartum hemorrhage** is based on the etiology. A vaginal delivery with greater than a 500 mL blood loss or a cesarean delivery associated with greater than a 1,000 mL blood loss is considered a postpartum hemorrhage. Other factors that can result in postpartum hemorrhage include uterine atony, retained placenta, lacerations of the genital tract, hematomas, inversion of the uterus, and subinvolution of the uterus. Treatments for a postpartum hemorrhage include a CBC, blood type and crossmatch, coagulation studies, establishment of venous access, and oxygen via a face rebreather mask.

If **uterine atony** is present, fundal massage is performed, after which the bladder is assessed for distension and emptied to attempt to resolve the issue. If uterine atony continues, uterotonic drugs are administered to attempt to resolve the atony. If a retained placenta is suspected, the health care provider will attempt to remove the retained fragments. The nurse will anticipate anesthesia to be administered to the client who requires removal of retained placenta and uterotonics.

If the client is unresponsive to any treatments to stop the bleeding, further surgical intervention is warranted. A client who has a laceration will have a firm fundus in the proper location at the expected height, but will continue to bleed actively. The health care provider will be required to locate and repair the laceration.

For any client—including the obstetrical client—who is actively hemorrhaging and is unstable with fluid resuscitation, blood replacement is required. Oxygen is administered by a non-rebreather face mask at 10–12 L/min. in conjunction with continuous pulse oximetry, keeping in mind that for a client who is experiencing significant hypovolemia, the measurements may not be accurate. The client may also require hemodynamic monitoring, which includes a central venous pressure or pulmonary artery catheter. Continuous electrocardiographic monitoring may be warranted, as is a urinary catheter with a urometer to allow for hourly urinary output assessments. Laboratory evaluation of hematocrit and hemoglobin levels, platelet counts, and coagulation studies are assessed due to the risk of disseminated intravascular coagulation. The nurse will continue to monitor the vital signs and the client's level of consciousness.

> **NOTE**
>
> It is important to understand that signs and symptoms of shock may not appear in a postpartum client until 30%–40% of her blood volume has been lost. Abnormal vital signs are a late symptom and may indicate the client is in the late stages of shock. Restoring the client's intravascular volume to promote oxygen delivery to the tissues is the primary goal of treatment.

Infectious Diseases

Treatment and care of the client with an infectious disease is specific to the client's clinical condition, source of infection, and symptoms. In addition to treatment, each type of infectious disease requires specific infection control precautions to prevent transmission. Treatments may include antipyretics, analgesics, antivirals, antibiotics, antiemetics, bed rest, and hydration. More serious treatments include respiratory support, such as oxygen or mechanical ventilation, and cardiovascular symptom management.

Clients experiencing illness from infectious diseases require education and information to make health care choices and should function as part of the health care team managing their condition. Nursing considerations before providing client education include assessment of the client's current knowledge, readiness to learn, health literacy, identifying cultural or religious beliefs that may not align with the treatment plan, and financial barriers.

Infectious diseases have specific signs, symptoms, and incubation periods. There are many infectious diseases, but the following are the most common.

Giardiasis

This protozoan is a common intestinal parasitic pathogen. The nonmotile stage of the protozoa can survive in the environment for months. Modes of transmission are person-to-person, animals, and food. Water such as lakes, streams, or swimming pools can be sources of contamination. The client may be asymptomatic or present with abdominal cramps or diarrhea.

Enterobiasis (Pinworms)

This is the most common helminthic infection in the United States. Transmission occurs where there are crowded conditions, such as daycare centers and classrooms. The eggs are either ingested or inhaled and can live in an indoor environment, contaminating anything with which they come into contact. Signs and symptoms of enterobiasis include intense rectal itching.

Gonorrhea

Gonorrhea is a bacterial disease that affects the mucous membranes of the reproductive tract, including the cervix, uterus, and fallopian tubes in women, and the urethra in men. The bacteria can also infect the mucous membranes of the mouth, throat, eyes, and rectum. Gonorrhea is spread through sexual contact and perinatally during childbirth. Men and women with gonorrhea may be asymptomatic. Signs and symptoms that may occur in men include dysuria or a white, yellow, or green urethral discharge that usually appears within 14 days after infection. The initial symptoms and signs in women include dysuria, increased vaginal discharge, or vaginal bleeding between periods. Rectal and pharyngeal infections may be asymptomatic; however, symptoms of rectal infection in both men and women may include discharge, anal itching, soreness, bleeding, or painful bowel movements. A sore throat may be associated with a pharyngeal infection.

Chlamydia

Chlamydia is a bacterial sexually transmitted infection that is predominantly asymptomatic in both women and men. Screening tests are generally relied upon for diagnosis. Acute salpingitis or pelvic inflammatory disease are the most serious complications for a female client.

Syphilis

Syphilis is an infection caused by a spirochete, which is thought to be transferred through microscopic abrasions in the subcutaneous tissue. The transmission of the spirochete can occur through sexual intercourse, kissing, biting, oral-genital sex, and transplacental transmission. Syphilis has very distinct stages and symptoms associated with each stage. Primary syphilis is characterized by a painless chancre appearing 5–90 days after infection and lasting 3–6 weeks before healing on its own. During the secondary stage, a red or brown rash may appear on the hands and feet or other parts of the body. The rash does not cause itching. Other symptoms may include fever, sore throat, muscle aches, fatigue, headaches, and hair loss. Secondary syphilis occurs six weeks to six months after the appearance of the chancre. During the latent stage of infection, the client is asymptotic, but the disease can be detected in the blood. Tertiary stage symptoms include neurologic, cardiovascular, musculoskeletal, or multiorgan system complications.

Human Papilloma Virus (HPV)

There are over 100 types of HPV virus, including two specific varieties that are highly oncogenic. HPV is transmitted through oral, vaginal, or anal sex. Lesions are typically 2–3 mm in diameter and 10–15 mm in height. They are found on the buttocks, vulva, vagina, anus, and cervix and appear as soft, papillary swellings that occur singularly or in clusters in the genital or anal area.

Trichomonas

Trichomonas is a protozoan that is almost always transmitted through intercourse. The infection may be asymptomatic, but women commonly experience a yellowish-to-greenish, frothy, mucopurulent, copious, malodorous vaginal discharge. Inflammation of the vulva and vagina may be present, as well as pruritis, dysuria, and dyspareunia.

Group B Streptococcus (GBS)

Group B streptococcus (GBS) may be considered normal vaginal flora in a nonpregnant client and is not associated with any symptoms; however, a GBS infection is associated with a poor perinatal outcome. GBS cultures are obtained during pregnancy. If GBS is present, the client is treated during labor based on the CDC guidelines, due to the risk of vertical transmission from the birth canal to the neonate. Exposure to GBS increases the risk of perinatal morbidity and mortality.

Herpes Zoster

Herpes is a viral infection caused by herpes simplex viruses type I or II. The virus is transmitted through contact with HSV in herpes lesions, mucosal surfaces, and genital and oral secretions. Most clients are asymptomatic or have very mild symptoms. The average incubation period after exposure to herpes is four days. The vesicles that form will break and leave painful ulcers that take 2–4 weeks to heal after the initial infection. The first outbreak of herpes is often associated with a longer duration of herpetic lesions; increased viral shedding; and systemic symptoms, including fever, body aches, swollen lymph nodes, or headache. Clients with recurrent outbreaks will have prodromal symptoms, such as localized pain, tingling, or shooting pains in the legs, hips, or buttocks, which occur hours to days before the eruption of herpetic lesions. These symptoms are often shorter in duration and less severe than the symptoms in the first outbreak.

Human Immunodeficiency Virus (HIV)

Human Immunodeficiency virus (HIV) is a virus that is spread by exposure to certain body fluids containing the virus that enter the body most commonly through anal or vaginal sex, sharing of needles, and—less commonly—childbirth, breastfeeding, or a needlestick with a contaminated sharp. There are other extremely rare situations in which HIV can be transmitted to another person. Seroconversion to HIV positivity usually occurs within 6–12 weeks. Although the client who has seroconverted may be asymptomatic, the seroconversion is often accompanied by a viremic, influenza-like response. Symptoms include fever, headache, night sweats, malaise, generalized lymphadenopathy, myalgias, nausea, diarrhea, weight loss, sore throat, and rash.

Hepatitis

The **hepatitis A** virus has an incubation period of approximately 28 days. Hepatitis A replicates in the liver and is shed in high concentrations in feces from 2–3 weeks before to 1 week after the onset of clinical illness. The risk for symptomatic infection is directly related to age, with more than 70% of adults having symptoms compatible with acute viral hepatitis and most children either asymptomatic or experiencing symptoms of unrecognized infection. Hepatitis A viral infections are primarily transmitted through the fecal-oral route, by either person-to-person contact or through consumption of contaminated food or water.

Hepatitis B is a viral infection with an incubation period from the time of exposure to the onset of the disease of 6 weeks to 6 months. Hepatitis B is transmitted by percutaneous or mucous membrane exposure to HBV-infected blood or body fluids, that contain HBV. The highest concentrations of HBV are found in blood, with lower concentrations found in other body fluids including wound exudates, semen, vaginal secretions, and saliva.

The **hepatitis C** virus is enveloped by a single strand of an RNA virus and is transmitted blood-to-blood, most commonly through illicit IV drug needle sharing, blood and blood products before 1992, needlestick injuries with contaminated needles, or unsanitary tattoo equipment. The average incubation period is seven weeks, and most clients are completely unaware they have the virus until tested or liver problems occur.

Tuberculosis

Tuberculosis is a highly contagious bacterial infection that is transmitted through the air. The incubation period may vary from about 2–12 weeks, and the client will remain infectious for as long as viable TB is present in the sputum. A client with active TB can transmit the droplets of bacteria—which may be inhaled by others—through coughing, laughing, sneezing, whistling, or singing. Signs and symptoms include coughing, chest pain, coughing up blood or sputum, weakness, fatigue, weight loss, chills, fever, and sweating at night.

Several types of prescriptions are used to treat TB. Treatment may include the use of isoniazid, which must be taken for at least six months, or a combination of isoniazid and rifapentine can be taken once a week for three months. There are also other antituberculotic drugs that can be used, and as with all prescribed treatment, the client's condition and age are taken into consideration when choosing the safest, most effective treatment. The success of a client's treatment is evaluated using bacteriologic evaluation of sputum, chest radiographic tests, and clinical evaluation.

Pertussis

Pertussis is a bacterial infection that is highly contagious and spread through the air by infected droplets. The incubation period of pertussis is commonly 7–10 days, with a range of 4–21 days. Pertussis is divided into the following three stages:

1. **Catarrhal stage:** This stage can last 1–2 weeks and is characterized by symptoms similar to a common cold. Signs and symptoms include a runny nose, sneezing, low-grade fever, and a mild cough.

2. **Paroxysmal stage:** Usually lasts 1–6 weeks, but can persist for up to 10 weeks. The cough is characterized by a high-pitched whoop (hence the name, "whooping cough"). Infants and young children often appear very ill and distressed and may turn blue and vomit. "Whooping" does not necessarily have to accompany the cough.

3. **Convalescent stage:** Usually lasts 2–6 weeks, but may last for months. The cough usually disappears after 2–3 weeks. Although the disease at this time is milder, the client is still able to transmit the disease to others, including unimmunized or incompletely immunized infants.

Varicella

Varicella is transmitted via contact or droplet and from contaminated objects. Signs and symptoms that may appear 1–2 days before the rash include fever, fatigue, loss of appetite, and headache. A rash will generally appear that turns into itchy, fluid-filled blisters and eventually into scabs. A client may develop chickenpox from 10–21 days after exposure and is contagious 1–2 days before the onset of the disease. The client remains contagious until all the chickenpox lesions have crusted (scabbed). The illness usually lasts 4–7 days.

Shingles

The **shingles** virus is spread by direct contact with fluid from the rash blisters. Approximately 1–5 days before the rash appears, the client will experience pain, itching, or tingling where the rash will develop. Other symptoms include fever, chills, headache, or nausea. The rash consists of blisters that typically scab over in 7–10 days. The rash usually clears up within 2–4 weeks.

Fifth disease

Fifth disease is a viral illness caused by parvovirus 19, which is found in respiratory secretions, such as saliva, sputum, and nasal mucous. The disease is spread through coughing and sneezing and can also be transmitted through blood and blood products. Symptoms appear within 4–14 days after acquiring the infection. Symptoms include fever, runny nose, headache, rash, and painful joints. A client may get an initial rash that resolves and then experience a second rash that usually resolves within 10 days, but can come and go for several weeks. The rash is itchy and appears most commonly on the face, though it may be found on the back, chest, buttocks, arms, legs, and soles of the feet. The client is most contagious during the initial symptoms (runny nose and fever) before the rash appears or the joint pain occurs.

Diphtheria

Diphtheria spreads from person to person through respiratory droplets or by contact with an object on which bacteria is present. The incubation period is 2–5 days or possibly longer; the period of communicability is usually 2 weeks, but can last up to 4 weeks. The bacteria produce a poison that causes symptoms such as weakness, sore throat, fever, and swollen glands. Also, dead tissue may form a thick, gray coating that can build up in the throat or nose. The poison may also get into the bloodstream, damaging the heart, kidneys, and nerves.

Influenza

Influenza viruses are spread through droplets from up to six feet away when persons with the flu talk, cough, or sneeze. Most clients are contagious one day before symptoms develop and 5–7 days after becoming sick. An immunocompromised client is infectious for longer than seven days. Most symptoms begin about two days after the virus enters the body. Clients may experience fever, chills, cough, sore throat, muscle or body aches, runny nose, headache, fatigue, nausea, and diarrhea.

Mumps

Mumps is a viral disease spread through direct contact with saliva or respiratory droplets from the mouth, nose, or throat. An infected client can likely spread mumps from a few days before their salivary glands begin to swell, and for up to five days afterward. Signs and symptoms of mumps include puffy cheeks; a tender, swollen jaw; fever; headache; muscle aches; and loss of appetite. Occasionally, severe symptoms may occur, such as encephalitis, meningitis, pancreatitis, oophoritis, orchitis, and mastitis. Symptoms typically appear 16–18 days after infection, but this period can range from 12–25 days after infection. Clients may experience very mild symptoms or may remain asymptomatic. The general recovery time is approximately two weeks.

Measles

Measles is a highly contagious virus that lives in the nose, throat, and mucous of an infected person and is spread through coughing and sneezing. The virus is also able to live up to two hours in the airspace. The client is contagious four days prior and four days after the rash appears. The symptoms of measles appear within 7–14 days after the client is infected and include high fever, cough, rhinitis, and conjunctivitis. Two to three days after symptoms begin, **Koplik's spots** may appear inside the mouth. In addition, 3–5 five days after the symptoms appear, a rash breaks out. The rash appears as flat red spots on the face, neck, trunk, arms, legs, and feet.

Rhinovirus

Rhinoviruses are the most common virus that can cause a cold. The virus is spread through the air and personal contact. Signs and symptoms of a rhinovirus infection typically appear after an incubation period of 12–72 hours and last 7–11 days, but may persist for longer. The initial symptom is nasal dryness or irritation, a sore throat, nasal discharge, congestion, and sneezing. Symptoms typically intensify over 2–3 days and include headaches, facial and ear pressure, coughing, hoarseness, and fever.

Chronic Illness

Clients with chronic illness require continuous treatment over an indefinite time to prevent their disease from becoming life-threatening. Chronic illness can be complex, as the condition is ongoing and there may be multiple illnesses the client must manage. A multidisciplinary team approach is useful for a client with chronic conditions, such as diabetes, heart failure, or kidney disease. A registered dietician can provide detailed dietary information to support the client, and a social worker can assist the client in securing food or other necessary resources to prevent complications.

Education for the client with a chronic illness includes safety and health promotion as well as management of psychosocial concerns. Safety considerations may consist of the environment, treatments, signs and symptoms to report, and follow-up laboratory testing. Health promotion and maintenance includes prescribed activity, medications, diet, and specific interventions to prevent complications. Psychosocial concerns may be addressed by including community support groups for the client or family members. Education for a client with a chronic illness is ongoing and will primarily focus on information that promotes independent functioning. Education also promotes psychological and psychosocial health, decreases the risk of complications, and allows the client to perform self-care independently or with minimal assistance.

Invasive Procedures

Nursing responsibility includes assisting with invasive procedures, such as the placement of a central line, thoracentesis, or a bronchoscopy. The health care facility's policy and procedures are reviewed and adhered to, providing guidance and maintaining the safety of the client. The nurse will provide client education, ensure the client has provided informed consent, assess the client for allergies, and ensure the correct treatments have been performed before a procedure. Treatments such as laboratory sampling, prescriptions, or IV placement are standard. The nurse also ensures that any necessary testing results, such as ECG readings or laboratory data, are reviewed, and that the client has been compliant with any restrictions, such as dietary or fluid intake. The nurse will obtain a baseline assessment and review the data for all clients before a procedure and will use that information to monitor for change after the procedure.

The nurse will ensure the supplies for the procedure are available and the client is positioned correctly. Before the procedure, a client verification process—which includes a time out—will be carried out according to the health care facility's policy and procedure. The nurse may be responsible for setting up a sterile field, and if a sterile field is required the nurse will ensure that sterile technique is maintained prior to and throughout the procedure. The client will be monitored throughout and after the procedure and is provided support and reassurance. All documentation is completed in a timely manner according to the health care facility's policy and procedures.

Phototherapy

Phototherapy may be used to treat other conditions but is primarily used to treat hyperbilirubinemia during the neonatal period. Phototherapy can be delivered through a lamp, blanket, or pad. The severity of the newborn's hyperbilirubinemia determines the type of device used to delivery phototherapy, the strength of light, duration of treatment, and the physical location in which the therapy is delivered. The overall effectiveness of phototherapy is related to the distance between the light, the neonate, and the surface area of skin that is exposed.

Implementation for safe, effective phototherapy includes the following considerations:

- Covering the newborn's eyes with an opaque eye shield to prevent retinal damage when using phototherapy lights

- Removing the eye covers every 4–6 hours for the assessment of discharge, infection, or injury. The eye covers are not to be removed when the newborn is under the lights. The assessment can be incorporated into feedings or general care.

- Dressing neonates in a diaper only and repositioning every 2–3 hours for maximum skin exposure

- Monitoring the neonate's vital signs and temperature according to the health care facility's policy and procedure

- Monitoring the neonate's weight every 24 hours

- Ensuring that a covering is placed between the infant's skin and the fiberoptic blanket (if used) to prevent burns

- Monitoring vital signs and temperature per the health care facility's policy and procedures

- Monitoring for signs of dehydration, hyperthermia, and hypothermia

- Promoting adequate feeding to prevent dehydration and promote bilirubin excretion. Monitoring hydration status through urinary output. Bilirubin is primarily excreted through stools; cleanse the area as soon as possible, providing meticulous skin care.

- Monitoring the infant's serum bilirubin levels as prescribed

Radiation Therapy

Radiation therapy is a commonly used treatment for clients with cancer. The overall goal of the treatment is to kill cancer cells using the least amount of radiation possible. The duration of radiation therapy is based on the size and location of the tumor, type of cancer, reason for treatment, the client's health, and other treatments the client is receiving. Radiation therapy may be delivered internally or externally, both of which require careful assessment of the client for adverse effects. Adverse effects are related to the part of a client's body that is treated and may be localized or systemic.

A client may experience acute adverse effects to radiation therapy, including the following:

- Alopecia

- Cerebral edema

- Nausea and vomiting

- Oral mucositis

- Altered taste

- Oral candidiasis
- Esophagitis
- Pharyngitis
- Anorexia
- Diarrhea
- Cystitis
- Vaginitis
- Fatigue
- Blurred vision
- Edema
- Dyspnea
- Infertility
- Sexual dysfunction
- Dental caries
- Acute xerostomia
- Skin reactions
- Conjunctival edema and tearing

Late adverse effects include the following:

- Radiation-induced fibrosis
- Brain necrosis
- Leukoencephalopathy
- Cognitive and emotional dysfunction
- Pituitary and hypothalamic dysfunction
- Xerostomia and dental caries
- Hypothyroidism
- Pulmonary fibrosis
- Osteoradionecrosis
- Pericarditis
- Cardiomyopathy
- Coronary artery disease
- Lymphedema
- Small and large bowel injury

Clients receiving radiation therapy require many interventions to address the adverse effects and side effects. Many clients experience treatment-related fatigue. The interventions to address the fatigue are primarily based on the underlying factors, but generally include balancing rest with activity, optimizing nutrition, implementing naps, conserving energy, hydration, exercise, and cognitive behavioral therapy.

Radiation therapy may also cause skin irritation. Approved products that hydrate the area of the skin can be recommended, but should be avoided two hours before radiation treatment; otherwise, they could exacerbate the irrigation area. The client should be instructed to avoid trauma or friction to the irritated site; wash the area with only lukewarm water using a mild soap; and avoid tight clothing, scratching, and very hot or cold temperatures over the treatment area. The client will also be instructed to avoid exposure to the sun for a prescribed amount of time—generally one year after treatment—to further protect the integrity of the skin.

Hair loss from radiation therapy is dependent on the area of the body being treated. A client's scalp may be tender after the initial hair loss. The client is instructed to protect the area from trauma and exposure to the sun.

A client undergoing radiation treatment may also experience problems with eating and digesting food. The overall goal is to maintain the client's nutrition and avoid weight loss. Recommending small frequent meals and eating a variety of foods is helpful. For clients with a loss of appetite or pain during chewing or swallowing, dietary powdered or liquid supplements will be introduced into the diet. Many clients may experience a change in the sense of taste. Trying different foods and adding tolerable spices or acceptable sweeteners may be helpful.

Mucositis generally occurs throughout the entire gastrointestinal tract, especially in the mouth. Mucositis in the mouth is referred to as **stomatitis**. The client is instructed to avoid mouthwashes with alcohol or glycerin. Spicy, salty, coarse foods, such as raw vegetables, nuts, or crackers can result in further irritation of the mucosa and should be avoided, as should smoking, chewing tobacco, alcohol, and hot liquids. If the client wears dentures, the nurse will instruct the client to wear them only during meals and to soak them in an antimicrobial solution when not wearing them. After soaking, the dentures should be thoroughly rinsed before insertion. Additional measures may include antimicrobial drugs, topical analgesics such as a mouthwash with lidocaine, and other medications. A client may experience **xerostomia** (dry mouth). The goal when treating a dry mouth is to relieve the discomfort and prevent complications. Recommended interventions include increasing fluid intake, mouth moisturizers, water-based lip moisturizer, sugar-free hard candy, frozen desserts, ice chips, and sugar-free gum.

A client receiving radiation therapy is at risk for oral infection and dental caries. Instruct the client to examine the mouth for sores, blisters, drainage, or fissures and to contact the health care provider if present. These areas will be cultured to identify a potential infection. An approved mouth rinse recipe may be recommended, such as one comprised of warm water, baking soda, and salt. The prevention of dental caries includes thorough care of the mouth. The client is instructed to avoid sugary snacks and to brush his or her teeth and tongue with a soft-bristled toothbrush or sponge in the morning, before bed, and after every meal. The client should also practice gentle flossing each day, if not at risk for bleeding. All full dental examinations and any necessary dental work should be completed before radiation therapy begins.

The client is at risk for bleeding due to the destruction of red blood cells and will be provided education on how to assess the skin and mouth daily for bruising, swelling, or petechiae.

Clients at risk for **thrombocytopenia** are instructed to protect themselves from injury by observing the following safety steps:

- Avoid activities in which the body may may be bumped, scratched, or scraped.

- Use electric razors.

- Use soft-bristled toothbrushes, as described above.

- Avoid aspirin or aspirin-containing products.

- Avoid trauma with intercourse.

- Use stool softeners.

- Avoid any trauma to the rectum, such as suppositories or an enema.

- Blow the nose gently.

- Avoid clothing and shoes that are too tight or that will rub against the skin.

Radiation therapy causes **neutropenia**, resulting in client immunosuppression. The client is at risk for infection and should be instructed to observe the following practices:

- Avoid crowds or others who may be ill.

- Practice thorough handwashing.

- Avoid drinking any fluids that have been standing out longer than one hour.

- Avoid reusing cups or glasses without washing them.

- Abstain from sharing any personal articles.

- Take his or her temperature daily if not feeling well.

- Clean the toothbrush thoroughly at least once a week, either in the dishwasher or with bleach, thoroughly rinsing afterward with hot water.

- Follow guidelines regarding eating fresh fruits, vegetables, meats, or eggs.

- Shower daily using an approved moisturizer to prevent further drying of the skin.

- Protect the skin from direct contact with pet bodily waste.

- Maintain clean household surfaces.

Body Temperature

The core body temperature remains relatively constant within the range of 97.6–99.6°F (36.5–37.5°C). Many factors can affect a client's temperature, including age, exercise, environment, circadian rhythms, stress, hormonal fluctuations, and smoking.

Extremes in a client's temperature can result in illness and death. **Hypothermia** is a core body temperature below 95°F (35°C) and is divided into the following three categories:

1. **Mild hypothermia:** 90–95°F (32–35°C), impaired cognition, dysarthria, shivering, decreased muscle coordination, and diuresis

2. **Moderate hypothermia:** 82.4–90°F (28–32°C), muscle weakness, increased loss of coordination, incoherence, decreased clotting, and acute confusion

3. **Severe hypothermia:** below 82.4°F (28°C), bradycardia, severe hypotension, decreased reflexes, dysrhythmias, decreased response to pain, acid-base imbalance, and bradypnea

Treatment for mild hypothermia includes the removal of all wet articles followed by external active or passive rewarming, such as with heaters, warm packs, or blankets. Treatment for moderate to severe hypothermia includes protecting the client from further heat loss by maintaining the airway, breathing, and circulation;

handling the client gently to prevent ventricular fibrillation; and implementing external and internal core measures to rewarm the client. Heated oxygen; warm IV fluids; heated peritoneal, gastric, or bladder lavage; and extracorporeal rewarming can be implemented for severe hypothermia.

Hyperthermia is defined as a body temperature higher than 104.0°F (40°C). The key to treatment is addressing the underlying cause, and the cooling measures implemented are based on the client's response to the hyperthermia. Signs and symptoms the nurse can anticipate include fever; hypotension; tachycardia; tachypnea; hot, flushed skin; malaise; weakness; and seizures. Treatment for hyperthermia may include cooling blankets, ice packs, fluid resuscitation, electrolyte replacement, adjustment of the environmental temperature, antipyretics, oxygen therapy, prescriptions to decrease shivering, cooling mattress, and peritoneal and gastric lavage.

Ventilation

The nurse will monitor, evaluate, and document the response of a client who requires ventilator assistance according to the health care facility's policy and procedure, health care provider's prescription, and the client's condition. The nurse will assess vital signs; auscultate bilateral breath sounds to ensure the endotracheal tube is in the correct place; assess the position of the tube; monitor capnography, pulse oximetry, and arterial blood gases to evaluate the effectiveness of the ventilator settings; and ensure that adequate gas exchange and effective ventilation is occurring.

Included in the assessment is the client's ability to synchronously breathe with mechanical ventilation. The client may require suctioning; this will be determined after interpreting the assessment data, which includes observing for secretions.

When assessing for ventilation, the area around the site of the endotracheal tube or tracheostomy is assessed for color, skin irritation, drainage, and tenderness. The ventilator settings are verified against the prescribed orders, and the level of water in the humidifier as well as the temperature in the system are assessed for safety. Condensation in the ventilator tubing is drained into the appropriate receptacle and emptied. All tubing is secured and free of any kinks. The nurse should be familiar with the types and causes of alarms and ensure that all alarms are activated and functioning. High-pressured alarms are activated when peak inspiratory pressure reaches the set alarm limit above the client's baseline. Secretions, water, kinks in the tubing, and a displaced airway or pneumothorax can increase peak inspiratory pressure. A low-pressure alarm is generally associated with a disconnection or leak in the ventilator circuit or a leak in the client's endotracheal or tracheal tube cuff.

Prevention of infection, as in the case of ventilator-assisted pneumonia, includes keeping the head of the bed elevated at 30 degrees, performing oral care and using an antimicrobial rinse as prescribed, preventing aspiration, and performing pulmonary hygiene. Other interventions include prescribed ulcer prophylaxis; maintaining nutrition, fluid, and electrolyte balance; maintaining muscle and joint strength; and interventions to prevent venous thrombus embolism.

A client who cannot communicate through speaking while on a ventilator will experience anxiety and will require an alternative method of communication.

Wound Care

A client may require a tube to facilitate drainage from a wound or incision or suctioning to remove secretions. The nurse is responsible for the assessment and documentation of the characteristics and amount of drainage and secretions from tubes, wounds, or suctioning. Included in the evaluation are the amount, color, consistency, and odor of the secretions, if applicable.

Clients with wounds are at risk for infection. There are additional factors besides impaired skin integrity that increase the chance for infection. Impaired circulation, respiratory disorders, anemia, poor nutrition, metabolic disorders, concurrent infections, stress, medications, and aging may increase the client's risk for wound infection. When monitoring a client's wound for infection, the nurse will include in the assessment an evaluation of laboratory data and assessment for signs and symptoms associated with infection. Laboratory data can consist of a CBC to evaluate the white blood cell count, wound cultures, and a comprehensive metabolic panel to help detect underlying conditions that may impair wound healing. Signs and symptoms associated with wound infection include fever, malaise, green or cloudy purulent fluid, inflammation, loss of function, delayed wound-healing, increased size or change of shape of the wound, increased or unrelieved pain, redness, swelling, and odor.

Before performing wound irrigation or a dressing change, the client will be assessed for pain and provided a prescription as needed. Some wound care and dressing changes may be painful and may also require interventions for the pain to decrease discomfort during the procedure. Irrigation of a wound may be required as part of wound care. Wounds are irrigated to remove debris, exudate, and bacterial colonization. A warm solution may be used to facilitate healing, or medications such as antibiotics may be administered into the wound using irrigation solutions.

When irrigating a wound, the appropriate solution, irrigation system, PPE, sterile kit, sterile gloves, and other resources, such as towels and basins, are obtained. The nurse will position the client, and—using clean gloves—remove the old dressing. The dressing is removed by holding the skin taut and pulling the tape toward the dressing, disposing of it into a biohazard bag. The nurse examines the area to ensure all of the adhesive from the tape has been removed. The nurse then assesses the perimeter of the wound, the color, tissue type, amount and characteristic of any drainage, odor, and any other signs or symptoms of infection. The nurse also measures the wound.

Before irrigating the wound, a basin and waterproof pad are placed below the wound to collect the fluid and protect the linens. A sterile field is established with normal saline or other ordered sterile solution, which is poured into a sterile container on a clean work field. The other items, such as gauze, are placed on the sterile field. After putting on sterile gloves, the nurse will fill the syringe with the solution and—holding the syringe one inch above the wound—irrigate the wound from the least contaminated to the most contaminated area until the solution is clear or the amount of prescribed solution has been used. The area around the wound will be dried with sterile gauze and the wound redressed according to the health care provider's prescription.

The health care provider may prescribe types of dressing changes ranging from wet or damp to dry dressing changes that may or may not include wound irrigation. When performing a dry dressing change, a sterile field is required as described above. If the wound does not require irrigation, the wound will be cleansed from the center toward the edges of the wound using full or half-circle motions at least one inch beyond the borders of the dressing. For each circle around the wound, a new applicator or gauze pad will be used. The size of the wound will determine which sterile item is used for cleansing. A cotton-tipped applicator may be used for a smaller wound, whereas gauze pads would be used for more extensive wounds.

After cleansing the wound, the area will be patted dry using sterile gauze, and the appropriate size gauze pad will be placed over the wound and secured with a dressing.

If the wound care is damp or wet-to-dry dressing, the same steps for preparation as discussed above will be performed. During this procedure, the gauze will be unraveled or counted and then placed in the ordered solution or normal saline. The excess fluid is squeezed out before packing the gauze gently and loosely into the wound using either sterile forceps or a sterile cotton-tipped applicator if the wound is tunneled. The gauze should not be hanging over the edges of the wound and, if necessary, cut the excess roll of gauze with sterile scissors. The primary dressing is applied over the area, followed by a secondary dressing to protect the wound. The sides of the dressing are secured with tape.

Drainage

A client may require a device or equipment to drain bodily fluids. Assessment of the drainage includes the amount, color, consistency, and odor. A client with a wound may have an open or closed drainage system; some drainage systems are sutured in place and require suture care. Closed drainage systems include the Jackson-Pratt and Hemovac systems, whereas T-tubes and Penrose drains are open systems.

The skin and surrounding site around the drain are assessed for signs and symptoms of infection, including erythema, warmth, pain, drainage, or damage. Drains that are associated with the stomach, small intestine, pancreas, and gall bladder contain drainage that can cause chemical damage to the skin surrounding the drain.

A client with a traumatic wound, a wound at high risk for infection, wounds that have dehisced, chronic wounds, or wounds that require reconstructive surgery may require negative pressure wound therapy. **Negative pressure wound therapy** is a vacuum-assisted wound closure that consists of a foam wound dressing system. The device continuously or intermittently applies negative pressure to promote health and closure of the wound. The wound is assessed as described above, in addition to confirming the unit is set to deliver the appropriate negative pressure. The foam around the wound site should be collapsed, the pressure seal intact, the tubing free of kinks, the alarm audible, batteries adequately charged, and the drainage chamber filling correctly and not overflowing. The nurse will instruct the client to avoid getting the device wet. If the device gets turned off, a moist dressing will be applied over the site and the health care provider will be notified.

When assessing a chest tube drainage system, the nurse will mark the quantity, time, and initials on the drainage system and note the type, color, and consistency of drainage. The dressing around the site is assessed for drainage and reinforced if needed.

Peritoneal Dialysis

A client requires **peritoneal dialysis** to remove excess fluids, maintain electrolyte balance, correct an acid-base imbalance, and allow the exchange of waste. There are several types of peritoneal dialyses that include continuous ambulatory, continuous cyclic, intermittent, and automated peritoneal dialysis. The type of peritoneal dialysis chosen is based on the client's condition, ability, and lifestyle. A client who is a candidate for peritoneal dialysis requires careful monitoring of weight, measurement and recording of abdominal circumference, and assessment of pertinent laboratory values, which include BUN, serum electrolytes, creatinine, pH, and CBC.

Before the procedure, the client will empty the bladder and baseline vital signs will be obtained. A prescribed amount of dialysate is warmed to the client's body temperature and infused by gravity through a primed catheter, which is connected to a catheter that has been surgically placed into the peritoneal space through the abdomen. The nurse will ensure the tubing is securely connected and free of kinks. The administration of fluid is referred to as **fill time**. The infused dialysate may require additives such as heparin, antibiotics, or potassium.

Once the dialysate is infused, the tubing is clamped and the fluid will remain for a prescribed amount of time in the peritoneum—this is referred to as **dwell time**. Throughout the infusion and dwell time the client will be assessed for symptoms of respiratory distress. If the client experiences symptoms such as dyspnea or tachypnea during the infusion, the client is positioned in a Fowler's or semi-Fowler's position and the rate of the infusion is decreased. When the prescribed dwell time is completed, the drainage tubing clamp is opened and the dialysate is drained out by gravity into a sterile container. The nurse will note the clarity, color, odor, and amount of fluid returned and obtain the client's vital signs, including the client's temperature. The client's BUN, creatinine, and serum electrolyte levels reflect the overall effectiveness of the peritoneal dialysis. **Peritonitis** is a major complication of peritoneal dialysis, so it is imperative that sterile technique is used when hooking up and handling the catheter and when changing the dressing around the site.

Tracheostomies

A client with a tracheostomy requires **tracheostomy suctioning** to maintain adequate ventilation and perfusion. Prior to suctioning an adult using an open system, the nurse will gather the necessary supplies, check that the bag mouth valve device has 100% oxygen flow, and don the appropriate PPE, such as a mask or shield, gown, and clean gloves. Placing the client in a semi-Fowler's or Fowler's position, the nurse will assess the respiratory system, put a pulse oximeter on the client, and set the pressure of the suction device to continuous 80–100 mmHg (60–80 mmHg for pediatric clients). The nurse prepares the items from the suctioning kit on a sterile field. With sterile gloves, the nurse grasps the sterile suction catheter that is on the sterile field and, with the clean hand, connects the tubing to the catheter. To test the function of the suction catheter the nurse uses the thumb to occlude the suction control port and carefully dips the sterile catheter into the sterile water, avoiding the edges of the container. The solution should collect in the suction canister, after which the nurse will release the thumb from the suction control port. If a tracheostomy oxygen mask was needed, the nurse uses the clean hand to remove the mask. If the bag valve mask is not contraindicated, the nurse uses the clean hand to provide 3–5 slow deep breaths with the device, timing the breaths based on the client's rate of inhalation.

To suction, the nurse ensures the suction port is opened and, with the client inhaling, inserts the catheter approximately 12–13 cm swiftly and gently into the tracheostomy. If resistance is met, the nurse pulls back the catheter 1 cm and begins withdrawing the catheter slowly while rotating it, providing intermittent suctioning by moving the thumb on and off the suction control port. The period of suctioning should not exceed 10 seconds. The client is hyperventilated, and, if suctioning more than once, the tracheostomy oxygen mask is replaced and the client is allowed to recover between suctioning attempts. During the procedure, the nurse will monitor the client's oxygen levels and heart rate to make sure the client is tolerating the procedure well.

When performing **oral or oropharyngeal suctioning**, the nurse follows the preparation information discussed above and tests the suction as describe in tracheostomy suctioning. For this procedure, the pressure suction device will be set to 120 mmHg. The suctioning is tested by connecting the catheter to the tubing and dipping the tip of the catheter in the center of the normal saline solution, avoiding the edges of the container and using the thumb to occlude the suction-control port on the catheter, ensuring the solution collects in the suction canister. With the client in a Fowler's or semi-Fowler's position, the nurse will hyperextend the neck if tolerated, remove the oxygen mask (if present; a nasal cannula may remain on the client), place the catheter in the client's mouth without applying suction, slide the catheter down the inner surface of the client's cheek toward the back of the throat, and then apply continuous suction. The nurse encourages the client to deep breath, cough, and expectorate. If using a Yankauer tube for suctioning, only the oral area is suctioned. The nurse replaces the oxygen mask on the client and repeats the procedure as tolerated. The client's respiratory and cardiac status will be assessed during the procedure.

For a client who requires **nasotracheal or nasopharyngeal suctioning**, the nurse sets up the sterile kit as described above, places the client in a Fowler's of semi-Fowler's position, and hyperextends the head, if tolerated. Using sterile technique, the nurse applies a water-soluble lubricant to the first 15 cm of the suction tip of the catheter and removes the nasal cannula or oxygen mask (if present) with the clean hand. The nurse instructs the client to inhale and inserts the catheter into a naris, slanting it downward and inserting it to the appropriate depth (15–20 cm for nasotracheal, 15–18 cm for nasopharyngeal). If resistance is met, the nurse pulls back the catheter 1 cm and begins withdrawing the catheter slowly while rotating it and providing intermittent suctioning by moving the thumb on and off the suction control port. The period of suctioning should not exceed 10 seconds. If suctioning more than once, the tracheostomy mask is replaced and the client is allowed to recover between suctioning attempts. During the procedure, the nurse will monitor the client's respiratory and cardiac status and heart rate to make sure the client is tolerating the procedure well.

Ostomies

Types of ostomies include a **urostomy** (e.g., neobladder, Indiana pouch, and intestinal diversion), an **ileostomy**, or a **continent bowel diversion** or a **colostomy**. The care and changing of the appliance is based on the type of ostomy and appliance. The ostomy may be a one- or two-piece system. The manufacturer's recommendation and the health care facility's policy and procedures are consulted before changing the appliance.

General instructions for the nurse include gathering all supplies and emptying the old pouch. Applying clean gloves, gently push the skin away from the pouch and—keeping the skin taut—the nurse will dispose of it according to the health care facility's policy and procedure. If the client is using an open-end pouch, emptying typically is performed over a graduated container, bedpan, or toilet. The nurse cleans the end of the pouch and reclamps it or replaces it if needed. The nurse removes and disposes of the gloves, performs hand hygiene, applies clean gloves, and gently cleans the skin around the area. The nurse should avoid soaps or baby wipes as these products can leave a residue that may interfere with the seal.

After cleansing the area, the nurse pats the skin dry and places a gauze over the stoma. The nurse then inspects the stoma and peristomal area for abnormalities and irritation. If a skin protectant has been ordered, the nurse applies it to a two-inch area around the stoma and allows it to dry. The nurse prepares the new pouch by cutting an opening for the stoma in the wafer, following the instructions on the ostomy measurement guide. (If a measurement guide is not available, the nurse centers the template over the wafer and cuts the hole 1/16–1/8 of an inch larger than the stoma.) If a one-piece system is used, the nurse removes the backing or applies the stoma adhesive, allowing it to dry. The nurse removes the gauze from the stoma, centers the opening of the appliance over the stoma, and secures the appliance in place (a two-piece system requires the placement of the wafer securely to the skin). The nurse then snaps on the pouch and assesses the seal.

Client education related to ostomies includes instructing the client to self-administer and maintain the ostomy site and includes gathering the correct supplies, explaining how to remove the old pouch, skin care around the area of the stoma, application of the ostomy pouch, frequency of pouch changes, when to drain the pouch, and overall lifestyle changes. Education also includes information regarding nutrition and fluid intake and addresses concerns about sexuality, odor, leakage, and activities such as swimming. The client will be instructed to notify the health care provider if he or she experiences vomiting, abdominal pain, fever, little or no waste flowing into the pouch, or an inability to pass gas or if the stoma appears pale, swollen, and begins to bleed.

A client with a tracheostomy requires monitoring for patency by keeping the tube free from secretions, preventing tissue damage, and providing wound care. When caring for a client with a tracheostomy, suctioning may be performed as described earlier. The equipment is assembled, and, after handwashing, the old dressings are removed. A sterile field is set up, and the inner cannula is removed and cleaned according to the health care facility's policy. If the cannula is disposable, it will be replaced with a new one. The stoma site and tracheostomy plate are cleaned according to policy and procedure. The tracheostomy ties will be replaced if soiled, securing new ties before replacing the old ones. If a knot is required, a square knot is tied and placed so it is visible at the side of the neck. Only one finger should be able to be slipped between the tie tape and the neck. The client is instructed on how to care for the tracheostomy tube, assess the skin site, and report any irregular heart rate, pain or discomfort, difficulty breathing that cannot be relieved by clearing secretions, or instances of mucous becoming thick and crusted.

Seizures

Seizure precautions are implemented according to the health care facility's policy and procedure. Precautions include having an Ambu bag, oxygen, and suctioning immediately available, and providing padded siderails for the client's bed. Clients at risk for a seizure who do not have an IV access may have a saline lock placed. Nursing management of a client who has experienced a seizure is based on the type of seizure the client has experienced. However, for all of the types of seizures, nursing interventions will include the following:

- Remaining with the client
- Calling for help
- Noting the time that the seizure started and the characteristics of the seizure
- Protecting the client from the surrounding area
- Lowering the bed to the lowest position
- Protecting the client's head by placing something soft under it
- Removing the client's glasses, if present
- Avoiding physical restrictions, but attempting to turn the client's head to the side to prevent aspiration
- Loosening tight clothing
- Initiating emergency medical measures as indicated by the client's status during the seizure

Following the seizure, nursing interventions include the following:

- Maintaining the client's airway
- Placing the client in a side-lying position
- Monitoring the client's vital signs and neurological status
- Observing the client for further seizures
- Providing emotional support
- Reorienting the client
- Cleaning the client if incontinence occurred
- Notifying the health care provider

Incentive Spirometry

Incentive spirometry is used to promote lung expansion and prevent respiratory problems such as atelectasis and pneumonia. There are many types of incentive spirometers, so it is essential to follow the manufacturer's recommendation and the health care facility's policy and procedure.

Chest physiotherapy includes the use of multiple positions to drain the lungs, vibration, percussion, deep breathing, and coughing. **Postural drainage** uses gravity to mobilize respiratory secretions and **percussion** helps drain the mucus into the larger airways, whereas **vibration** is used to shake the secretions into the larger airways. Deep breathing is encouraged to help move the loosened mucus and may result in coughing. Coughing helps clear secretions that have accumulated in the trachea. The nurse will monitor the client during and after treatment, receiving postural drainage for hypoxemia, increased intracranial pressure, hypotension, bronchospasms, pain, cardiac dysrhythmias, and musculoskeletal injury. A client's condition may be contraindicated with certain positions used for postural drainage or treatments. The therapeutic evaluation includes improved conditions evidenced by the amount of sputum production, vital signs, chest x-ray, arterial blood gas values, oxygen saturation, ventilation settings, breath sounds, and subjective response to therapy.

Removal of Sutures or Staples

The removal of staples requires sterile technique. After handwashing and preparation of a sterile field, the dressing (if present) is removed and the wound inspected to determine that it has healed sufficiently to remove the staples. If the wound appears sufficiently healed and no complications—such as infection—are noted, the incision site is cleaned according to the health care facility's policy and procedure, after which the area is allowed to dry.

The lower tip of the staple extractor is placed beneath the second staple and the handle depressed. When activating the staple extractor, it is important to avoid pulling upward. When both ends of the staple are visible, the nurse moves the staple on the staple extractor away from the skin and places it on the sterile piece of gauze by releasing the staple handles on the extractor. The nurse then proceeds to remove every second staple to the end of the incision line and, using sterile technique, places the steri-strips over the site of every removed staple. The nurse removes the remaining staples as described above, followed by the application of a steri-strip over each stapled area. A sterile dressing is applied over the incision site (or exposed to air if irritated by clothing) according to the health care provider's prescription. The staples are counted and disposed of in the sharps container. The procedure is documented, including the number of staples removed.

The process for removing sutures requires a sterile field as described above, followed by lifting and clipping each knot with sterile scissors. When the sutures are removed, the area is cleansed and steri-strips are applied over the incision.

Acquired Immune Deficiency Syndrome (AIDS)

A client with acquired immune deficiency syndrome (AIDS) may remain asymptomatic after the initial infection or may experience flu-like symptoms. More severe symptoms occur a few months after exposure to the infection when seroconversion occurs. Symptoms include diarrhea, fever, enlarged liver or spleen, headache, muscle pain, nausea and vomiting, sore throat, thrush, or neurological symptoms. The symptoms can be mistaken for viral infection and usually disappear over a short period. The client may remain asymptomatic for many years and begin to experience severe symptoms months or many years later.

As the client's immune system weakens, other complications affect a variety of systems, including the immune, integumentary, respiratory, gastrointestinal, and central nervous systems. Opportunistic infections occur as a result of the client's immunosuppression, including protozoal, fungal, bacterial, and viral infections. The client is also at risk for malignancies, including lymphoma and Kaposi sarcoma, as well as lung cancer, gastrointestinal cancer, and other cancers. The client is at risk for HIV-associated dementia characterized by cognitive, motor, and behavioral impairment. The disease—or side effects of the medications—can result in neuropathies and myopathies. Altered metabolism from the infection or cancer can result in AIDS wasting syndrome, causing the client to appear emaciated. The client is also at risk for kidney and endocrine problems, as well as skin changes.

Evaluation of the client's treatment is based on the response to **highly active antiretroviral therapy (HAART)**. HAART is a lifelong prescriptive therapy used to prevent the virus from replicating, thereby reducing the viral load and the complications and morbidity associated with HIV. The therapy also works to restore and preserve immunological function and prevent HIV transmission. The classification of drugs used in HAART therapy target a different step in the viral life cycle of the virus as it infects a CD4 T lymphocyte or other target cells.

FLUID AND ELECTROLYTE IMBALANCES

An imbalance of fluids and electrolytes can become life-threatening if not corrected. Fluid and electrolyte imbalances can occur due to illness, chronic disease, hormonal imbalance, prescriptions, or environmental exposure. When caring for all clients with a fluid and electrotype imbalance, the nurse will perform the following interventions:

- Adhere to the health care facility's policy and procedure.

- Refer to the facility's laboratory parameters.

- Maintain the safety of the client through the prevention of seizures and falls.

- Assess the physiological systems affected.

- Monitor and trend laboratory findings.

- Assess vital signs.

- Assess intake and output.

- Maintain the safety of the equipment used to monitor the client.

All interventions and treatments will be evaluated for effectiveness as evidenced by restoration of the fluid and electrolyte imbalance and absence of physiological and phycological pathology associated with the imbalance.

Dehydration

Dehydration is a fluid imbalance that can be the result of the loss of water or the loss of water and electrolytes, referred to as **isotonic dehydration**. Diagnosis of the type of dehydration is dependent upon the client's history, symptoms, and laboratory evaluation.

Causative factors associated with a fluid imbalance or water deficit include the following:

- Burns

- Fever

- Diuretics

- Diarrhea

- Vomiting

- Diaphoresis

- Hemorrhage

- Decreased oral fluid intake

- Third space shifting of fluid

Treatment is based on the condition of the client and includes oral and IV replacement of fluid. Nursing care for a client experiencing a fluid deficit includes fall precautions as well as monitoring of intake and output, changes in condition, and laboratory data. Many of the following symptoms associated with dehydration, if not corrected, can lead to hypovolemic shock, organ failure, and death:

- Thirst

- Anuria

- Oliguria

- Headache

- Weight loss

- Tachycardia

- Hypotension

- Constipation

- Dysrhythmias

- Poor skin turgor

- Muscle weakness

- Concentrated urine

- Slow capillary refill

- Postural hypotension

- Altered mental status

- Abnormal electrolytes

- Sunken appearing eyes

- Weak and thready pulses

- Dry oral mucous membranes

- Elevated BUN and creatinine

- Elevated urine specific gravity

- Low hemoglobin and hematocrit

Fluid Overload

Fluid overload results from excessive fluid in the extracellular fluid space and can be caused by many different factors, such as excessive fluid intake, inadequate excretion of fluids, and physiological disease processes.

Causative factors associated with a fluid overload include the following:

- SIADH

- Cirrhosis

- Renal disease

- Heart failure

- Respiratory disorders

- Neurological disorders

- Excessive sodium intake

- Excessive IV fluid intake

- Elevated aldosterone or steroid levels

Symptoms are based on the severity of fluid overload. Treatment of the symptoms may include the administration of diuretics; restriction of sodium; dialysis, if needed; daily weights; monitoring intake and output; and treatment for electrolyte imbalances including hyponatremia, hypophosphatemia, hyperglycemia, and hypomagnesemia; as well as treatment for complications for overcorrection. Nursing care for a client experiencing a fluid overload is based on the client's clinical condition and will include monitoring intake and output, change in condition, and laboratory data.

Nursing assessment associated with fluid overload includes the following:

- Coma
- Rales
- Edema
- Ascites
- Lethargy
- Oliguria
- Dyspnea
- Crackles
- Seizures
- Azotemia
- Irritability
- Headache
- Confusion
- Orthopnea
- Tachypnea
- Paresthesia
- Tachycardia
- Weight gain
- Pale cool skin
- Increased CVP
- Bounding pulses
- Visual disturbances
- Electrolyte changes
- Distended neck veins
- Increased GI motility
- Pulmonary congestion
- Elevated blood pressure
- Engorged varicose veins

- Decreased pulse pressure
- Skeletal muscle weakness
- Altered level of consciousness
- Decreased urine specific gravity
- Pitting edema in dependent areas
- Decreased hemoglobin and hematocrit

Electrolytes

Electrolytes are minerals that dissolve in the body's water and carry either a positive or negative electric charge. Most electrolytes have different concentrations within the intracellular and extracellular fluid to maintain membrane excitability and allow for the transmission of nerve impulses. Electrolytes function to balance the amount of water in the body, manage acid-base balance, move nutrients into the cells and waste out of the cells, transmit nerve impulses, and generate energy.

Potassium

The normal potassium level is 3.5–5.0 mEq/L. Potassium is required for normal cell function because of its role in maintaining intracellular fluid volume and transmembrane electrochemical gradients. Potassium has a strong relationship with sodium, which is the main regulator of extracellular fluid volume, including plasma volume.

Factors that place a client at risk for **hypokalemia** (low level of potassium in the blood serum) include the following:

- TPN
- Cirrhosis
- Diuretics
- Diarrhea
- Vomiting
- Alkalosis
- Alcoholism
- Heart failure
- Kidney disease
- Insulin therapy
- Hyperalimentation
- Water intoxication
- Anorexia nervosa
- Cushing's disease
- Fasting or starvation
- Hyperaldosteronism

- Excessive diaphoresis
- Prolonged NG suction
- Magnesium deficiency
- Wound drainage (especially GI)
- Inappropriate use of digitalis, corticosteroids, or diuretics

Signs and symptoms associated with hypokalemia are based on the severity of the deficit and may include the following:

- Coma
- Nausea
- Anxiety
- Lethargy
- Polyuria
- Tiredness
- Vomiting
- Confusion
- Tachypnea
- Constipation
- Tachycardia
- Dysrhythmia
- ECG changes
- Disorientation
- Paralytic ileus
- Flaccid paralysis
- Abdominal distention
- Weak, thready pulses
- Skeletal muscle weakness

Treatment is based on the severity of the deficit and may include the following:

- Oral potassium replacement
- IV potassium replacement for serious deficits
- Dietary intake of potassium-rich foods
- Potassium
- Diuretics

- Monitoring
  - Continuous ECG monitoring
  - Monitoring of apical pulse
  - Monitoring of IV site for infiltration
  - Monitoring of respiratory rate and breathing effectiveness
  - Monitoring of ability to cough
  - Oxygen saturation
  - Serum potassium level
  - Intake and output
  - Prevention from falls and injury

Hyperkalemia (elevated level of potassium in the blood serum) may be caused by the following:

- Burns
- Acidosis
- Hemolysis
- Renal disease
- Crush injuries
- Chemotherapy
- Salt substitutes
- ACE inhibitors
- Adrenal insufficiency
- A bolus of IV potassium
- Oral potassium chloride
- Potassium-sparing diuretics
- Uncontrolled diabetes mellitus
- Transfusions of whole blood or packed RBCs
- Over-ingestion of potassium-containing foods
- Rapid infusion of potassium-containing IV solutions

Signs and symptoms associated with hyperkalemia are based on the severity of the elevation. Neuromuscular changes associated with hyperkalemia include early signs of skeletal muscle twitching, burning, and tingling sensations, followed by paresthesia in the hands and around the mouth. As the hyperkalemia worsens, muscle weakness occurs, moving from the hands and feet to the arms and legs, followed by flaccid paralysis. When the potassium levels are lethal, the client's respiratory muscles will be affected.

Other signs and symptoms of hyperkalemia include the following:

- Diarrhea
- Irritability
- Bradycardia
- Hypotension
- Dysrhythmia
- ECG changes
- Abdominal cramping
- Cardiac arrest with rapid IV infusion of potassium

Treatment of hyperkalemia includes restricting oral and IV potassium intake. Drug therapy can be used to enhance potassium excretion or promote the movement of potassium from the extracellular fluid into the cell through the use of IV fluids containing glucose and insulin. IV calcium gluconate, Kayexalate, and dialysis are used to treat severe cases. Cardiovascular changes are the most common cause of death in clients with hyperkalemia. The client requires ECG monitoring as well as respiratory monitoring of the client's breathing rate and effectiveness, ability to cough, oxygen saturation, serum potassium level, and intake and output. Because of the progressive muscle weakness, the client is at risk for falls and injury.

Sodium

The serum sodium levels influence the water balance, and usually remain within the normal range of 135–145 mEq/L. The hormones aldosterone, antidiuretic hormone (ADH), and natriuretic peptide influence the kidneys' regulation of the serum sodium balance by either excreting or retaining fluid.

Factors placing a client at risk for **hypernatremia** include the following:

- Fever
- Diarrhea
- Vomiting
- Dehydration
- Renal failure
- Corticosteroid use
- Cushing's disease
- Diabetes insipidus
- Excessive sweating
- High sodium intake
- Hyperaldosteronism
- Increased water loss
- Excessive amounts of hypertonic IV solution
- Overcorrection of acidosis with sodium bicarbonate

The signs and symptoms of hypernatremia are based on the severity of the imbalance. Skeletal muscle changes in a mild case of hypernatremia are characterized by muscle twitching and irregular contractions, whereas in a worsening case, the muscles and nerves are less able to respond to stimuli and the muscles become progressively weaker, characterized by reduced or absent deep tendon reflexes and the risk for respiratory ineffectiveness. A client experiencing hypervolemia will have an increased pulse rate, whereas a client with hypernatremia will exhibit slow to normal, but bounding pulses.

Other symptoms include the following:

- Thirst
- Fever
- Nausea
- Polyuria
- Seizures
- Anorexia
- Agitation
- Vomiting
- Confusion
- Tachycardia
- Restlessness
- Dry flushed skin
- Sticky tongue or mucous membranes

Treatment for hypernatremia includes drug and nutritional therapies, or—if the levels are life-threatening—the client may require hemodialysis. IV infusion may be needed to restore fluid volume if the imbalance is due to fluid loss. The infusions should be prescribed at a slow rate to prevent cerebral edema, brain damage, and death. Diuretics may be prescribed to promote sodium excretion. The client will be carefully monitored for overhydration, seizure precautions, neurological changes, and oral hygiene care. Other interventions may include dietary restriction of sodium; ensuring the client has an adequate fluid intake; monitoring of intake and output, vital signs, and weight; and prevention of injury from falls.

Factors that place the client at risk for **hyponatremia** include the following:

- Burns
- SIADH
- Diarrhea
- Anorexia
- Cirrhosis
- Vomiting
- Heart failure
- Renal disease

- Hyperglycemia

- Hyperlipidemia

- Adrenal insufficiency

- Excessive diaphoresis

- Diuretics (high ceiling)

- Psychogenic polydipsia

- Wound drainage (especially GI)

The signs and symptoms of hyponatremia are based on the severity of the imbalance. Signs and symptoms include the following:

- Coma

- Death

- Fatigue

- Nausea

- Dry skin

- Seizures

- Vomiting

- Headache

- Tachycardia

- Hypotension

- Disorientation

- Abdominal cramps

- Behavioral changes

- Weak, thready pulses

- Dry mucous membranes

- Muscle cramps and weakness

- Decreased deep tendon reflexes

Treatment is based on the type of sodium deficit and the underlying cause. A client may require dosage adjustments for existing prescriptions that cause or increase hyponatremia or the implementation of prescriptions to treat conditions associated with the imbalance. IV saline infusions may be used to restore both water and sodium volume. If hyponatremia has occurred as a result of fluid excess, drug therapy may be used to promote excretion of water; if due to Addison's disease, a hormone replacement is required. Nutritional therapy may be used for the treatment of mild hyponatremia. When fluid overload has caused hyponatremia or when kidney fluid excretion is impaired, the client may require fluid restriction. Nursing interventions include seizure precautions as well as the monitoring of intake and output, weight, and lab values, which include electrolytes and glucose. The client will be assessed for signs of excessive fluid loss, hypokalemia, and hyperkalemia.

Calcium

Calcium is necessary for bone mineralization, neuromuscular processes, activating enzymes, skeletal and cardiac muscle contraction, nerve impulse transmission, and blood clotting. The normal range for calcium is 9.0–10.5 mg/dL.

Causative factors associated with **hypercalcemia** include the following:

- Cancer
- Immobility
- Dehydration
- Osteoporosis
- Renal failure
- Steroid therapy
- Thiazide diuretics
- Hyperparathyroidism
- Prolonged immobilization
- Excessive intake of calcium or vitamin D

The signs and symptoms of hypercalcemia are based on the severity of the imbalance. The client with hypercalcemia will be monitored closely for cardiovascular changes, such as dysrhythmias. Prolonged hypercalcemia is associated with depressed electrical conduction. Mild hypercalcemia is associated with increased heart rate and blood pressure.

Signs and symptoms associated with hypercalcemia include the following:

- Coma
- Nausea
- Polyuria
- Anorexia
- Vomiting
- Constipation
- Mood swings
- Kidney stones
- Increased thirst
- Abdominal pain
- Impaired memory
- Pathological fractures
- Dry mucous membranes

Treatment of hypercalcemia is based on the severity of the disorder and includes cardiac monitoring, IV normal saline to restore fluid and increase calcium excretion, and drug therapy to lower calcium levels. Calcium reabsorption inhibitors such as calcitonin, bisphosphonates, prostaglandin synthesis inhibitors (ASA, NSAIDS), loop diuretics, or glucocorticoids may be administered. The client may require hemodialysis or parathyroid removal. Thiazide or vitamin D supplements are discontinued. Ongoing assessment includes the client's circulatory status and monitoring for blood clots; intake and output; ECG rhythms; gastrointestinal, renal, and neuro status; and limiting calcium-rich foods. Client education should include avoiding smoking and alcohol. Weight-bearing and strength exercises should be encouraged according to the health care provider's prescription.

Causative factors associated with **hypocalcemia** include the following:

- Diarrhea
- Immobility
- Alcoholism
- Pancreatitis
- Steatorrhea
- Renal disease
- Lactose intolerance
- Hyperphosphatemia
- Hypoparathyroidism
- Vitamin D deficiency
- Inadequate dietary intake
- Calcium chelators or binders
- Wound drainage (especially GI)
- Removal or destruction of parathyroid glands
- Malabsorption disorders, such as celiac sprue or Crohn's disease

The signs and symptoms of hypocalcemia are based on the severity of the imbalance and may include the following:

- Tetany
- Seizures
- Irritability
- Bone pain
- Osteoporosis
- Osteomalacia
- Rickets (children)
- Pathological fractures
- Tingling and numbness

- Respiratory distress, bronchospasm

- Cardiac dysrhythmias, ECG changes

Treatment of hypocalcemia is based on the degree of deficiency. Drug therapy includes oral replacement or replacement by IV; use of drugs that enhance absorption or raise the serum calcium levels; vitamin D (enhances absorption); and aluminum hydroxide, which may increase serum levels.

If IV calcium is prescribed, the nurse monitors the IV site carefully and maintains seizure precautions, which include decreasing environmental stimuli and ensuring oxygen and suction are immediately available. The nurse monitors dysrhythmias; assesses vital signs; observes the range of joint motion; and assesses for depressions over the bony areas, which could indicate a bone fracture. The client is assessed for continued hypocalcemia by testing for the Trousseau sign or the Chvostek sign. Client education is provided as needed regarding increasing calcium dietary intake.

Magnesium

Magnesium plays an essential role in skeletal contraction, vitamin activation, blood coagulation, carbohydrate metabolism, and protein synthesis. It also affects the absorption of sodium, phosphorus, calcium, and potassium. The normal serum level is 1.5–2.5 mEq/L.

Causative factors associated with **hypermagnesemia** include the following:

- Renal disease

- IV magnesium replacement

- Overtreatment of hypomagnesemia

- Overuse of a magnesium-based laxative

- Antacids such as Milk of Magnesia, Epsom salt, or Riopan

The signs and symptoms of hypermagnesemia are based on the severity of the imbalance and may include the following:

- Coma

- Diarrhea

- Flushing

- Lethargy

- Vomiting

- Bradycardia

- Diaphoresis

- Hypotension

- ECG changes

- Hallucinations

- Slurred speech

- Muscle weakness

- Respiratory depression

- Cardiac and respiratory arrest
- Decreased deep tendon reflexes

Treatment is focused on decreasing the serum level of magnesium and correcting the underlying cause. High-ceiling loop diuretics or IV fluid free of magnesium can be used to reduce the magnesium levels. In emergency situations, calcium gluconate can be administered to reverse the effects of the magnesium, and hemodialysis may be implemented as well. The client will be educated about the excessive use of laxatives and antacids. The client requires frequent monitoring of vital signs, intake and output, ECG data, and neurological status, as well as assessment of deep tendon reflexes.

Causative factors associated with **hypomagnesemia** include the following:

- Polyuria
- Diarrhea
- Vomiting
- Steatorrhea
- Alcoholism
- NG drainage
- Malnutrition
- Hypokalemia
- Hyperaldosteronism
- Malabsorption syndrome
- Citrate used in blood transfusion
- GI disorders (Crohn's disease, celiac disease)

Signs and symptoms of hypomagnesemia include the following:

- Nausea
- Fatigue
- Cramps
- Tremors
- Seizures
- Anorexia
- Vomiting
- Confusion
- Constipation
- Memory loss
- Hyperactive reflexes

- Ventricular fibrillation

- Painful muscle contractions

- Premature ventricular contractions

Treatment for hypomagnesemia is based on the severity of the deficit. Hypomagnesemia often occurs with hypocalcemia, so the interventions will also include restoring the imbalance of calcium. The primary focus is on correcting the underlying cause and restoring the imbalance with the IV magnesium sulfate, oral supplements, and dietary intake. Any medications that have high amounts or phosphorus will lower the magnesium level and should be discontinued. The client who is receiving IV magnesium sulfate is monitored closely for signs of hypermagnesemia as described above. In the presence of severe hypomagnesemia, the client is at risk for seizures and paralytic ileus. The client may be positive for the Chvostek sign and Trousseau sign if the hypomagnesemia occurs with hypocalcemia. Seizure precautions must be implemented, as well as close monitoring of intake and output, as the renal system excretes magnesium.

Phosphorus

The majority of phosphorus in the human body is found in the bones, where it assists with cell growth and metabolism, formation of energy supplies, activation of vitamins and enzymes, and the homeostasis of calcium and acid-base balance. The normal serum phosphorus range is 2.5–4.5 mEq/L.

Physiological systems tolerate hyperphosphatemia. Any physiological problems caused by hyperphosphatemia are a result of hypocalcemia. Phosphorus has an inverse relationship with calcium; when the phosphorus level is increased, the calcium level is decreased. Tetany can occur if hypocalcemia is present, and for clients experiencing chronic kidney disease, soft tissue calcifications can occur, as well as major vessels lined with calcification. Managing hyperphosphatemia requires the management of hypocalcemia, as previously discussed. Phosphate restriction and binders, as well as dialysis, may be necessary.

Factors that can result in **hyperphosphatemia** include the following:

- Crush injuries

- Renal insufficiency

- Systemic infections

- Diabetic ketoacidosis

- Tumor lysis syndrome

Causative factors associated with **hypophosphatemia** include the following:

- TPN

- Burns

- Alkalosis

- Diuretics

- Anorexia

- Alcoholism

- Malignancy

- Renal failure
- Hypokalemia
- Malabsorption
- Hypercalcemia
- Hyperglycemia
- Cushing's disease
- Hypomagnesemia
- Refeeding syndrome
- Hyperparathyroidism
- Uncontrolled diabetes mellitus
- Phosphate binding aluminum antacids
- Use of aluminum hydroxide and magnesium-based antacids

The effect of hypophosphatemia is most evident in the musculoskeletal, cardiac, hematological, and central nervous system changes. The muscle weakness that can accompany severe hypophosphatemia includes **rhabdomyolysis**. Chronic hypophosphatemia leads to decreased bone density, placing the client at risk for fractures.

The signs and symptoms of hypophosphatemia are based on the severity of the imbalance and may include the following:

- Coma
- Death
- Seizures
- Osteomalacia
- Rhabdomyolysis
- Muscle weakness
- Respiratory failure
- Hemolytic anemia
- Impaired leucocyte and platelet function

Treatment is based on the severity of the deficit. The focus of treatment is correcting the underlying cause of the deficiency. Oral phosphate with vitamin D and IV phosphate may be administered. Nutritional therapy is implemented, and drugs and foods associated with the loss of phosphate should be avoided. Client care includes implementing fall safety precautions and monitoring the respiratory, neurological, and cardiovascular systems, as well as muscle strength and hematological reports. Serum electrolyte levels are monitored, especially phosphate and calcium, as these electrolytes have an inverse relationship.

Chloride

Chloride is essential for the formation of hydrochloric acid in the stomach. The normal serum range of chloride is 98–106 mEq/L. Imbalance of chloride is usually associated with other electrolyte imbalances. However, a client who has excessive vomiting or prolonged gastric suctioning is at risk for **hypochloremia**. The imbalance is corrected by addressing the underlying cause.

HEMODYNAMICS

Cardiac output is based on the heart rate times the stroke volume. Many factors can affect the client's cardiac output, including cardiovascular disease, decreased oxygenation, impaired cardiac contractility, increased afterload or decreased preload, prescriptions, and any alteration in the heart rhythm, rate, or conduction system.

Findings associated with decreased cardiac output include the following:

- Pallor
- Edema
- Fatigue
- Dyspnea
- Syncope
- Chest pain
- Orthopnea
- Tachypnea
- Palpitations
- Diaphoresis
- Weight gain
- Hypotension
- ECG changes
- Cool extremities
- Oliguria or anuria
- Decreased peripheral pulses
- Decreased oxygen saturation
- Altered level of consciousness

Identifying **cardiac rhythm strip abnormalities** begins with an understanding that one completed cardiac cycle on the tracing includes the P wave; T wave; and Q, R, and S waves, which comprise the QRS complex. The **P wave** reflects atrial depolarization (cardiac contraction), the **QRS Complex** reflects ventricular depolarization and atrial repolarization, and the **T wave** is the resting phase of the cardiac cycle, which occurs during ventricular repolarization.

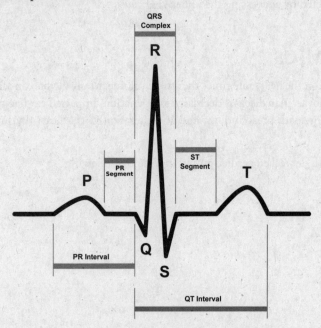

The recording speed is typically set at 25 mm/sec; the time is measured on the horizontal access. The ECG is printed on graph paper with each small block measuring 1 mm × 1 mm, representing 0.04 seconds. One large 5 mm × 5 mm block, which is defined by dark bold lines, represents 0.20 seconds. Five large blocks represent 1 second, and 30 large blocks represent 6 seconds.

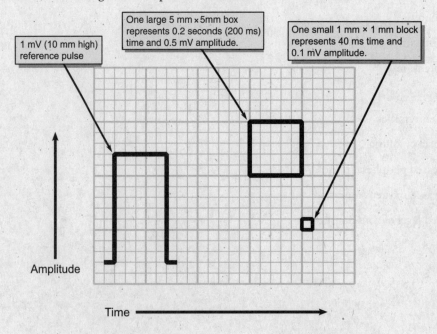

All strips are read from right to left, and it is critical to remember to always assess the client first. Using a five-step approach, the nurse must assess the following:

- Heart rate

- Heart rhythm

- P wave

- PR interval

- QRS complex

To assess the **atrial rate**, the P waves are counted; to determine the **ventricular rate**, the number of QRS complexes are counted. Using the 6-second method, the number of QRS complexes occurring within a 6-second interval are counted and multiplied by 10 to determine the **heart rate**. A rate determination chart can also be used, which is a more accurate method.

The **heart rhythm** is determined by assessing the interval between the R waves and classified as either regular or irregular. If the intervals vary by less than 0.06 seconds, the rhythm is considered regular. The P wave is the first deviation from the isoelectric line, and it should be round and upright. It is important to determine if the P waves are present, regular, accompany every QRS complex, smooth, or look similar. The **PR interval** is measured from the onset of the atrial contraction to the onset of the ventricular contraction. A normal interval is 0.12–0.20 seconds. It is important to determine if the PR interval is greater than 0.20 or less than 0.12 seconds, and if the intervals are consistent across the strip.

The **QRS complex** represents depolarization of the ventricles. The Q wave should have a downward negative deflection. The R wave in the complex should move upward and positive; it should be the tallest waveform. The S wave has a sharp negative downward deflection following the R wave. The normal interval is 0.06–0.12 seconds. The U wave—which is not usually visible, but will typically follow the T wave—may appear much smaller, rounded, and upright as a positive deflection. The origin is not fully understood, but it may indicate the client is hypokalemic.

Sinus Bradycardia

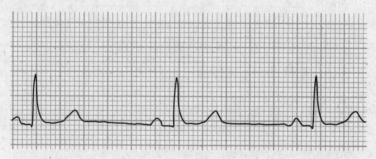

Sinusbradylead2.JPG: James Heilman, MDderivative work: Mysid (using Perl and Inkscape)
[CC BY-SA 3.0 (https://creativecommons.org/licenses/by-sa/3.0)]

Sinus bradycardia is defined as a heart rate that is 60 beats or less. Causes of sinus bradycardia include hypoglycemia, hypothermia, previous cardiac history, hypothyroidism, medications, toxic exposure, and inferior wall myocardial infarction. Not all clients are symptomatic; however, if the client is symptomatic, he or she may experience syncope, confusion, hypotension, dizziness, weakness, diaphoresis, shortness of breath, exercise intolerance, and chest pain. The client may require atropine, IV fluids, and oxygen. If treatment is unsuccessful, the client will need a pacemaker.

Premature Ventricular Contractions

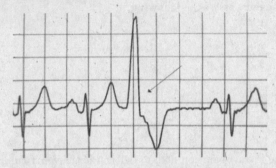

James Heilman, MD [CC BY-SA 3.0 (https://creativecommons.org/licenses/by-sa/3.0)]

A **premature ventricular contraction (PVC)** is an ectopic beat arising from an irritable site in the ventricles and is not considered a rhythm. The contractions appear in different patterns and have different shapes. When a contraction occurs with every other beat, it is referred to as **ventricular bigeminy**; if it occurs with every third beat, it is **ventricular trigeminy**, and with every fourth beat, it is called a **ventricular quadrigeminy**. When two PVCs appear next to each other, they are referred to as **couplets**. Three or more PVCs in a row are considered **runs of ventricular tachycardia**.

Causes of PVCs include exercise, stress, caffeine, electrolyte imbalances (hypokalemia and hypomagnesemia), hypoxia, tricyclic antidepressants, COPD, anemia, nicotine, digitalis toxicity, and heart disease, including myocardial infarction, congestive heart failure, and mitral valve prolapse.

Signs and symptoms associated with PVCs include palpitations, dizziness, weakness, and hypotension. Treatment is focused on identifying the cause, providing oxygen, and managing drug administration (including lidocaine or procainamide).

Ventricular Tachycardia

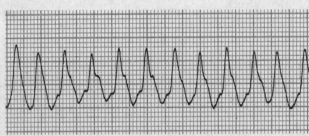

Ventricular tachycardia occurs when abnormal electric ventricular signals result in a rate of 100 beats or more per minute, either intermittently or sustained. The beats originate from the ventricles.

Causative factors for ventricular tachycardia include the following:

- Myocardial ischemia or infarction
- Rheumatic heart disease
- Heart failure
- Cardiomyopathy
- Valvular heart disease
- Some electrolyte imbalances
- Medication toxicity with digitalis

- Procainamide

- Epinephrine

- Quinidine

- Steroids

- Hypotension

- Acid-base imbalance

- Hypoxia

A client with three or more PVCs in a row is at risk for ventricular tachycardia. Clinical manifestations are based on the rate.

Symptoms associated with ventricular tachycardia include the following:

- Lightheadedness

- Dizziness

- Palpitations

- Loss of consciousness

- Chest pain

- Dyspnea

- Cardiac arrest

Treatment for ventricular tachycardia includes the following:

- Cardioversion

- CPR

- Oxygen

- Medications, including amiodarone, lidocaine, and magnesium sulfate

In addition, an internal pacemaker or radiofrequency catheter ablation may be necessary. The client will require ongoing monitoring of the rhythm, airway, breathing, circulation, and level of consciousness.

Atrial Fibrillation

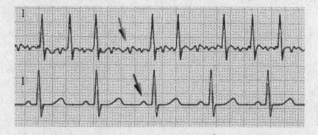

J. Heuser [CC BY-SA 3.0 (http://creativecommons.org/licenses/by-sa/3.0/)]

Atrial fibrillation is characterized by multiple disorganized impulses from the atria at a rate of 350–600 BPM. The rhythm is chaotic, the P waves are unclear, the atria are unable to contract, and the ventricles have a rapid and irregular response. The ventricular filling is reduced, affecting cardiac output and impairing the perfusion of the heart. During atrial fibrillation, the blood cannot be pumped out of the heart, placing the client at risk for thrombus formation, which may result in pulmonary emboli, stroke, or deep vein thrombus.

Risk factors for atrial fibrillation include the following:

- Heart disease
- Diabetes
- Smoking
- Hypertension
- Obesity
- Older age
- Congestive heart failure
- Thyroid disease
- Lung disease
- Sleep apnea
- Systemic infection
- Excessive alcohol
- Use of stimulants

Symptoms include nausea, dizziness, a fluttering sensation in the chest, and weakness. Treatment is based on the severity of the problem and the client's response. Drug therapy includes calcium channel blockers, such as diltiazem, or, if difficulty ensues, amiodarone. Beta blockers may be used to slow the ventricular response and include metoprolol and esmolol. Other treatments include anticoagulation therapy, cardiac glycosides, cardioversion (ensure oxygen is off during the procedure), ablation, and a pacemaker. Following cardioversion, airway patency is maintained, oxygen is administered, level of consciousness is monitored, drug therapy is administered as prescribed, skin integrity of the chest is assessed, and emotional support is provided. Cardiac enzymes and labs associated with anticoagulation therapy will be monitored, and the client will be provided education on symptoms of a stroke.

Ventricular Fibrillation

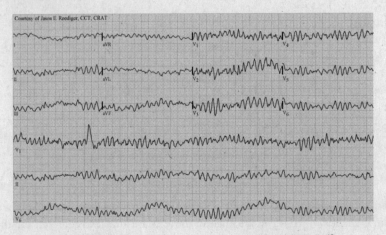

Jer5150 [CC BY-SA 3.0 (https://creativecommons.org/licenses/by-sa/3.0)]

Ventricular fibrillation appears as a chaotic rhythm with a wavy baseline. The contraction of the ventricles is disorganized and ineffective. Both the P waves and the QRS complex are absent.

Causes of ventricular fibrillation include the following:

- Myocardial ischemia or infarction
- Cardiomyopathy
- Heart failure
- Coronary artery disease
- Drug toxicity (including digitalis, procainamide, epinephrine, quinidine)
- Drug overdose
- Untreated ventricular tachycardia
- Electrolyte imbalances
- Hemorrhage
- Shock
- Hypothermia
- Trauma

Signs and symptoms include absent pulse and loss of consciousness. The client requires immediate defibrillation and CPR.

Clients with decreased cardiac output have a minimal amount of oxygen reserve to meet physiological demands. Nursing interventions are focused on reducing the client's cardiac workload. The client may require assistance with activities of daily living (ADL) and is encouraged to rest frequently between activities. Active and passive ranges of motion can be implemented to maintain strength and mobility and prevent complications. A dietary consult is essential, as the client requires dietary and fluid intervention based on the diagnosis. Eating several small meals throughout the day and avoiding any straining will decrease the cardiac workload and improve cardiac output. Other interventions include monitoring weight daily, providing prescription information, and educating the client regarding signs and symptoms to report to the health care provider.

For clients experiencing **cardiac arrhythmias**, the nurse will adhere to the health care agency's policy and procedure, protocols, and Advanced Cardiovascular Life Support (ACLS) and CPR standards of practice to improve the client's condition. A client may require a temporary or permanent pacemaker to initiate myocardial contractions in an emergency. Temporary pacing options are chosen based on the client's condition. Transcutaneous and transvenous pacing can be programmed as a fixed rate or as flexible demand pacing. The health care facility's protocol or the health care provider will provide the direction on the rate, amount of output, and chamber to be paced.

The location of the capture on the rhythm strip is dependent on which chamber the pacemaker is placed. The client who requires placement of a permanent pacemaker will have an x-ray to confirm the lead placement. During the initial postoperative period, the left arm is positioned for comfort and movement is minimized to prevent dislodging the wires. The nurse will assist the client with range of motion exercises as prescribed and monitor the function of the pacemaker by performing client cardiac output assessments and ECGs. Potential complications related to the pacemaker include failure to pace, failure to capture, improper sensing, runaway pacemaker, dysrhythmias, and battery failures. Postoperatively, the client is at risk for bleeding, myocardial perforation, cardiac tamponade, pneumothorax, hemothorax, emboli, infection at the site, as well as endocarditis. The surgical site will be monitored for signs and symptoms of infection.

A client may require an **arterial line**, which is placed in the radial, brachial, or femoral artery to continuously monitor hemodynamic pressures or obtain arterial blood gases and blood samples. Following placement of the catheter, the client is monitored for complications, which include infection, hematoma, hemorrhage, infiltration, catheter migration, and occlusion of the catheter lumen or arterial. The assessment consists of the evaluation of the extremity for warmth, sensation, pulse, and capillary refill. Obtaining accurate monitoring requires that the transducer be placed at the level of the right atrium.

Most health care facilities have specially trained telemetry technicians to monitor clients who require telemetry. Each health care facility's guidelines and protocols for monitoring a client will be consulted to delineate the roles in ECG interpretation. The nurse remains responsible for client assessments, interventions, and communication. The client's baseline ECG and any significant changes should be interpreted by viewing an actual printed strip, with alarm parameters on the monitor verified and audible.

A client with chronic kidney disease that has become life-threatening and is no longer manageable by conventional therapy may require hemodialysis or peritoneal dialysis. Hemodialysis can be performed in many settings, including the home in which a skilled partner is available to assist in the procedure.

Hemodialysis requires anticoagulation through the blood circuit pump, so the client should be monitored during and immediately after the procedure for bleeding. Any invasive procedures should be avoided. Vascular access is required for hemodialysis and may be permanent or temporary. An **AV fistula** or **AV graft** provides permanent vascular access, while a dialysis catheter or subcutaneous device allows

> **NOTE**
>
> Peritoneal dialysis is discussed in the "Alterations of Body Systems" section of this chapter.

for temporary access. The nurse will assess the sites for complications, such as infection, and will ensure the permanent vascular access sites are functioning. The distal pulses and capillary refill of the arm with the fistula or graft are auscultated for a bruit and palpated for a thrill over the site.

Before performing hemodialysis, the nurse will record the client's weight, obtain baseline vital signs, assess laboratory values, and collaborate with the health care provider regarding which prescriptions will be held, as many drugs can be partially removed through dialysis. Post-dialysis, the client will be closely monitored for several hours for common problems, such as hypotension, nausea, vomiting, dizziness, muscle cramps, and headache. The client's weight will be obtained and blood pressure, pulse, respirations, temperature, and intake and output will also be monitored.

ILLNESS MANAGEMENT

Identifying client data that needs to be reported immediately requires nursing judgment based on critical thinking. The inability to recognize pertinent data or clinical findings results in a delay of care for the client, which may result in further physiological or psychological decline and death.

The nurse is accountable for adhering to the health care facility's policy and procedures regarding specific protocols when monitoring a client.

The nurse is responsible for gathering a client's baseline data assessment, which includes not only physical assessment findings, but laboratory and testing results. Assessments are based on the client's condition, and it is essential that the nurse recognize early signs and symptoms of pathological change from the client's baseline or when treatments, interventions, and medications have been ineffective or produce unexpected responses. Specific conditions may require adherence to a protocol and the use of specific tools to monitor the client for change, such as the Glasgow Coma Scale. Tools for communication are also frequently used, such as the SBAR, to ensure the effectiveness of communication. Many health care facilities identify "critical" labs for which the nurse is immediately notified. The nurse is accountable for the immediate reporting of any suspected change in condition, abnormal laboratory or testing results, and any adverse response to treatment or medications that compromise the client's physiological and psychological state. The nurse will follow the health care facility's policy and procedure regarding events that require internal reporting in addition to the immediate notification of the health care provider.

Education regarding the management of illness is based upon many factors, which include the client's physiological and psychological condition, developmental age, available family and community support, socioeconomic state, culture, and religion. Interventions required to manage a client's recovery from illness require a fundamental understanding of the client's condition or illness. The interventions the nurse will implement are specific to the client's condition and are focused on the promotion of the client's recovery.

Gastric lavage may be prescribed for a client as a therapeutic or diagnostic treatment. Gastric lavage can be performed using closed system irrigation or an intermittent open system. Both procedures require the insertion of a nasogastric tube, and after verification of tube placement (when performing a closed system irrigation), the prescribed solution—warmed to room temperature—will be infused through the nasogastric tube using a Y connector. The drainage or suction tubing will be connected to the other arm of the Y connector. After emptying the stomach, the nurse clamps the drain or turns off the suction and allows the prescribed amount of fluid to flow into the stomach by gravity. After stopping the flow of the solution, the nurse allows it to drain by gravity or suctions the fluid out. The treatment is repeated until the fluid returns light pink or clear and absent of clots. The nurse measures the amount of drainage, subtracting the amount of irrigant instilled, and records the gastric output.

Intermittent open system irrigation requires manual administration and removal of the solution using a 50 mL syringe. The solution is withdrawn manually, and the treatment is repeated until the fluid returns light pink or clear and absent of clots. The nurse will monitor the client's vital signs and tolerance of the procedure, notifying the health care provider of the client's ability or inability to tolerate the procedure or if the color of aspirate does not change over the prescribed amount of fluid and time. The nurse adheres to the health care facility's policy and procedures.

A client's ventilation and oxygenation can be affected by many factors. Clients who experience ventilatory failure are unable to move the oxygen they inhale in and out of the lungs, which results in the buildup of carbon dioxide.

Factors associated with **ventilatory failure** include:

- Stroke
- COPD
- Meningitis
- Sleep apnea
- Pneumothorax
- Kyphoscoliosis
- Pulmonary edema
- Pulmonary embolism

> **NOTE**
>
> The nurse plays a pivotal role as a liaison between the health care team and the client to promote and provide continuity of care in the management of the client's illness. The concepts of client management, continuity of care, and referrals are discussed in the "Safe and Effective Care Environment Review" section of Chapter 3.

- Chemical depression
- Neuromuscular disorders
- Increased intracranial pressure
- External obstruction or constriction
- Acute respiratory distress syndrome
- Spinal cord injuries affecting nerves to the intercostal muscles

Impaired gas exchange occurs at the alveolar-capillary membrane level, in which there is poor diffusion of oxygen into the arterial blood and carbon dioxide is retained.

Factors associated with **poor oxygenation** include:

- Pneumonia
- High altitudes
- Pleural effusion
- Hypoventilation
- Smoke inhalation
- Pulmonary edema
- Hypovolemic shock
- Abnormal hemoglobin
- Carbon monoxide poisoning
- Acute respiratory distress syndrome

A client may experience both ventilatory failure and oxygen failure, which occur with cystic fibrosis, asthma attack, chronic bronchitis, or emphysema. Recognizing the causative factor or risk factors and the signs and symptoms associated with impaired ventilation and oxygenation, understanding the diagnostic testing, performing the appropriate nursing assessments, and implementing the proper interventions will prevent the client's clinical condition from further deteriorating. Restoration of ventilation and oxygenation includes correcting the underlying cause of the impairment to avoid respiratory failure hypoxemia and hypercapnia. Other treatments consist of supplemental oxygenation, medications, laboratory assessments, and procedures.

Clients experiencing an acute decline in ventilation and oxygenation require emergency intervention, which includes respiratory support with supplemental oxygen, mechanical ventilation, oxygen saturation monitoring, and arterial blood gas monitoring, and, based on the underlying cause, may consist of medications such as diuretics, steroids, and other treatments, as well as laboratory evaluations. Treatment for a client experiencing chronic hypoxemia includes treating the underlying condition and providing supplemental oxygen and nutritional support.

The final step of the nursing process allows for the nurse to evaluate the effectiveness of the treatment plan for a client with an acute or chronic diagnosis and to determine if the goals and outcomes for the client have been met.

PATHOPHYSIOLOGY AND MEDICAL EMERGENCIES

Identifying and understanding the pathophysiology related to acute or chronic conditions entails an understanding of the etiology of the condition, the disease process, signs and symptoms of the condition, how the condition is diagnosed, treatment options, prognosis, and how these elements relate to the client. General principles of pathology include tissue injury and repair, immunity, and cellular structure.

Tissue injury and repair occur in four overlapping phases. The first phase is **homeostasis**. During homeostasis, the body works to stop the bleeding through vasoconstriction, thrombin, and platelet formation. Fibrin strands begin to adhere, and a fibrin mesh is formed. The thrombus that forms keeps the platelets and blood cells trapped in the wound.

During the second phase—the **inflammatory phase**—the inflammatory process occurs in which the neutrophils destroy the bacteria and remove the debris. Macrophages will also arrive and clean up the wound debris. This phase is characterized by edema, redness, heat, and pain and usually lasts 4–6 days.

Phase three is the **proliferative phase**, which can last from four days to three weeks. During this time, granulation occurs, filling the wound bed with new connective tissue and new blood vessels. The margins of the wound begin to contract and pull toward the center of the wound bed. Epithelial cells from the wound migrate across the wound until it is covered with epithelium.

The fourth phase, the **maturation phase**, lasts from three weeks up to two years and is characterized by the reorganization of collagen fibers as the tissue remodels and matures.

The **immune function** includes inflammation, antibody-mediated immunity, and cell-mediated immunity. Inflammation is a nonspecific short-term body response to invasion or injury, but it does not provide true immunity. The following are five cardinal manifestations of inflammation:

1. Warmth

2. Redness

3. Swelling

4. Pain

5. Decreased function

It is important to note that the timing of the stages may overlap with each other. **Antibody-mediated immunity** involves antigen-antibody interactions that occur after the sensitization of the B lymphocyte to foreign cells and lymphocytes. The antigen-antibody interactions neutralize, eliminate, or destroy foreign proteins and provide long-lasting immunity against a specific toxin or organism. This type of immunity can be acquired actively or passively. Cell-mediated immunity does not produce an antigen-antibody interaction, but instead involves the T cells. The T cells enhance immune activity through secretion of various factors, cytokines, and lymphokines.

The cellular structure includes a plasma membrane, which acts as a protective coating, and a cytoskeleton, which provides a structural framework for the cell shape, movement, organelle movement, and cell division. The cellular structure also contains the cytoplasm and the genetic material.

The **cytoplasm** contains dissolved nutrients, helps break down waste products, and moves material around the cell. It also contains many salts and is an excellent conductor of electricity. The genetic materials DNA and RNA reside within the cytoplasm.

Normal cells divide slowly or not at all and do not migrate. They have specific morphologic features, a smaller nucleus-to-cytoplasm ratio, many differentiated functions, a tight adherence, well-regulated growth, a diploid number of chromosomes, and a low mitotic index. A **benign tumor cell** has all the characteristics of a normal cell except its cell division is continuous or inappropriate and growth is expanded.

Malignant cells are abnormal and rapidly or continuously divide and can migrate and invade. They are anaplastic in appearance and have a larger nucleus-to-cytoplasm ratio, little or no differentiated function, loose adherence, aneuploid chromosomes, and a high mitotic index.

Medical Emergencies

An understanding of pathophysiology is necessary for the use of critical thinking and clinical reasoning when caring for a client in an emergency. This understanding allows for complications to be anticipated and for the use of accurate clinical judgment. Caring for a client in an emergency situation not only requires the knowledge of pathophysiology, but necessitates adherence to the health care facility's policy and procedures, protocols, and the facilitation of accurate and timely communication among the health care team managing the client.

When caring for a client with a medical emergency, safety is a priority. Safety considerations during a medical emergency include the following:

- Client identification

- Injury prevention for both the client and the staff

- Decreasing the risk for errors and adverse events

- Providing emotional support to the client

- Explaining all emergency interventions

The nurse will promptly notify the primary health care provider about all adverse responses to treatment and unanticipated changes in condition. Basic emergency care procedures are carried out according to the health care facility's policy and procedures, protocols, and the health care provider's prescription, always maintaining the safety of the client and staff. Advanced emergency procedures can be provided by nurses who have obtained certification for Advanced Cardiac Life Support (ALS), Pediatric Advanced Life Support (PALS), and Neonatal Resuscitation (NRP). All client responses to emergency interventions are documented according to the health care facility's policy and procedures.

A client with wound dehiscence or evisceration requires emergency care. Risk factors for wound dehiscence or evisceration include wound infection, a poorly healing wound, anemia, diabetes, and obesity. Signs and symptoms of wound dehiscence include suture margins that are separated at any point along the incision line, broken sutures, redness, or an increase in unrelieved pain at the incision site. A disruption in the healing process as evidenced by edema, bleeding, or exudate from the incision site may also indicate the wound will dehisce. A client may experience partial- or full-thickness dehiscence. A full-thickness wound dehiscence may be further complicated by evisceration in which the abdominal organs protrude from the incision.

Emergency interventions for a client with wound dehiscence and evisceration include remaining with the client, applying a sterile nonadherent or saline dressing over the site, and requesting that the health care provider be notified immediately. The client will be instructed to avoid coughing. The nurse will maintain the client in a position no higher than 20 degrees, with the knees flexed. If evisceration has occurred, the nurse will not attempt to push the organs back through the wound. The client is monitored for shock and frequent vital signs are obtained as well as other interventions according to the health care facility's policy and procedure until the health care provider arrives.

Unexpected Response to Therapies

Nearly all treatments, therapies, prescriptions, and interventions have risks and complications. The risks for an unexpected adverse response to therapy is based on the condition of the client and the treatment and procedures. For example, a client who has had surgery or given birth is at risk for hemorrhage. Some prescriptions place a client at risk for increased intracranial pressure. The nurse is responsible for implementing preventative measures and monitoring the client based on the health care facility's policy and procedures. Understanding the potential adverse response to prescribed treatments and interventions will help the nurse identify the early signs and symptoms in a client and help with monitoring the client accordingly, intervening in a timely manner with the appropriate interventions to prevent further harm to the client. Clients may experience an unexpected response to therapy, such as the client who requires a urinary catheter and then develops a urinary tract infection. The nurse caring for clients who experience an unexpected response to therapy will promote their recovery through collaboration with the health care team and the utilization of the nursing process.

SUMMING IT UP

- The focus of the **physiological integrity** NCLEX-RN Client Needs category is to assess the nurse's ability to promote physical health and wellness by providing care and comfort, reducing client risk potential, and managing health alterations.

- A **primary nursing goal** is assessing a client for pain, intervening as appropriate, and providing nonpharmacological comfort measures.

- The nurse may collaborate with other professionals when caring for clients who require **assistive devices** such as crutches, canes, walkers, wheelchairs, and prostheses.

- The nurse will assess for changes in **sensory conditions** of all clients who have risk factors such as disease processes or clients who are receiving prescriptions that place them at risk for impaired communication, speech, vision, or hearing problems. The nurse will also assess for changes in a client's elimination, mobility, chewing, swallowing, ability to perform personal hygiene, rest, and sleep.

- Common **altered elimination findings** include urinary retention, urinary incontinence, and bowel incontinence.

- There are many different types of **traction**, including running traction, balanced suspension, skeletal traction, and skin traction. Traction involves the use of various weights and pully systems to apply tension on a limb, bone, or muscle, thereby allowing reduction, alignment, immobilization, prevention or correction of deformities, and decreased muscle spasms.

- Nursing **interventions** may be necessary for clients experiencing pain. The location and intensity of the pain, as well as the client's age, gender, race, genetics, and culture, are integral to the **pain assessment**.

- The focus of the NCLEX-RN **pharmacological and parenteral therapies** subcategory is to assess the nurse's ability to provide care related to the administration of medications and parenteral therapies. Part of the nursing role when administering medications includes providing client education and preparation. The nurse must also be knowledgeable about the client's medical and prescription history, current condition, and prescribed medical treatments with which a newly prescribed medication may interact.

- **Traditional and complementary alternative medicine (TM/CAM)** is commonly used in combination with conventional medicine. Throughout treatment or use of TM/CAM, the nurse will evaluate the outcomes of the therapy.

- Understanding pain will assist the nurse in evaluating the client during a **comprehensive pain assessment**. Data gathered in the assessment includes identifying the location and intensity of the pain.

- The nurse may be required to **administer blood or blood products** to replace blood or lost blood components.

- When providing education about medications for a client, the nurse may have to include additional discussion and demonstration for **self-administration** of medication.

- Medications include **oral, buccal, ophthalmic, and otic medications** and may be administered using metered dose inhalers, nasogastric tubes, topical prescriptions, and transdermal patches. The nurse may also have to administer suppositories and analgesics and provide **subcutaneous, intramuscular, or intravenous** medication injections.

- The nurse must educate the client about the need for **total parenteral nutrition (TPN)** before initiating TPN.

- **Enteral feedings** are required when the client is unable to meet nutritional needs adequately through the oral intake of food, inability to swallow, or refusal to eat. Examples of enteral feeding tubes include **nasogastric, nasojejunal, nasoduodenal, jejunostomy,** and **PEG tubes**.

- Type O (negative) blood is referred to as a **universal donor**, while type AB (positive) is considered a **universal recipient**.

- The focus of the NCLEX-RN **reduction of risk potential** subcategory is to assess the nurse's ability to reduce the likelihood that clients will develop complications or health problems related to existing conditions, treatments, or procedures. This assessment is accomplished through the nurse's ability to do the following:

  - Assess accurately

  - Respond efficiently to changes or trends in a client's vital signs

  - Perform diagnostic testing

  - Monitor the test results

  - Intervene appropriately

- The nurse must be aware of changes in a client's **vital signs** such as pulse, respiratory rate, oxygen saturation, and blood pressure.

- The nurse may use a variety of **testing and monitoring methods**, including the following:

  - Direct pressure monitoring

  - Central venous pressure monitoring

  - Fetal heart rate monitoring

  - Intra-arterial blood pressure monitoring

  - ECG testing

  - Blood glucose testing

  - Venous blood sampling

  - Urinalysis

  - Stool analysis

  - Ultrasound

  - Cultures, such as sputum, throat, or wound cultures

- Diagnostic tests, treatments, or procedures may cause complications, such as bleeding, abnormal circulation distal to the extremities, and various types of **shock**.

- The nurse may have to monitor the client's response and recovery from **anesthesia**.

- The focus of the **physiological adaptation** NCLEX-RN subcategory is to assess the nurse's ability to do the following:

  - Manage and provide care for clients with acute, chronic, or life-threatening physical health conditions

- Understand how to assist with **invasive procedures**
- Implement and monitor a client who requires **phototherapy**
- Maintain the optimal temperature of the client
- Monitor and care for clients with **impaired ventilation or oxygenation**

- The nurse must help a client cope with **alterations in his or her body systems**, which includes illness and disease, and identify client attributes of coping, such as health-sustaining habits, life satisfaction, social supports, and effective and healthy response to stress.

- The nurse must be prepared to assist a client experiencing such **obstetrical complications** as seizure, precipitous labor, postpartum hemorrhage, uterine atony, shock, and hemorrhaging.

- The nurse must take special measures when caring for a client with a potentially life-threatening **fluid and electrolyte imbalance**.

- The nurse must be vigilant for findings associated with **decreased cardiac output**.

- The nurse must use **critical thinking skills** to identify client data that needs to be reported; the inability to do so results in a delay of client care, which may result in further physiological or psychological decline and death.

- The nurse is accountable for adhering to the health care facility's policy and procedures regarding specific protocols when monitoring a client.

- The nurse identifies and understands the pathophysiology related to acute or chronic conditions by understanding the **etiology** of the condition, the disease process, signs and symptoms of the condition, how the conditions are diagnosed, treatment options, prognosis, and how these elements relate to the client.

- General principles of pathology include **tissue injury and repair, immunity, and cellular structure**.

- Because the risks for an unexpected adverse response to therapy are based on the condition of the client and the treatment and procedures, the nurse is responsible for the following:

  - Implementing **preventative** measures
  - Monitoring the client based on the health care facility's policy and procedures
  - Understanding the **potential adverse response** to prescribed treatments and interventions

PRACTICE QUESTIONS: PHYSIOLOGICAL INTEGRITY

Directions: The following are examples of the types of questions you will encounter on the NCLEX-RN exam. Read each question carefully and choose the best answer unless otherwise directed. Check your answers against the answer key and explanations that follow.

1. The nurse is caring for a client with delirium. For which type of incontinence should the nurse anticipate monitoring the client?

   1. Total
   2. Mixed
   3. Overflow
   4. Transient

2. Which prescription should the nurse recognize as a possible contributing factor to the significant weight gain of a client?

   1. Glucagon
   2. Corticosteroid
   3. Bulk-forming laxative
   4. Gastrointestinal lipase inhibitor

3. Which statement made by a client indicates an understanding of a full liquid diet?

   1. "I will be able to strain a creamed soup."
   2. "The liquids I can drink will be thickened."
   3. "I can drink orange juice without the pulp."
   4. "I can only drink fluids that I can see through."

4. The health care provider has prescribed 10 mg of ketorolac. The nurse has available ketorolac 15 mg/mL. How many mL will the nurse administer? **Round your answer to the nearest tenth.**

   _____ mL

5. The health care provider has prescribed 500 mL normal saline to infuse over 3 hours. The infusion set has a drop factor of 15 gtt/mL. Calculate the drips per minute. **Round to the nearest whole number.**

   _____ gtt/min.

6. The health care provider has prescribed 2 g ampicillin in 100 mL of normal saline to be infused over 30 minutes IVPB. Using an infusion pump, for how many mL per hr. will the nurse program the pump?

   _____ mL/hr.

7. The nurse observing a fetal heart rate tracing notes a client is experiencing early decelerations. For which classification category should the nurse document the finding?

   1. I
   2. II
   3. III
   4. IV

8. Which finding for a client who is using a sequential compression device should be of concern to the nurse?

   1. The compression delivered to the sleeves is cycling.
   2. The client is ambulating with the SCD sleeves in place.
   3. The client is wearing anti-embolism stockings under the SCD sleeves.
   4. The nurse can place two fingers between the SCD sleeves and the client's leg.

Practice Questions

9. The nurse is preparing to care for a newborn delivered to a client with type I diabetes. For which complication should the nurse monitor the neonate?

    1. Hyperthermia
    2. Hypothermia
    3. Hypoglycemia
    4. Hyperglycemia

10. The nurse notes a client's serum sodium is 132 mEq/L. Which assessment findings should the nurse anticipate? **Select all that apply.**

    1. Vomiting
    2. Tachycardia
    3. Hypotension
    4. Disorientation
    5. Chvostek sign
    6. Increased deep tendon reflexes

ANSWER KEY AND EXPLANATIONS

1. 4	3. 1	5. 167 gtt/min.	7. 1	9. 3
2. 2	4. 0.7 mL	6. 200 mL/hr.	8. 2	10. 1, 2, 3, 4

1. **The correct answer is 4.** Clients with delirium may experience transient incontinence. Transient incontinence occurs when there is a loss of cognitive functioning or loss of awareness that urination is to happen in a socially unacceptable place. Total incontinence (choice 1) is a continuous, unpredictable loss of urine without distention or awareness of bladder fullness. Mixed incontinence (choice 2) is a combination of stress and urge incontinence. Overflow incontinence (choice 3) results from incomplete bladder emptying.

2. **The correct answer is 2.** Corticosteroids can cause an increase in appetite and affect the client's metabolism, resulting in weight gain. Glucagon (choice 1) and bulk-forming laxatives (choice 3) can cause a loss of appetite, resulting in weight loss, rather than weight gain. Gastrointestinal lipase inhibitors (choice 4) reduce the absorption of fat and can result in weight loss.

3. **The correct answer is 1.** The client may have strained creamed soup. A full liquid diet is provided for clients who cannot tolerate mechanical soft diets and includes foods that may become liquid at room or body temperature. A full liquid diet does not entail thickening liquids (choice 2), the client may have orange juice with pulp (choice 3), and the fluids do not have to be clear (choice 4).

4. **The correct answer is 0.7 mL.**

$$\frac{10 \text{ mg}}{15 \text{ mg/mL}} = 0.66 \text{ mL}$$

Rounded to the nearest tenth = 0.7 mL

5. **The correct answer is 167 gtt/min.**

3 hours × 60 minutes = 180 minutes

$$\frac{2,000 \text{ mL}}{180 \text{ min.}} \times \frac{15 \text{ (gtt)}}{\text{mL}} = \frac{30,000}{180}$$
$$= 166.66$$
$$= 167 \text{ gtt/min.}$$

6. **The correct answer is 200 mL/hr.**

$$\frac{100 \text{ mL}}{30 \text{ min.}} \times \frac{60 \text{ min.}}{1 \text{ hr.}} = \frac{6,000}{30} = 200 \text{ mL/hr.}$$

7. **The correct answer is 1.** Early decelerations is a normal finding and does not warrant concern. When documenting the fetal heart rate pattern, a three-tiered fetal heart rate classification system is used. Category I is reflective of normal findings. Category II (choice 2) reflects indeterminant results, and category III (choice 3) reflects abnormal findings. There is not a category IV classification (choice 4).

8. **The correct answer is 2.** Ambulating with SCD sleeves in place puts the client at risk for falling; the sleeves should be removed if the client is going to ambulate. Choice 1 is not concerning, since the compression device is intended to cycle. It is acceptable for a client to wear anti-embolism stockings under the SCD sleeves (choice 3). The nurse should be able to place two fingers between the SCD sleeves and the client's legs (choice 4), so this finding is expected.

9. **The correct answer is 3.** A neonate born to a type I diabetic mother is at risk for hypoglycemia. Maternal type I diabetes is not associated with neonatal hyperthermia (choice 1), hypothermia (choice 2), or hyperglycemia (choice 4).

10. **The correct answers are 1, 2, 3, 4.** The range for normal serum sodium levels is 135–145 mEq/L. A client with serum sodium of 132 mEq/L is experiencing hyponatremia. Assessment findings for hyponatremia include vomiting, tachycardia, hypotension, and disorientation. A Chvostek sign (choice 5) is associated with hypocalcemia, not hyponatremia. The deep tendon reflexes are decreased with hyponatremia, rather than increased (choice 6).

Answers Practice Questions

PART IV
PRACTICE TESTS

Practice Test 2

Practice Test 3

ANSWER SHEET: PRACTICE TEST 2

1. ① ② ③ ④ ⑤ ⑥
2. ① ② ③ ④
3. ① ② ③ ④
4. ① ② ③ ④ ⑤ ⑥
5. ① ② ③ ④
6. ① ② ③ ④
7. ① ② ③ ④
8. ① ② ③ ④ ⑤ ⑥
9. ① ② ③ ④
10. ① ② ③ ④
11. ① ② ③ ④
12. ① ② ③ ④ ⑤ ⑥
13. ① ② ③ ④
14. ① ② ③ ④
15. ① ② ③ ④ ⑤ ⑥
16. ① ② ③ ④
17. _____
18. ① ② ③ ④ ⑤ ⑥
19. ① ② ③ ④
20. ① ② ③ ④
21. ① ② ③ ④ ⑤ ⑥
22. ① ② ③ ④
23. ① ② ③ ④
24. ① ② ③ ④
25. ① ② ③ ④

26. ① ② ③ ④ ⑤ ⑥
27. ① ② ③ ④
28. ① ② ③ ④
29. ① ② ③ ④ ⑤
30. _____
31. ① ② ③ ④
32. ① ② ③ ④
33. ① ② ③ ④
34. ① ② ③ ④
35. ① ② ③ ④
36. ① ② ③ ④
37. ① ② ③ ④
38. ① ② ③ ④
39. ① ② ③ ④ ⑤ ⑥
40. ① ② ③ ④
41. ① ② ③ ④
42. ① ② ③ ④
43. ① ② ③ ④
44. ① ② ③ ④ ⑤ ⑥
45. ① ② ③ ④
46. ① ② ③ ④
47. ① ② ③ ④
48. ① ② ③ ④
49. ① ② ③ ④
50. ① ② ③ ④ ⑤

51. ① ② ③ ④ ⑤ ⑥
52. ① ② ③ ④
53. ① ② ③ ④ ⑤ ⑥
54. _____
55. ① ② ③ ④
56. ① ② ③ ④
57. ① ② ③ ④ ⑤ ⑥
58. ① ② ③ ④
59. ① ② ③ ④
60. ① ② ③ ④ ⑤ ⑥
61. ① ② ③ ④ ⑤ ⑥
62. ① ② ③ ④ ⑤
63. _____
64. ① ② ③ ④
65. ① ② ③ ④
66. ① ② ③ ④
67. ① ② ③ ④
68. ① ② ③ ④
69. ① ② ③ ④
70. ① ② ③ ④ ⑤
71. _____
72. ① ② ③ ④
73. ① ② ③ ④ ⑤ ⑥
74. ① ② ③ ④ ⑤
75. ① ② ③ ④ ⑤ ⑥

76. ① ② ③ ④
77. ① ② ③ ④
78. _____
79. ① ② ③ ④
80. ① ② ③ ④
81. ① ② ③ ④
82. ① ② ③ ④ ⑤ ⑥
83. ① ② ③ ④ ⑤ ⑥
84. ① ② ③ ④
85. ① ② ③ ④
86. ① ② ③ ④ ⑤ ⑥
87. ① ② ③ ④ ⑤
88. ① ② ③ ④
89. ① ② ③ ④
90. ① ② ③ ④
91. ① ② ③ ④
92. ① ② ③ ④ ⑤ ⑥
93. ① ② ③ ④
94. ① ② ③ ④ ⑤
95. ① ② ③ ④
96. ① ② ③ ④
97. ① ② ③ ④
98. ① ② ③ ④
99. ① ② ③ ④ ⑤ ⑥
100. ① ② ③ ④

Answer Sheet

Practice Test 2

100 Questions – 150 minutes

Directions: This test matches the current NCSBN NCLEX-RN test plan. You may encounter the following types of questions:

1. **Multiple-choice** questions that will have only one correct answer.
2. **Multiple-answer** questions that will have more than one correct answer.
3. **Fill-in-the-blank** questions that will require math calculations.
4. **Hot spot** questions, where you will mark a very specific location on an image.

Each item will require you to perform critical thinking. It is important that you identify exactly what the question is asking before moving on to the answer choices. For multiple-choice and multiple-response questions, read all the answer choices, choose the best answer(s), and fill in the corresponding circle(s) on the answer sheet. Take care to not just pick the first answer that makes sense. For fill-in-the-blank questions, use the appropriate math calculation and fill in the correct answer in the blank provided. For hot spot questions, follow the directions provided in the question to indicate the correct answer. An answer key and explanations follow the practice test.

1. Which techniques should the nurse include before inserting a peripheral IV? **Select all that apply.**

   1. Wear clean gloves for IV insertion.
   2. Maintain aseptic technique for insertion.
   3. Wipe the visibly soiled area with a skin antiseptic.
   4. Allow the antiseptic to dry before dressing the site.
   5. Clean the IV site with a skin antiseptic using a circular motion.
   6. Avoid palpating the insertion site after the antiseptic is applied.

2. Which is the correct interpretation of the ECG tracing?

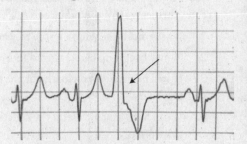

   1. Atrial tachycardia
   2. Ventricular tachycardia
   3. Premature atrial contraction
   4. Premature ventricular contraction

Practice Test 2

3. The nurse has provided teaching for a client prescribed light therapy. Which statement made by the client indicates further instruction is required?

   1. "I may experience a headache."
   2. "I will plan on receiving treatment in the evening."
   3. "Irritability sometimes occurs with the treatment."
   4. "This treatment will help suppress the secretion of melatonin."

4. Which should the nurse ensure the postoperative client is able to do before implementing the use of an incentive spirometer? **Select all that apply.**

   1. Exhale fully.
   2. Hold the device.
   3. Inhale spontaneously.
   4. Splint during the treatment.
   5. Hold his or her breath for 10 seconds.
   6. Seal the lips around the mouthpiece.

5. The nurse has reviewed postprocedural care with a client scheduled for a bronchoscopy. Which statement made by the client indicates further teaching is required?

   1. "I will most likely have a sore throat."
   2. "I may cough up blood-tinged mucous."
   3. "I will be monitored closely for the first few hours."
   4. "I can have ice chips after the sedation has worn off."

6. Which reason should the nurse include in the client teaching when discussing the position for a thoracentesis?

   1. "The position widens the space between your ribs."
   2. "The position helps identify your thoracic vertebrae."
   3. "The position provides the best exposure to your back."
   4. "The position flattens the posterior surface of your lungs."

7. The nurse has received an arterial blood gas report with the following values: pH 7.48, $PaCO_2$ 50, and an HCO_3 of 28. Which should the nurse interpret from the results?

   1. Fully compensated metabolic alkalosis
   2. Fully compensated metabolic acidosis
   3. Partially compensated metabolic alkalosis
   4. Partially compensated respiratory alkalosis

8. Which laboratory findings should the nurse associate with a client suspected of refeeding syndrome? **Select all that apply.**

   1. Sodium—145 mEq/L
   2. Magnesium—0.9 mEq/L
   3. Chloride—104 mEq/L
   4. Phosphate—1.8 mg/dL
   5. Potassium—3.2 mEq/L
   6. Calcium—8.7 mEq/dL

9. Which should the nurse instruct the client to do in the process of collecting a stool sample for a culture?

   1. Place a small sample in a clean container.
   2. Obtain the sample as early in the morning as possible.
   3. Void before obtaining a stool sample.
   4. Use toilet paper sparingly.

10. The nurse is reviewing the laboratory results for a client scheduled for a procedure requiring the use of iodinated contrast medium. Which laboratory finding should be of **most** concern to the nurse?

    1. Platelet count—30,000
    2. Creatinine—2.1 mg/dL
    3. Potassium—4.7 mEq/L
    4. Blood urea nitrogen—18 mg/dL

11. To ensure the reading is accurate, which assessment should the nurse include when initiating pulse oximetry for a client with a suspected arrhythmia?

 1. Obtain the client's pulse rate.

 2. Obtain the client's blood pressure.

 3. Place the client on an ECG monitor.

 4. Place the oximeter on the left extremity.

12. Which factors should the nurse recognize may **decrease** the accuracy of a pulse oximeter reading? **Select all that apply.**

 1. Pneumonia

 2. Hyperthermia

 3. PaO$_2$ 40 mmHg

 4. PaCO$_2$ 39 mmHg

 5. Hemoglobin 9 g/dL

 6. Carbon monoxide poisoning

13. After reviewing the following ECG tracing of a newborn infant, which action should the nurse take?

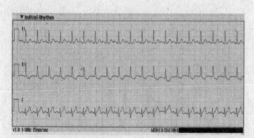

User:MoodyGroove [CC BY-SA 3.0 (https://creativecommons.org/licenses/by-sa/3.0)]

 1. Apply oxygen.

 2. Assess the newborn.

 3. Continue monitoring.

 4. Notify the health care provider.

14. Which technique should the nurse include when obtaining a blood sample from a PICC line?

 1. Discard the first 10 mL of blood.

 2. Use a mask during the procedure.

 3. Use a vacuum tube system to obtain the sample.

 4. Flush the PICC line before collecting the sample.

15. Which serum laboratory tests should the nurse anticipate evaluating for a client who has received a computed tomography with contrast? **Select all that apply.**

 1. Protein

 2. Glucose

 3. Uric acid

 4. Bilirubin

 5. Creatinine

 6. Glomerular filtration rate

16. The nurse has completed the education for a client with an ileostomy. Which statement made by the client indicates an understanding of the teaching?

 1. "I will increase my intake of insoluble fiber."

 2. "If I get constipated, I can irrigate my ostomy."

 3. "I will try to only take enteric-coated prescriptions."

 4. "I will increase the amount of sports drinks when I lose fluids."

Practice Test 2

17. Which anatomical location will the nurse identify as the site for the stoma for a client scheduled for an ileostomy? **Draw an arrow to the correct spot.**

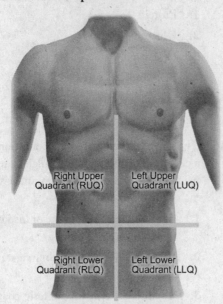

Abdominopelvic Quadrants

Blausen.com staff (2014). "Medical gallery of Blausen Medical 2014";. WikiJournal of Medicine 1 (2). DOI:10.15347/wjm/2014.010. ISSN 2002-4436. [CC BY 3.0 (https://creativecommons.org/licenses/by/3.0)]

18. Which should the nurse instruct the client with an ileostomy to avoid to help limit flatulence? **Select all that apply.**

1. Caffeine
2. Chewing gum
3. Dairy products
4. Carbonated beverages
5. Processed food products
6. Drinking through a straw

19. Which is the nursing **priority** for a newborn with esophageal atresia who becomes cyanotic?

1. Apply oxygen.
2. Suction the oropharynx.
3. Reposition the infant laterally.
4. Prepare for endotracheal tube intubation.

20. The nurse is caring for a newborn suspected of having a congenital heart defect. For which diagnostic procedure should the nurse prepare the neonate?

1. Chest x-ray
2. Echocardiogram
3. Electrocardiogram
4. Magnetic resonance imaging

21. The nurse is caring for a client who has experienced hypotonic fluid volume excess. Which laboratory values should the nurse plan on monitoring? **Select all that apply.**

1. BUN
2. Albumin
3. Creatinine
4. Hematocrit
5. Serum sodium
6. Urine specific gravity

22. Which statement made by the parent of a newborn requiring phototherapy lights for the treatment of jaundice indicates further teaching is needed?

1. "I can take the mask off while I feed the baby."
2. "I will close my newborn's eyes before placing the mask."
3. "I will reposition my baby under the lights every two hours."
4. "I will rub some lotion on my baby's dry skin before phototherapy."

23. Which should the nurse include in the care of a client receiving radiation therapy for breast cancer?

1. Limit visitors to 30 minutes per day.
2. Cover the area with loose-fitting clothing.
3. Ensure a lead container is available in the client's room.
4. Wear a dosimeter film badge while caring for the client.

24. The nurse is preparing to care for a client returning from an open lung biopsy. Which treatment should the nurse anticipate during post-procedural care?

    1. CPAP
    2. Ventilator
    3. Chest tube
    4. Blood transfusion

25. Using the SBAR tool (situation, background, assessment, and recommendation), which information communicated by the nurse to the health care provider reflects the client's situation?

    1. "Mr. Smith was admitted yesterday with acute pancreatitis."
    2. "Mr. Smith would benefit from a higher dosage of pain medication."
    3. "Mr. Smith has not experienced relief of pain from the prescription."
    4. "I see that Mr. Smith was admitted a month ago for treatment of alcohol abuse."

26. Which are safe practices for newborn identification? **Select all that apply.**

    1. Using ID band barcoding
    2. Using two body-site identification
    3. Using a distinct naming system
    4. Using the number on the infant's alarm band
    5. Ensuring the information on the band is legible
    6. Placing the mother's room number on the crib

27. An inpatient client treated for substance abuse frequently verbally abuses other clients in the dining area. Which is the **most** effective nursing intervention to address the client's actions?

    1. Redirection
    2. Limit setting
    3. Modeling behavior
    4. Behavioral contract

28. The educator has reviewed the procedure for irrigating a client's eye. Which statement made by the nurse indicates further teaching is needed?

    1. "I will apply pressure to keep the client's eye open."
    2. "After I complete the irrigation, I will pat the orbit of the eye dry."
    3. "The client will be instructed to look up prior to irrigating the eye."
    4. "The flow of irrigation is directed from the inner to the outer canthus."

29. A client with a baby tells the nurse her car does not have a back seat. Which information regarding car seat safety should the nurse recommend? **Select all that apply.**

    1. "Turn the front airbag off."
    2. "Place your infant facing forward."
    3. "Place the infant facing backward."
    4. "Position the car seat at a 45° angle."
    5. "Tuck the shoulder belt under the seat."

30. The health care provider prescribes 1,000 mL of normal saline to infuse over six hours. The IV infusion set drop factor is 15 gtt/mL. For how many mL/hr. will the nurse set the infusion pump? **Round to the nearest whole number.**

    _____mL/hr.

31. Which finding is associated with the **highest** suicidal risk for a client who expresses a desire to hurt himself?

    1. Feelings of hopelessness
    2. Accessibility to weapons
    3. History of a suicide attempt
    4. A family member who committed suicide

Practice Test 2

32. Which statement made by the nurse demonstrates an understanding of conducting a performance improvement project?

   1. "The findings of the quality initiative can be published."

   2. "We can gather the data for the project using randomization."

   3. "Based on the initial data, we can make changes to the project."

   4. "We can form a hypothesis to help predict the outcome of the project."

33. A member of the nursing staff states to the manager, "I am frustrated with this new staffing pattern." Which **initial** action should the nurse manager consider?

   1. Review the department's expenditures.

   2. Clarify the nurse's feelings of frustration.

   3. Review the intended goals for the change.

   4. Explain the practicality of the staffing pattern.

34. A client post-mastectomy tells the nurse that she is embarrassed about the way she looks. Which response should the nurse provide?

   1. "It is normal to have difficulty coping with this change."

   2. "I am concerned about your inability to cope with this change."

   3. "Would you like to talk more about your feelings of embarrassment?"

   4. "Would you like to discuss some solutions that may address your concerns?"

35. Which food should the nurse recommend for the client prescribed a renal diet?

   1. Ham

   2. Pastrami

   3. Roast beef

   4. Grilled cheese

36. For which situation should the pediatric nurse intervene?

   1. The door to a child's room is open.

   2. The side rails of a child's bed are raised.

   3. A parent is pulling a child with an IV in a wagon.

   4. An infant is laying on the daybed with a parent.

37. After extubating a client from a ventilator, which assessment finding requires **immediate** attention?

   1. Stridor

   2. Copious oral secretions

   3. Hoarseness

   4. Difficulty speaking

38. A client seeking treatment tells the nurse he does not want his medical information released to the insurance company. Which response should the nurse provide the client?

   1. "Your insurance company can only view certain portions of your record."

   2. "Your insurance company is not allowed to share your personal information."

   3. "Your insurance company requires your permission to obtain your medical information."

   4. "Your insurance company has the right to all of your medical information to review the claims."

39. Which principle information will the nurse use to identify clients who are at high risk of adversely reacting to a prescription? **Select all that apply.**

   1. History

   2. Assessment

   3. Physical activity

   4. Laboratory data

   5. Socioeconomic status

   6. Adherence to treatment

40. The nurse has provided client education regarding expected body changes in the third trimester of pregnancy. Which client statement indicates further teaching is needed?

   1. "I may have difficulty sleeping at night."
   2. "I may experience vaginal leakage of fluid."
   3. "I may experience leakage of colostrum."
   4. "I may begin to notice Braxton Hicks contractions."

41. Which information will the nurse include in the education of two-part breathing for a client experiencing anxiety?

   1. The focus is on slow deep breathing and relaxing your muscles.
   2. The focus is on deep inhalations and imagining a peaceful scene.
   3. The focus is on abdominal breathing and interrupting your thoughts.
   4. The focus is on relaxing your muscles and interrupting your thoughts.

42. The nurse is preparing to make room assignments for several clients who are to be admitted to the unit. Which client should be assigned to a room by the nursing station?

   1. A client with anorexia nervosa
   2. A client with bipolar disorder experiencing mania
   3. A client with a depersonalization-derealization disorder
   4. A client with schizophrenia who believes her food is poisoned

43. The nurse is obtaining a medication history from a client who received prescriptions from another country. Which should the nurse take into consideration?

   1. The generic name of prescriptions are different in other countries.
   2. Prescriptions with identical brand names contain different active ingredients.
   3. Prescriptions from other countries are classified differently than in the United States.
   4. The prescription dosages are prescribed using a different measurement system.

44. Which newborn wake states will the nurse discuss with the parents of a newly delivered infant? **Select all that apply.**

   1. Crying
   2. Drowsy
   3. Irritable
   4. Light sleep
   5. Quiet alert
   6. Active alert

45. The nurse has verified the client has provided informed consent for a procedure. Which ethical principle has the nurse demonstrated?

   1. Fidelity
   2. Veracity
   3. Autonomy
   4. Beneficence

46. The nurse is reviewing the medication history of a client with a protein deficiency. For which prescription should the nurse be concerned?

   1. Atenolol
   2. Folic acid
   3. Phenelzine
   4. Doxycycline

Practice Test 2

47. Which principles of drug therapy should the nurse recognize as **increasing** the risk to the infant of a breastfeeding client?

    1. Use of sustained-release formulations

    2. Use of the lowest effective dosage of medication

    3. Avoidance of medications that have a long half-life

    4. Taking medications immediately after breastfeeding

48. Which statement made by an adolescent client should concern the nurse?

    1. "None of the boys in my class are cute."

    2. "Everyone has started their period except me."

    3. "I don't like wearing a bra; it is uncomfortable."

    4. "All of the changes I am experiencing are confusing."

49. Which **initial** intervention should the nurse perform for a client experiencing a postpartum hemorrhage?

    1. Initiate an IV line.

    2. Administer oxygen.

    3. Perform fundal massage.

    4. Place the client in Trendelenburg.

50. A client states to the nurse, "I do not understand how a 12-step treatment plan can help me with my gambling addiction." Which information should the nurse provide the client? **Select all that apply.**

    1. "You will be offered the option of participating in group therapy."

    2. "You can attend as many meetings as you would like for support."

    3. "You will learn how to stop gambling through the support of others."

    4. "You can locate and attend meetings in whichever location is convenient."

    5. "You will be assigned a sponsor for support while you work through the 12 steps."

51. Which areas of focus are **essential** for the nurse to address throughout adolescence? **Select all that apply.**

    1. Risk reduction

    2. Emotional well-being

    3. Cognitive development

    4. Community affiliations

    5. Violence and injury prevention

    6. Social and academic competence

52. Which ethical principle is the nurse practicing when implementing safety measures to prevent client injury?

    1. Justice

    2. Fidelity

    3. Beneficence

    4. Nonmaleficence

53. For which **initial** interventions should the nurse prepare to educate a 28-year old female client who is experiencing stress incontinence? **Select all that apply.**

    1. Fluid management

    2. Increased dietary fiber

    3. Bladder training program

    4. Pelvic floor strengthening

    5. Intermittent catheterization

    6. Pharmacological treatment

54. A client has heparin infusing at 30 mL/hr. on an infusion pump. There are 20,000 units of heparin in 500 mL of D5W. How many units of heparin per hour is the client receiving? _____units/hr.

55. The nurse has provided education on the prevention of reinfection for the parent of a child with enterobiasis. Which statement made by the parent indicates an understanding of the information?

    1. "I will throw away my child's bedding."

    2. "I will spray the air with a disinfectant."

    3. "I will keep my child's fingernails short."

    4. "I will make sure I bathe my child daily."

56. Which statement made by the nurse reflects the correct way to remove a client's staples?

    1. "I will start removing the staples from the middle of the incision."

    2. "I will remove every other staple starting with the second staple."

    3. "I will place steri-strips over the incision after removing all of the staples."

    4. "I will cleanse the incision site after I completely remove the staples."

57. Which tasks should the nurse delegate to the UAP? **Select all that apply.**

    1. Removing a client's surgical dressing

    2. Removing a client's SCDs before ambulation

    3. Transporting a client to the radiology department

    4. Notifying housekeeping to refill the hand sanitizer

    5. Reassessing a client who has been medicated for pain

    6. Preparing a room for a client who will be admitted with kidney stones

58. Which client should the charge nurse assign to the nurse from the pediatric unit?

    1. The client with hypokalemia receiving a KCL infusion

    2. The client with congestive heart failure due for furosemide

    3. The client with sickle cell anemia receiving a blood transfusion

    4. The client with chronic pancreatitis who requires discharge teaching

59. The nurse has provided a client with insomnia education on sleep promotion. Which statement made by the client indicates further teaching is needed?

    1. "I will try and drink warm milk before I go to bed."

    2. "I will go to the gym in the evening so that I will tire out."

    3. "I will spend some time journaling before I try to sleep."

    4. "I will maintain the same sleep schedule on the weekends."

60. The nurse is preparing to care for a child who is experiencing salicylate toxicity. Which assessment findings should the nurse anticipate? **Select all that apply.**

    1. Tinnitus

    2. Confusion

    3. Bradycardia

    4. Hyperthermia

    5. Hypertension

    6. Respiratory depression

61. Which vaccinations are recommended for a healthy older adult? **Select all that apply.**

    1. Flu vaccine

    2. Meningococcal

    3. Shingles vaccine

    4. Pneumococcal vaccine

    5. Tetanus and diphtheria booster

    6. Tetanus, diphtheria, pertussis vaccine

62. A parent tells the nurse her child has been exposed to pertussis. For which **initial** symptoms will the nurse instruct the parent to monitor the child? **Select all that apply.**

    1. Fever

    2. Coughing

    3. Lacrimation

    4. Flushed cheeks

    5. Protruding tongue

63. The health care provider has ordered a continuous infusion of nitroprusside 5 mcg/kg/minute for a client weighing 210 lbs. Nitroprusside is available in a solution of 200 mg in 250 mL D5W. How many mL/hr. will the nurse program the infusion pump for in order to deliver the prescribed rate? **Round to the nearest tenth.**

_____mL/hr.

64. Which home health client is a **priority** for the nurse to visit?

   1. A client with a stage III wound who requires wound care

   2. A client with diabetes who needs a hemoglobin A1c drawn

   3. A client with rheumatoid arthritis experiencing unrelieved pain

   4. A client with CHF reporting a weight gain of 2 lbs. within 48 hours

65. Which is **most** essential for the home health nurse to consider when providing client care?

   1. The health care facility's fiscal budget

   2. The budget allocated to staffing hours

   3. The health care facility's capital expenditure

   4. Familiarity with insurance reimbursement

66. The nurse reviewing a male client's records notes he has been taking saw palmetto for the past few months. Based on this finding, which question should the nurse include in the assessment?

   1. "Are you experiencing urinary frequency?"

   2. "Are you experiencing premature ejaculation?"

   3. "Are you having difficulty obtaining an erection?"

   4. "Are you experiencing a significant loss of urine?"

67. The nurse has provided a client education about the treatment of narcolepsy. Which statement made by the client indicates further teaching is required?

   1. "I will make sure I get daily exercise."

   2. "I will avoid taking naps during the day."

   3. "I will avoid heavy meals before bedtime."

   4. "I will lower the temperature before I go to sleep."

68. A client placed in seclusion after throwing chairs in the dining area asks the nurse when she can come out. Which response should the nurse provide?

   1. "We need to talk about your behavior."

   2. "You can come out if you take your medication."

   3. "We need to talk about how you are feeling right now."

   4. "You can come out after I speak to your health care provider."

69. Which physical assessment finding should the nurse be concerned with for the client receiving treatment to correct hypokalemia?

   1. Decreased reflexes

   2. Weak, thready pulse

   3. Abdominal distension

   4. Numbness in the extremities

70. Which statements indicate the nurse is participating directly in health care cost-effectiveness? **Select all that apply.**

   1. "The clients on this unit do not need the new equipment."

   2. "I have discussed the projected costs of treatment with my client."

   3. "The staffing design should be changed to provide more efficient care."

   4. "I am concerned that the clients cannot afford the prescribed medication."

   5. "Social services has been assisting the clients with obtaining community resources."

71. A health care provider orders acetaminophen 480 mg per mouth. The nurse has available acetaminophen 160 mg/5 mL.

    How many mL will the nurse administer?
    _____mL

72. The nurse has provided safety education for a client with a wound vac therapy unit. Which statement made by the client indicates further teaching is required?

    1. "I will cover the unit when I shower."

    2. "I will avoid using an extension cord with the unit."

    3. "I will avoid plugging in the cord in areas where people walk."

    4. "If I see a sudden increase in blood in the tubing, I will turn the unit off."

73. The nurse has received handoff on a surgical client who required cryoprecipitate in the post-anesthesia recovery unit. Which laboratory data does the nurse anticipate reviewing to evaluate the **initial** effectiveness of the treatment? **Select all that apply.**

    1. aPTT

    2. Platelets

    3. Fibrinogen

    4. Red blood cells

    5. Hemoglobin and hematocrit

    6. Internationalized normal ratio

74. The nurse educator is preparing to discuss with the nursing staff coping skills for clients who are experiencing hopelessness. Which skills should the educator include? **Select all that apply.**

    1. Personalization

    2. Emotional reasoning

    3. Cognitive reframing

    4. Assertiveness training

    5. Problem solving skills

75. Which will the nurse manager include in a discussion with the nursing staff about the variable costs of the unit? **Select all that apply.**

    1. Utilities

    2. Medications

    3. Unit supplies

    4. Nursing personnel

    5. Administrative salaries

    6. Minimal staffing to keep the unit open

76. Which **initial** treatment should the nurse anticipate for the client with the following ECG tracing?

    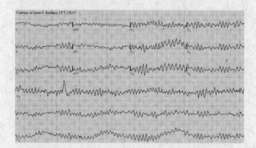

    Jer5150 [CC BY-SA 3.0 (https://creativecommons.org/licenses/by-sa/3.0)]

    1. Initiate CPR.

    2. Initiate defibrillation.

    3. Initiate an IV.

    4. Administer oxygen.

77. After notification of a toxic chemical spill in the community, which statement made by a nurse prepared in disaster management should concern the nurse manager?

    1. "I will have triage set up."

    2. "I will familiarize myself with the disaster plan."

    3. "I will have the list of community resources ready."

    4. "I will obtain the personal protective equipment."

78. When discussing a cardiac cycle reflected on an ECG tracing, which will the nurse identify as associated with the repolarization of the ventricles? **Draw an arrow to the correct spot on the diagram.**

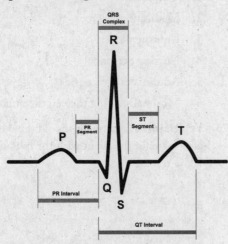

79. The nurse caring for a deteriorating client has been unable to reach the health care provider. Which **initial** action should the nurse take?

   1. Alert risk management.
   2. Notify the director of nursing.
   3. Follow the chain of command.
   4. Notify the emergency department provider.

80. The nurse is participating in triaging a mass casualty situation. Which client will the nurse classify as **urgent**?

   1. The client with a sprained ankle.
   2. The client with an airway obstruction.
   3. The client with an open tibial fracture.
   4. The client with myocardial infarction.

81. The nurse notes the following ECG rhythm for a type I diabetic client. Which is the nurse's **priority** assessment?

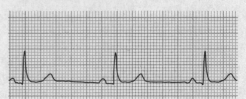

Sinusbradylead2.JPG: James Heilman, MDderivative work: Mysid (using Perl and Inkscape) [CC BY-SA 3.0 (https://cre-ativecommons.org/licenses/by-sa/3.0)]

   1. Pulse
   2. Blood glucose
   3. Blood pressure
   4. Level of consciousness

82. The nurse is preparing to provide education for a client prescribed warfarin. Which should the nurse instruct the client to limit to small amounts? **Select all that apply.**

   1. Garlic
   2. Ginger
   3. Cloves
   4. Grape juice
   5. Apple juice
   6. Cranberry juice

83. When assessing the milestones of an 18-month old client, which parental questions will the nurse include in the assessment? **Select all that apply.**

   1. "Can your child say single words?"
   2. "Can your child drink from a cup?"
   3. "Can your child scribble with a crayon?"
   4. "Does your child separate easily from you?"
   5. "Does your child point to objects he wants?"
   6. "Does your child understand words like 'in' and 'under?'"

84. Which statement made by the client reflects a therapeutic effect of levothyroxine?

    1. "My heart does not beat as fast."
    2. "My weight gain has slowed down."
    3. "I do not need much sleep anymore."
    4. "I feel like I have much more energy."

85. A client with cataracts requires a referral to an orthopedic health care provider. Which statement reflects the nurse's facilitation of the client's referral?

    1. "I will give you a list of orthopedists to choose from."
    2. "I will call an orthopedic office and make your appointment."
    3. "I will obtain a referral from your primary health care provider."
    4. "I will copy your medical records for you to take to an ophthalmologist."

86. Which interventions will the nurse implement to promote the nutritional intake for an older client? **Select all that apply.**

    1. Decrease environmental noise.
    2. Check on the client during mealtimes.
    3. Provide adequate nonglaring lighting.
    4. Ensure the client is toileted before meals.
    5. Remove emesis basins, bedpans, or urinals.
    6. Ensure the head of the bed is in a high-Fowler's.

87. Which referrals can the nurse make for a client? **Select all that apply.**

    1. Social services
    2. Laboratory testing
    3. Crisis intervention
    4. Closer access to care
    5. Physical therapy consult

88. The nurse has provided education for a client with type I diabetes prescribed insulin glargine (U-300). Which statement made by the client indicates an understanding of the information?

    1. "I can expect this type of insulin to be cloudy."
    2. "I am glad I only have to take the insulin once a day."
    3. "I will store the unopened pens in a dark, cool place."
    4. "I am happy that I will no longer need short-acting insulin."

89. The nurse has received a referral to conduct a home visit to assess an elderly man's ability to care for himself. Which **initial** activity should the nurse take during the initiation phase of the home visit?

    1. Schedule the home visit.
    2. Introduce herself and provide professional identity.
    3. Clarify the source of the referral with the client.
    4. Determine the family's willingness for a home visit.

90. An older client states to the nurse, "I don't understand why my electricity got turned off because I give my nephew money to pay my bills." Which suspected form of abuse would the nurse reference when notifying the social worker?

    1. Neglect
    2. Emotional
    3. Economic
    4. Psychological

91. Which is the nurse assessing when evaluating pupillary accommodation?

    1. Pupillary size
    2. Pupillary shape
    3. Pupillary reflexes
    4. Pupillary reactivity

92. Which will the nurse recognize as factors that increase the risk for child abuse? **Select all that apply.**

    1. Nonbiological caregiver
    2. Single income household
    3. Single parent household
    4. Children with chronic illness
    5. Younger than four years of age
    6. Presence of congenital abnormalities

93. After assessing the laboratory data of assigned clients, which client should the nurse assess **first**?

    1. A client receiving heparin with an aPTT of 25 seconds
    2. A client post appendectomy with a platelet count of 130,000
    3. A client receiving brachytherapy with a temperature of 100.1°F and WBC count of 8,000
    4. A client with a femur fracture with a hemoglobin of 15 g/dL and hematocrit of 41%

94. Which aids should the nurse anticipate using for a client with Parkinson's disease to promote independence when eating? **Select all that apply.**

    1. Insulated dish
    2. Handleless cups
    3. Grip scoop dish
    4. Sectional plates
    5. Weighted utensils

95. Which environmental finding should be of **most** concern to the nurse on the pediatric unit?

    1. Unplugged IV pumps
    2. An empty hand sanitizer dispenser
    3. A housekeeping cart in the hall
    4. A child's bed with several stuffed animals

96. The educator has reviewed insulin safety with the nursing staff. Which statement made by a nurse indicates an understanding of the information?

    1. "U-100 insulin syringes can be used for U-500 insulin."
    2. "Long-duration insulins can be administered more than twice a day."
    3. "NPH is the only insulin that can be mixed with short-acting insulins."
    4. "A short-duration slower-acting insulin cannot be administered intravenously."

97. Which statement made by the nurse indicates an understanding of evidence-based practice?

    1. "We can use the current evidence-based practice to help address the rate of falls in the unit."
    2. "I should be careful using evidence-based practice because it is not always research-based."
    3. "I will research the most current evidence-based practice before performing a dressing change for my client."
    4. "We should review new evidence-based practice before choosing the performance improvement indicators."

98. In which situation should the nurse intervene when observing a client bottle-feed her newborn baby?

    1. Stroking the newborn's cheek before a feeding
    2. Encouraging the newborn to finish the formula in the bottle
    3. Laying the newborn semi-upright in her lap during a feeding
    4. Placing a small amount of formula on the nipple before the feeding

99. Which integumentary findings may be related to poor personal hygiene? **Select all that apply.**

    1. Odor
    2. Rash
    3. Scales
    4. Pallor
    5. Dryness
    6. Coolness

100. Which **initial** action should the nurse take when concerned that a UAP is not meeting performance expectations?

    1. Document the actual observation.
    2. Report the findings to the manager.
    3. Discuss the observations with the UAP.
    4. Create an employee improvement plan.

ANSWER KEY AND EXPLANATIONS

1. 1, 2, 4, 6	**21.** 1, 4, 5, 6	**41.** 3	**61.** 1, 3, 4, 5	**81.** 4
2. 4	**22.** 4	**42.** 2	**62.** 1, 2, 3	**82.** 1, 2, 3, 6
3. 2	**23.** 2	**43.** 2	**63.** 36 mL/hr.	**83.** 1, 2, 3, 5
4. 3, 6	**24.** 3	**44.** 1, 2, 5, 6	**64.** 3	**84.** 4
5. 4	**25.** 3	**45.** 3	**65.** 4	**85.** 3
6. 1	**26.** 1, 2, 3, 5	**46.** 4	**66.** 1	**86.** 1, 3, 4, 5
7. 3	**27.** 4	**47.** 1	**67.** 2	**87.** 1, 3
8. 2, 4, 5	**28.** 1	**48.** 2	**68.** 3	**88.** 2
9. 3	**29.** 1, 3, 4, 5	**49.** 3	**69.** 4	**89.** 3
10. 2	**30.** 42 mL/hr.	**50.** 2, 3, 4, 5	**70.** 1, 3, 4, 5	**90.** 3
11. 1	**31.** 3	**51.** 1, 2, 5, 6	**71.** 15 mL	**91.** 3
12. 3, 5, 6	**32.** 3	**52.** 3	**72.** 1	**92.** 1, 4, 5, 6
13. 3	**33.** 2	**53.** 1, 2, 3, 4	**73.** 1, 3, 6	**93.** 1
14. 3	**34.** 3	**54.** 1,120 units/hr.	**74.** 3, 4, 5	**94.** 1, 3, 4, 5
15. 5, 6	**35.** 3	**55.** 3	**75.** 2, 3, 4	**95.** 3
16. 4	**36.** 4	**56.** 2	**76.** 1	**96.** 3
17. Arrow points to right lower quadrant	**37.** 1	**57.** 2, 3, 4, 6	**77.** 2	**97.** 1
	38. 3	**58.** 3	**78.** Arrow pointing to "T"	**98.** 2
18. 2, 4, 6	**39.** 1, 2, 4	**59.** 2	**79.** 3	**99.** 1, 2, 3, 5
19. 2	**40.** 2	**60.** 1, 2, 4, 6	**80.** 3	**100.** 1
20. 2				

1. **The correct answers are 1, 2, 4, and 6.** Clean gloves are applied after hand hygiene. The antiseptic is applied to the area of IV insertion for a minimum of 30 seconds using a back and forth scrubbing motion rather than a circular motion (choice 5), after which the area is allowed to dry. The site is to remain aseptic throughout the insertion and securement of the IV site. Visibly soiled skin is washed with soap and water, not a skin antiseptic (choice 3), before preparing the site for IV insertion.

2. **The correct answer is 4.** The QRS complex reflects ventricular depolarization.

Premature ventricular contractions occur as a result of increased irritability of the ventricular cells, which causes the ventricles of the heart to beat prematurely.

3. **The correct answer is 2.** If the client indicates that he will plan on receiving treatment in the evening, then further instruction is required. Light therapy is the first-line treatment for seasonal affective disorder (SAD). This type of therapy is most effective when it is done early in the morning after the client first wakes up. The statements made in choices 1, 3, and 4 indicate that the client understands that he may experience a

headache as well as irritability and that the treatment is used to help suppress the secretion of melatonin.

4. **The correct answers are 3 and 6.** Incentive spirometry is used to prevent atelectasis. Before initiating the treatment, the client must be able to inhale spontaneously and seal the lips around the mouthpiece. Exhaling fully (choice 1), holding the device (choice 2), and splinting during the therapy (choice 4) do not directly affect the client's ability to use a spirometer. The client should be able to hold his or her breath for at least 3 seconds for effective treatment. It is not necessary to hold the breath for 10 seconds (choice 5).

5. **The correct answer is 4.** Further teaching is required if the client indicates that she can have ice chips or liquids after the sedation has worn off. The client can have ice chips or liquids after the gag reflex has returned. The effects of the sedation make the client sleepy, but do not affect the client's gag reflex. The client will have a sore throat (choice 1), may cough up blood-tinged mucous (choice 2), and will be monitored closely for the first few hours (choice 3).

6. **The correct answer is 1.** The nurse should let the client know that the position for a thoracentesis widens the space between the ribs. A client is placed in a sitting position with the arms and head resting and supported on an adjustable, anchored bedside table. This position helps to enlarge the intercostal space to insert the needle. The position is not specifically initiated to identify thoracic vertebrae (choice 2) or provide the best exposure to the back (choice 3). The positioning during a thoracentesis does not flatten the posterior surface of the lungs (choice 4).

7. **The correct answer is 3.** The normal ranges for pH, $PaCO_2$, and HCO_3 are as follows:

- Normal pH range: 7.35–7.45
- Normal $PaCO_2$ range: 35–45
- Normal HCO_3 range: 22–26

The client's pH is alkalotic and the HCO_3 (bicarbonate) is elevated, which reflects a metabolic alkalotic state. The $PACO_2$, which is acid, is elevated to try and compensate for the alkalotic environment. Since the pH has not been corrected, the result is a partially compensated metabolic alkalosis.

8. **The correct answers are 2, 4, and 5.** Hypomagnesemia, hypophosphatemia, and hypokalemia are all associated with refeeding syndrome. The sodium level in choice 1 is at the high end of normal, while the chloride and calcium levels in choices 3 and 6, respectively, are within a normal range.

9. **The correct answer is 3.** The nurse should request that the client void before obtaining a stool sample to avoid contaminating the specimen with urine. The nurse is responsible for placing a small sample in a clean container (choice 1), not the client. It is not necessary to obtain a sample in the morning (choice 2). Choice 4 is incorrect because toilet tissue can be used, but the nurse should instruct the client to not contaminate the specimen with toilet tissue.

10. **The correct answer is 2.** A serum creatinine that is 2.1 mg/dL is significantly elevated. Administering iodinated contrast media places the client at risk for acute kidney injury. The platelet count shown in choice 1 is below normal but does not pose the most significant risk of harm to the client. The potassium and BUN levels shown in choices 3 and 4, respectively, are within normal ranges.

11. **The correct answer is 1.** Cardiac arrhythmias, which result in low perfusion, may interfere with the pulse oximetry readings. To verify the readings are accurate, the nurse will palpate the client's pulse and confirm that it correlates with the reading on the electrocardiographic waveform. It is not necessary to obtain blood pressure (choice 2) or an ECG (choice 3) or to place the pulse oximeter probe on the left extremity (choice 4) to validate a pulse oximeter reading.

12. **The correct answers are 3, 5, and 6.** A PaO_2 of 40 mmHg is associated with severe hypoxia. A pulse oximetry reading is inaccurate in severely hypoxic clients. Pulse oximetry can provide incorrect information for clients with carbon monoxide poisoning as it does not detect carbon dioxide levels, and it may not accurately help identify a hypoxic situation for a client with anemia. Pulse oximetry is useful for clients with pneumonia (choice 1) and hyperthermia (choice 2). A $PaCO_2$ 39 mmHg (choice 4) is normal.

13. **The correct answer is 3.** The nurse should continue monitoring. The heart rate on the ECG tracing is about 150 beats per minute, which is within the normal baseline for a newborn. There is no need to apply oxygen (choice 1), further assess the newborn (choice 2), or notify the health care provider (choice 4).

14. **The correct answer is 3.** A vacuum tube system should be used to obtain the sample to prevent having to transfer blood from a syringe to a tube. It is necessary to discard only the first 3–5 mL of blood, not the first 10 mL as choice 1 indicates. The nurse is not required to use a mask (choice 2) during the procedure. The PICC line should be flushed with 10–20 mL of normal saline after obtaining the sample, but not before as choice 4 indicates.

15. **The correct answers are 5 and 6.** A client receiving contrast dye is monitored for contrast-induced kidney damage. Serum creatinine and the glomerular filtration rate reflect the function of the kidney. Serum protein (choice 1), glucose (choice 2), uric acid (choice 3), and bilirubin (choice 4) are not used to assess the renal system for damage.

16. **The correct answer is 4.** The statement by the client that she will increase the amount of sports drinks when losing fluids indicates an understanding of the nurse's teaching. A client with an ileostomy is at risk for electrolyte imbalance. Sports drinks can help replace lost electrolytes during times of fluid loss. Enteric-coated or time-released prescriptions (choice 3) may not be adequately absorbed in clients with proximal ileostomies. A client with an ileostomy should avoid the intake of a high amount of insoluble fiber (choice 1) to prevent obstruction. An ileostomy should not be irrigated (choice 2), as it can increase the risk for dehydration.

17. **The correct answer is shown below.** An ileostomy is a procedure in which the small intestine is usually diverted through the lower right quadrant of the abdominal wall.

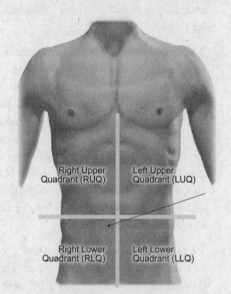

Abdominopelvic Quadrants

18. **The correct answers are 2, 4, and 6.** Chewing gum, carbonated beverages, and drinking through a straw are some of the actions that contribute to flatulence. Caffeine (choice 1) can cause dehydration. Dairy products (choice 3) and processed foods (choice 5) are not specifically associated with flatulence for a client with an ileostomy.

19. **The correct answer is 2.** The overflow of saliva into the larynx from the proximal esophageal pouch causes a laryngeal spasm resulting in cyanosis. The secretions should

be immediately suctioned from the oro-pharynx to prevent aspiration. Administering oxygen (choice 1) will not resolve the cyanosis. The infant should be repositioned in a supine position with the head elevated at least 30° after suctioning the secretions, rather than being repositioned laterally (choice 3). It is not necessary to prepare for endotracheal intubation (choice 4).

20. **The correct answer is 2.** An echocardiogram is used to evaluate the size, structure, and movement of the heart and is most useful in assessing cardiac defect. Chest radiography (choice 1), an electrocardiogram (choice 3), and an MRI (choice 4) are not used to evaluate a newborn for a congenital heart defect.

21. **The correct answers are 1, 4, 5, and 6.** Laboratory results that are monitored for a client experiencing hypotonic fluid volume excess include BUN, hematocrit, serum sodium, and urine specific gravity. These laboratory values are decreased due to the hemodilution that has occurred. Albumin (choice 2) and creatinine (choice 3) are not specifically monitored for hypotonic fluid volume excess.

22. **The correct answer is 4.** The statement from the parent that she will rub some lotion on the baby's dry skin before phototherapy indicates that further teaching is needed. Lotion or creams on a newborn's skin places the newborn at risk for burns because the lotions or creams can absorb heat. The mask can be removed during feedings (choice 1). The eyes are closed before putting a mask over them (choice 2) to avoid corneal abrasion. The newborn should be repositioned at least every two hours (choice 3) to maximize skin exposure.

23. **The correct answer is 2.** The area being treated can be covered with soft, loose clothing. Radiation therapy for breast cancer does not pose a risk to others; therefore, it is not necessary to limit visitors to 30 minutes per day (choice 1) or wear a dosimeter film badge while caring for the client

(choice 4). There is no need to make sure a lead container is available in the client's room (choice 3).

24. **The correct answer is 3.** The client with an open lung biopsy will have a chest tube placed to remove air and fluid so the lung can be reinflated. A CPAP (choice 1) is not used for the treatment of a client who has had a lung biopsy. Neither a ventilator (choice 2) nor a blood transfusion (choice 4) is an anticipated treatment for a client with an open lung biopsy.

25. **The correct answer is 3.** The assessment portion of the SBAR tool reflects findings such as vital signs, laboratory findings, clinical impressions, or concerns. Providing information such as the admission diagnosis (choice 1) and history (choice 4) reflects the client's background, and suggesting interventions (choice 2) is a recommendation.

26. **The correct answers are 1, 2, 3, and 5.** Safe practices for newborn identification include the use of ID band barcoding, two body-site identification, a distinct naming system, and ensuring the information on the band is legible. Using the number on the infant alarm band (choice 4) and placing the mother's room number on the newborn's crib (choice 6) are not appropriate methods for newborn identification.

27. **The correct answer is 4.** A behavioral contract is a client-centered approach that may be useful when a client experiences ongoing undesirable behavior. Redirection (choice 1) is used after undesirable behavior to re-engage the client in a more appropriate action, but does not address the actual behavior. Limit setting (choice 2) is preferably done in advance before the problem behavior. Modeling behavior (choice 3) is a method of learning behaviors through observation but does not address the client's actual behavior.

28. **The correct answer is 1.** Applying pressure when opening the eye should be avoided. The client is instructed to look up (choice 3)

to expose the conjunctiva. As soon as the eye is thoroughly flushed, the orbit of the eye is gently patted dry (choice 2), carefully avoiding the area over the eye. The flow of irrigation will be directed from the inner to outer canthus (choice 4) to prevent further contamination or injury to the eye.

29. **The correct answers are 1, 3, 4, and 5.** The airbags must be turned off, the infant rear-facing, the car seat placed at a 45° angle to prevent slumping and airway obstruction, and all shoulder belts must be tucked under the seat or somewhere away, so they do not cross over the infant's face or body. The infant should never be placed facing forward (choice 2), especially in the front seat of a car with an airbag, due to a serious injury that can be caused if the airbag deploys.

30. **The correct answer is 42 mL/hr.**

$$6 \text{ hrs.} \times 60 \text{ minutes} = 360 \text{ minutes}$$

$$\frac{1,000 \text{ mL}}{360 \text{ min}} \times \frac{15 \text{ (gtt)}}{1 \text{ mL}} = \frac{15,000}{360}$$
$$= 41.6$$
$$= 42 \text{ mL/hr.}$$

31. **The correct answer is 3.** A client expressing the desire to hurt himself who has a history of a suicide attempt has the highest risk for suicide. Feelings of hopelessness (choice 1), accessibility to weapons (choice 2), and a client with a family member who has committed suicide (choice 4) are risk factors but not the highest ones.

32. **The correct answer is 3.** The nurse's statement that based on initial data, changes can be made to the project indicates an understanding of conducting a performance improvement project. Publishing data (choice 1), randomization (choice 2), and forming a hypothesis to advance general knowledge (choice 4) reflect the components of a research project.

33. **The correct answer is 2.** Frustration is a stage of the conflict that requires clarification. Reviewing the department's

expenditures (choice 1) and intended goals for the change (choice 2) or explaining the practicality of the staffing pattern (choice 4) do not directly address the nurse's feelings of frustration.

34. **The correct answer is 3.** A mastectomy places the client at risk for difficulty coping with her body image. Offering the client the opportunity to discuss her feelings conveys support and will provide further information to help the nurse identify the appropriate interventions that may be helpful to the client. Telling the client that it is normal to experience difficulty with coping (choice 1) minimizes the client's feelings. Responding to the client about the concern for her inability to cope with the change (choice 2) is an assumption and may block any further communication. Solutions or interventions can be offered (choice 4) after the nurse has gathered more information through the exploration of the client's feelings.

35. **The correct answer is 3.** Clients who require a renal diet should avoid or limit foods high in sodium. Roast beef has the least amount of sodium. Ham (choice 1), pastrami (choice 2), and grilled cheese (choice 4) are all high in sodium.

36. **The correct answer is 4.** An infant laying on the daybed with a parent is at risk for falling. Preventing injuries for a pediatric client includes leaving the door of a child's room open (choice 1) and keeping the side rails of a child's bed raised (choice 2). A parent pulling a child with an IV in a wagon (choice 3) is not a safety risk unless the client is too young or has a condition that prohibits the activity.

37. **The correct answer is 1.** Stridor is a symptom of a narrowed airway and requires immediate intervention. Hoarseness (choice 3) and a sore throat are common after extubating a client. Difficulty speaking (choice 4) may be the result of vocal cord irritation or a sore throat and requires further assessment, but does not require the most

immediate attention. It is usual for large amounts of oral secretions (choice 2) to be present immediately after extubating a client for which oral suctioning may be needed to protect the airway.

38. **The correct answer is 3.** The nurse should let the client know that the insurance company requires that the client provide permission to obtain medical information. A client must sign a consent to release medical records to a third-party payer, such as an insurance company. With a client's permission, the insurance company may acquire the medical record for review of claims (choice 4). The insurance company does not have an automatic right to any client's medical records (choice 1) without the client's consent. While it is true that the insurance company cannot share personal information, this is not the best answer, as it provides no supporting information.

39. **The correct answers are 1, 2, and 4.** The principle information the nurse will use to identify the clients at risk of adversely reacting to a prescription include history, assessment, and laboratory data. Physical activity (choice 3), socioeconomic status (choice 5), and adherence to treatment (choice 6) are not associated with a high risk of reacting adversely to a prescription.

40. **The correct answer is 2.** Further teaching is needed if the client indicates that she may experience vaginal leakage of fluid. The client should be instructed to report any vaginal fluid leakage as this may indicate the amniotic sac has ruptured. The client may have difficulty getting comfortable, and sleep is interrupted by the need to urinate frequently (choice 1). The leakage of colostrum occurs (choice 3), and Braxton Hicks contractions (choice 4) are noticeable in the third trimester.

41. **The correct answer is 3.** Two-part breathing exercises focus on abdominal breathing and interrupting thoughts. Slow deep breathing and relaxing the muscles (choice 1),

deep inhalations and imagining a peaceful scene (choice 2), and relaxing the muscles and interrupting thoughts (choice 4) are not the correct combinations used in two-part breathing for anxiety.

42. **The correct answer is 2.** The client experiencing mania should be placed by the nursing station because she is at most risk for injury. A client with anorexia nervosa (choice 1), depersonalization-derealization disorder (choice 3), or schizophrenia (choice 4) with delusions of her food being poisoned are not at the most risk for injury and therefore do not require a room by the nursing station.

43. **The correct answer is 2.** Products with the identical brand name may have different active ingredients. Brand names in one country are different from brand names used in another country. Generic names of drugs in other countries may also be different (choice 1). The differences in the classification of the prescription (choice 3) or the measurement systems (choice 4) is irrelevant.

44. **The correct answers are 1, 2, 5, and 6.** Newborn wake states include crying, drowsy, quiet alert, and active alert. Irritable (choice 3) is not considered a wake state. Light sleep (choice 4) is a sleep state.

45. **The correct answer is 3.** Autonomy promotes the personal freedom and self-determination of the client. Fidelity (choice 1) is keeping one's promises or commitments. Veracity (choice 2) is concerned with telling the truth. Beneficence (choice 4) refers to the actions one takes to promote the good of the client.

46. **The correct answer is 4.** Malnutrition can result in decreased levels of plasma protein which reduces the protein binding activity of drugs. Plasma protein binding affects the time the drug stays in the body and the drug's efficacy. Doxycycline is a high plasma protein binding medication which may be ineffective in treating a client with a decreased level of plasma protein. Phenelzine (choice 3) is a monoamine oxidase inhibitor,

and atenolol (choice 1) is a beta-blocker. Both are water-soluble drugs, as is folic acid (choice 2), which do not require a significant amount of plasma protein to be present.

47. **The correct answer is 1.** The use of sustained-released formulations should be avoided. The client should take the lowest effective dosage of medication (choice 2) and avoid medications with a long half-life (choice 3). Taking medication immediately after breastfeeding (choice 4) will minimize the drug concentration in the milk with the next feeding.

48. **The correct answer is 2.** The client's statement about everyone else starting their period should raise some concern. If an adolescent does not enter puberty at the same time as her peers, considerable inner conflict may occur. It is normal for adolescents to show interest in appearances and attractiveness (choice 1). There is nothing concerning regarding the client's comments about adjusting to wearing a bra (choice 3) or experiencing confusion about the physical changes (choice 4) that occur during adolescence. Confusion regarding body changes is expected.

49. **The correct answer is 3.** Performing fundal massage stimulates uterine contractions and allows for an initial assessment to help determine the source of bleeding, which most frequently occurs from uterine atony. Starting an IV line (choice 1), administering oxygen (choice 2), and placing the client in Trendelenburg (choice 4) are not the initial interventions for a client experiencing a postpartum hemorrhage.

50. **The correct answers are 2, 3, 4, and 5.** The nurse should let the client know that he may attend as many meetings as needed, the 12-step program can help to stop the gambling through the support of others, and that the client can obtain a sponsor for support while he works through the 12 steps of the program. Gamblers Anonymous is a 12-step program that is a self-help group; it does not

offer group therapy, so choice 1 would be incorrect information to relay to the client.

51. **The correct answers are 1, 2, 5, and 6.** Risk reduction, emotional well-being, violence and injury prevention, and social and academic competence are areas that are important for the nurse to address throughout adolescence. Cognitive development (choice 3) and community affiliations (choice 4) are not areas of focus that are necessary to address during adolescence.

52. **The correct answer is 3.** Beneficence refers to the actions one takes to promote the good of the client. The principle of justice (choice 1) refers to treating others with equitability and fairness. Fidelity (choice 2) is keeping one's promises or commitments, and nonmaleficence (choice 4) means doing no harm to the client.

53. **The correct answers are 1, 2, 3, and 4.** Fluid management such as overhydrating, consuming alcohol, or drinking caffeinated beverages can contribute to stress incontinence. Increased dietary fiber will decrease constipation, which can cause urinary leakage. A bladder training program and pelvic floor strengthening are recommended to increase the amount of urine that can be held in the bladder and strengthen the muscles which are weakened. Intermittent catheterization (choice 5) and pharmacological treatment (choice 6) are not initial interventions for a female client experiencing stress incontinence. Topical vaginal estrogen may be useful for clients nearing menopause or who are postmenopausal.

54. **The correct answer is 1,120 units/hr.**

$$\frac{20,000 \text{ units}}{500 \text{ mL}} = 40 \text{ units/mL}$$

$$40 \text{ units} \times 30 \text{ mL/hr.} = 1,120 \text{ units/hr.}$$

55. **The correct answer is 3.** Enterobiasis causes intense perianal rectal itching. The child's nails should be kept short to minimize the chance of reinfection as ova can collect under the child's fingernails when scratching. The

child's bedding should be washed in hot water but does not need to be thrown away (choice 1). Spraying disinfectant in the air (choice 2) will not eradicate the eggs. Bathing (choice 4) increases the risk of reinfection; the child should shower daily.

56. **The correct answer is 2.** The staples should be removed, starting with the second staple and then removing every other staple to prevent wound dehiscence. The staples should not initially be removed from the middle of the incision (choice 1). Aseptic technique is used to clean the incision site before and after removal of the staples (choice 4) and prior to placing steri-strips over the area where the staple has been removed (choice 3).

57. **The correct answers are 2, 3, 4, and 6.** The UAP can remove a client's SCDs prior to ambulation, transport a stable client to the radiology department, notify housekeeping to refill the hand sanitizer, and prepare a room for a client who will be admitted with kidney stones. The nurse will remove the surgical dressing (choice 1) to assess the incision and reassess a client's pain (choice 5).

58. **The correct answer is 3.** The client with sickle cell anemia receiving a blood transfusion is the most appropriate assignment for the pediatric nurse. Sickle cell anemia occurs in infancy, childhood, and adolescence. The client with hypokalemia (choice 1) is at risk for cardiac arrhythmias. The client with congestive heart failure due for furosemide (choice 2) and the client with chronic pancreatitis (choice 4) who requires discharge teaching are not the most appropriate clients to assign the pediatric nurse.

59. **The correct answer is 2.** If the client indicates that he will go to the gym in the evening so that he will tire out, then further teaching is needed. Strenuous activities in the evening can perpetuate insomnia. Milk (choice 1) contains L-tryptophan, which promotes sleep. Journaling (choice 3) may help the client relieve stress. Maintaining the same sleep schedule (choice 4) helps establish a sleep-wake pattern.

60. **The correct answers are 1, 2, 4, and 6.** Tinnitus, confusion, hyperthermia, and respiratory depression are signs and symptoms associated with salicylate toxicity. Bradycardia (choice 3) and hypertension (choice 5) are not associated with salicylate toxicity.

61. **The correct answers are 1, 3, 4, and 5.** Vaccinations recommended for the older adult include the flu vaccine, shingles vaccine, pneumococcal vaccine, and the tetanus and diphtheria booster. The meningococcal vaccine (choice 2) is not included in the recommendations. The tetanus, diphtheria, pertussis vaccine (choice 6) should only be administered if the client did not receive the vaccine as an adolescent; otherwise, the tetanus-diphtheria booster is recommended every ten years for an older adult.

62. **The correct answers are 1, 2, and 3.** The first stage of pertussis is the catarrhal stage, which begins with symptoms of an upper respiratory tract infection—fever, coughing, and signs of coryza such as lacrimation. Flushed cheeks (choice 4) and a protruding tongue (choice 5) occur during the paroxysmal stage.

63. **The correct answer is 36 mL/hr.**

Convert pounds to kilograms:

$$\frac{210 \text{ lb.}}{2.2 \text{ kg}} = 95.45 \text{ kg} = 95.5 \text{ kg}$$

Calculate the micrograms:

$$95.5 \text{ kg} \times 5 \text{ mcg/kg/min} = 477.5 \text{ mcg/min}$$

Calculate the micrograms per hour:

$$477.5 \text{ mcg/min} \times 60 \text{ min/hr.} = 28,650 \text{ mcg/hr.}$$

Convert the micrograms to milligrams and calculate the hourly rate:

$$28,650 \text{ mcg/hr.} = \frac{28.65 \text{ mg}}{200 \text{ mg}} \times 250 \text{ mL}$$
$$= 35.81$$
$$= 36 \text{ mL/hr.}$$

64. **The correct answer is 3.** The priority for the nurse is to visit the client with rheumatoid arthritis experiencing unrelieved pain. A client with a stage III wound (choice 1) is not urgent. A hemoglobin A1c (choice 2) can be drawn at any time throughout the day. Weight gain of 2 lbs. in 48 hours is not significant for a client with CHF (choice 4).

65. **The correct answer is 4.** The nurse must be familiar with the contractual constraints of the insurance that is reimbursing the health care organization for the client's care. There are different rules regarding different costs related to the types of services covered. Nurses should be knowledgeable about the health care agency's fiscal budget (choice 1), staffing budget (choice 2), and capital expenditure (choice 3) to practice cost-conscious nursing.

66. **The correct answer is 1.** Saw palmetto is used to reduce the symptoms of an enlarged prostate, which includes urinary frequency. Saw palmetto is not used to treat premature ejaculation (choice 2) or erectile dysfunction (choice 3). Dribbling of urine (choice 4) is a symptom associated with an enlarged prostate.

67. **The correct answer is 2.** If the client indicates that he will avoid taking naps during the day, then further teaching may be required. The client should plan naps to sustain alertness, but no later than midday to avoid disruption of sleep at night. Daily exercise (choice 1), avoiding heavy meals before bedtime (choice 3), and lowering the environmental temperature (choice 4) will promote sleep.

68. **The correct answer is 3.** The nurse should respond by telling the client that they need to talk about how the client is feeling. This will enable the nurse to assess the client's current mental state to ensure that she will demonstrate safe behavior before releasing her from seclusion. Initially telling the client that her behavior will need to be discussed (choice 1) may cause a defensive reaction. Advising the client that she can come out of the seclusion room if she takes her medication (choice 2) is unethical and can result in intentional tort. Using the health care provider as a delay in releasing the client from seclusion (choice 4) is inappropriate and may further agitate the client.

69. **The correct answer is 4.** Numbness in the extremities is a symptom of hyperkalemia and may indicate overtreatment has occurred. Expected findings associated with hypokalemia include decreased reflexes (choice 1); a weak, thready pulse (choice 2); and abdominal distension (choice 3).

70. **The correct answers are 1, 3, 4, and 5.** The statements that reflect direct participation in health care cost-effectiveness include acknowledging new equipment is not necessary and examining staffing designs to provide more efficient care. The concern about the client's ability to obtain prescriptions and social services assisting clients in obtaining community resources will decrease the chance of the client being readmitted to the health care facility. Discussing projected costs of treatment (choice 2) includes the client in the decision making process and provides the client information needed to make health care decisions, but is not directly related to cost-effectiveness.

71. **The correct answer is 15 mL.**

$$\frac{480 \text{ mg}}{160 \text{ mg}} \times 5 \text{ mL} = \frac{2,400}{160} = 15 \text{ mL}$$

72. **The correct answer is 1.** The nurse will need to further educate the client who indicates that he will cover the unit when he showers. The client must be disconnected from the wound vac therapy system before showering. The other statements communicate to the nurse that the client understands the provided safety education. A cord plugged in areas where people are walking (choice 3) can result in an accident. The use of extension cords (choice 2) should be avoided, and the unit automatically turns off if there is a sudden increase in blood in the tubing or cannister (choice 4).

73. The correct answers are 1, 3, and 6. Cryoprecipitate is used for the replacement of fibrinogen for a client who is at risk for bleeding or who has lost blood. The specific laboratory results used to evaluate treatment with cryoprecipitate include an aPTT, fibrinogen, and an internationalized normal ratio. Platelets (choice 2), red blood cells (choice 4), and hemoglobin and hematocrit (choice 5) are not initially affected by the administration of cryoprecipitate but are influenced by the restoration of hemostasis.

74. The correct answers are 3, 4, and 5. Cognitive reframing assists a client in viewing a situation differently, problem solving skills enable the client to actively participate and improve his situation, and assertiveness training allows the client to make decisions for himself proactively. Personalization (choice 1) and emotional reasoning (choice 2) are not coping skills; they are cognitive distortions.

75. The correct answers are 2, 3, and 4. Variable costs are directly correlated with client volume or acuity and include medications, unit supplies, and nursing personnel. Fixed costs of a unit are those that do not change, including utilities (choice 1), administrative salaries (choice 5), and the minimum staffing required to keep the unit open (choice 6).

76. The correct answer is 1. The ECG rhythm denotes the client is experiencing ventricular fibrillation, which requires emergent treatment. CPR should immediately begin until defibrillation is initiated (choice 2). The client is ventilated with 100% oxygen (choice 4), and an IV is started (choice 3).

77. The correct answer is 2. A nurse prepared for disaster training should be familiar with the facility's disaster plan. Disaster management includes setting up triage (choice 1), knowing who to call in the community for further resources (choice 3), and knowledge of the personal protective equipment (choice 4) needed to manage the situation.

78. The correct answer is shown below. The T wave reflects the repolarization of the ventricles in the cardiac cycle.

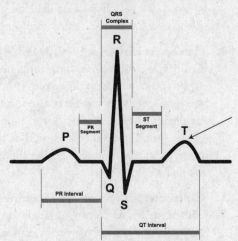

79. The correct answer is 3. The chain of command reflects the line of authority in a health care facility. The nurse will follow the health care facility's chain of command to resolve the issue. The director of nursing (choice 2) may not be formally identified as the initial contact in the health care facility's chain of command, so it is essential to adhere to the organizational chart that delineates who is to be immediately notified. The incident will be reported to the risk management department (choice 1), but the initial action is aimed at protecting the client. The emergency department provider (choice 4) may not be identified as the first contact in the chain of command.

80. The correct answer is 3. An open tibial fracture is classified as urgent. The classification of urgent includes a client who has a significant injury requiring treatment within 30 minutes to two hours. A sprained ankle (choice 1) is considered non-urgent. Airway obstruction (choice 2) and myocardial infarction (choice 4) are emergent, as they are an immediate threat to the client's life.

81. The correct answer is 4. The initial nursing assessment is the client's level of consciousness, as many clients with bradycardia are asymptomatic. Symptoms associated with hypoglycemia do include a change in the level of consciousness, so this initial assessment is important. The client's pulse (choice 1), blood glucose (choice 2), and blood pressure (choice 3) can be assessed accordingly.

82. **The correct answers are 1, 2, 3, and 6.** Garlic, ginger, and cloves have antiplatelet effects and can increase the client's risk for bleeding. Cranberry juice may also increase the client's risk of bleeding. Grape juice (choice 4) and apple juice (choice 5) do not interact with warfarin or place the client at risk for bleeding.

83. **The correct answers are 1, 2, 3, and 5.** Most toddlers at 18 months can say single words, drink from a cup, scribble with a crayon, and point to objects they want. An 18-month-old toddler may cling to caregivers in new situations and may not separate easily (choice 4) and is not expected to understand words like *in* and *under* (choice 6).

84. **The correct answer is 4.** Levothyroxine is used to treat hypothyroidism, which is associated with a decreased amount of energy. A therapeutic effect of levothyroxine is an increase in energy. Tachycardia is not a symptom of hypothyroidism, so choice 1 does not apply. The client should not continue to gain weight (choice 2), as this is a symptom of hypothyroidism. Little need for sleep (choice 3) may be an indication the client's dosage of levothyroxine is too high.

85. **The correct answer is 3.** The primary care provider refers clients to specialists such as orthopedic providers. The need for a referral of a medical nature indicates the client is experiencing a health care deficit and requires treatment from a medical or nurse practitioner. Many insurance companies require a referral. Referrals also contain information another clinician may need, which increases the chance the client will follow through with treatment. Providing the client with a list of orthopedic clinicians to choose from (choice 1) or calling an office to make an appointment (choice 2)

are not appropriate unless a referral has been obtained. The nurse cannot copy the client's medical records without consent, and copying the records does not facilitate a referral (choice 4).

86. **The correct answers are 1, 3, 4, and 5.** Decreasing distraction, such as environmental noise, promotes a relaxing environment. Adequate nonglaring lighting is provided; the client is toileted before meals; and all emesis basins, bedpans, or urinals should be placed in the bathroom. Interruptions during mealtimes should be avoided, so frequent checks (choice 2) should be avoided. The client should sit in a chair at mealtimes, rather than being positioned in bed (choice 6).

87. **The correct answers are 1 and 3.** The nurse cannot order treatments or consultations unless there is a standing prescription or protocol granting that authority to the RN. The nurse may make social services and or crisis intervention referrals. Laboratory testing (choice 2), ongoing medical treatment, access to care that is geographically closer (choice 4), or a physical therapy consult (choice 5) all require a referral by a health care practitioner.

88. **The correct answer is 2.** Insulin glargine U-300 is three times as concentrated as insulin glargine U-100 and the duration of action is more than 24 hours. Therefore, the client will only need to take the insulin once a day. Glargine is a clear insulin, so it will not appear cloudy (choice 1). Unopened pens with insulin glargine should be stored in the refrigerator (choice 3). The client will still require short-acting insulin (choice 4) before or right after eating a meal.

89. **The correct answer is 3.** During the initiation phase of a home visit, the initial nursing activity includes the initial clarification of the source of the referral with the client. During the pre-visit phase, the nurse will schedule the home visit (choice 1) and determine the family's willingness for a home visit (choice 4). When conducting the

actual in-home visit, the nurse will introduce herself and provide her professional identity (choice 2).

90. **The correct answer is 3.** Economic abuse occurs when a person in charge of a client's finances fails to utilize the funds appropriately. Neglect (choice 1) occurs when physical and medical care are not provided. Emotional abuse (choice 2) is systematic malicious manipulation through nonphysical acts. Psychological abuse (choice 4) is an attempt to distort another person's reality.

91. **The correct answer is 3.** Accommodation is the eye's ability to focus on near objects. When assessing the pupillary reflexes, the nurse is evaluating accommodation. Pupillary size (choice 1), shape (choice 2), and reactivity (choice 4) are not assessed during the evaluation of pupillary accommodation.

92. **The correct answers are 1, 4, 5, and 6.** Factors that increase the risk of child abuse include a nonbiological caregiver, children with chronic illness or the presence of congenital abnormalities, and a child younger than four years of age. A single income (choice 2) or single parent household (choice 3) does not specifically increase the risk of child abuse.

93. **The correct answer is 1.** The client receiving heparin with an aPTT of 25 seconds is at risk for bleeding. The acceptable range of an aPTT for a client receiving heparin is 30–40 seconds. The client with a platelet count of 130,000 (choice 2) is not at risk for bleeding. The client receiving brachytherapy with a temperature of 100.1°F and a WBC of 8,000 (choice 3) has a WBC count that is within an acceptable range and does not require an immediate assessment. The hemoglobin and hematocrit for the client with a femur fracture (choice 4) is within acceptable limits.

94. **The correct answers are 1, 3, 4, and 5.** An insulated dish will help keep food at the proper temperature as the client will need more time to eat. Grip scoop dishes and sectional plates prevent the dish from sliding away and can help with pushing food onto the utensils. Weighted utensils can help stabilize tremors. The cups should have wide handles for the client to grasp and lids to prevent spillage. A handleless cup (choice 2) would not be appropriate.

95. **The correct answer is 3.** The nurse should be most concerned with a housekeeping cart in the hall because the cart may have accessible cleaning chemicals that can be ingested by a child. This cart should be removed immediately. Unplugged IV pumps (choice 1) or an empty hand sanitizer dispenser (choice 2) are not the most immediate environmental concerns. A child can have stuffed animals in the bed (choice 4) as long as it is not contraindicated based on his or her condition.

96. **The correct answer is 3.** NPH is the only insulin that can be mixed with short-acting insulins. Only U-500 syringes should be used when drawing up U-500 insulin (choice 1). Long-duration insulins (choice 2) cannot be administered more than twice a day. A short-duration slower-acting insulin (choice 4) can be administered intravenously.

97. **The correct answer is 1.** The use of evidence-based practice allows the nurse to evaluate the current research and use it to problem solve and make decisions to improve the quality of care for the clients. Evidence-based practice is based on research (choice 2), but does have different levels of evidence. The nurse will adhere to the health care facility's policy and procedures (choice 3) or take a quality improvement approach by presenting evidence-based research to support making changes in the current policy and procedure. Performance improvement indicators are identified based on factors associated with the health care facility such as client outcomes, client feedback, length of stay, readmissions, increased length of stay, near misses, and sentinel events. Generally, researching evidence-based practice takes place after the performance improvement indicators have been identified (choice 4).

98. **The correct answer is 2.** A term newborn may consume 1 to 2 ounces of formula during a feeding and should not be overfed. Stroking the newborn's cheek (choice 1) or placing a small amount of formula on the nipple before feeding (choice 4) can entice the newborn to feed. The newborn can be laid in the mother's lap in a semi-upright position during a feeding (choice 3).

99. **The correct answers are 1, 2, 3, and 5.** Integumentary findings associated with poor hygiene include odor, rash, scales, and dryness. Pallor (choice 4) and coolness (choice 6) are not related to poor personal hygiene.

100. **The correct answer is 1.** The nurse will document the actual observation or instances where there is a concern. The documentation allows the nurse the opportunity to have a framework of reference when discussing the observations with the UAP (choice 3) and will allow the nurse to provide specific feedback. Also, the documented information can be provided to the manager (choice 2). The manager's role includes creating employee improvement plans (choice 4).

ANSWER SHEET: PRACTICE TEST 3

1. ① ② ③ ④	26. ① ② ③ ④	51. ① ② ③ ④	76. ① ② ③ ④
2. ① ② ③ ④	27. _____	52. ① ② ③ ④	77. ① ② ③ ④
3. ① ② ③ ④	28. ① ② ③ ④	53. ① ② ③ ④	78. ① ② ③ ④
4. ① ② ③ ④ ⑤ ⑥	29. ① ② ③ ④	54. ① ② ③ ④	79. ① ② ③ ④
5. ① ② ③ ④	30. _____	55. ① ② ③ ④	80. ① ② ③ ④
6. ① ② ③ ④	31. ① ② ③ ④	56. _____	81. ① ② ③ ④
7. ① ② ③ ④	32. ① ② ③ ④	57. ① ② ③ ④	82. ① ② ③ ④
8. ① ② ③ ④	33. ① ② ③ ④	58. _____	83. ① ② ③ ④
9. ① ② ③ ④ ⑤ ⑥	34. _____	59. ① ② ③ ④ ⑤ ⑥	84. ① ② ③ ④ ⑤ ⑥
10. ① ② ③ ④	35. ① ② ③ ④	60. ① ② ③ ④	85. ① ② ③ ④ ⑤ ⑥
11. ① ② ③ ④ ⑤ ⑥	36. ① ② ③ ④ ⑤ ⑥	61. ① ② ③ ④	86. _____
12. ① ② ③ ④	37. ① ② ③ ④	62. ① ② ③ ④	87. ① ② ③ ④
13. ① ② ③ ④	38. ① ② ③ ④ ⑤ ⑥	63. ① ② ③ ④	88. ① ② ③ ④
14. ① ② ③ ④	39. ① ② ③ ④ ⑤ ⑥	64. ① ② ③ ④	89. ① ② ③ ④
15. ① ② ③ ④	40. ① ② ③ ④	65. _____	90. ① ② ③ ④
16. ① ② ③ ④	41. ① ② ③ ④ ⑤ ⑥	66. ① ② ③ ④	91. ① ② ③ ④
17. ① ② ③ ④ ⑤ ⑥	42. ① ② ③ ④ ⑤ ⑥	67. ① ② ③ ④	92. ① ② ③ ④ ⑤ ⑥
18. ① ② ③ ④	43. _____	68. ① ② ③ ④ ⑤ ⑥	93. ① ② ③ ④
19. ① ② ③ ④ ⑤ ⑥	44. ① ② ③ ④	69. ① ② ③ ④	94. ① ② ③ ④
20. ① ② ③ ④	45. ① ② ③ ④	70. ① ② ③ ④	95. _____
21. ① ② ③ ④ ⑤ ⑥	46. ① ② ③ ④	71. ① ② ③ ④	96. ① ② ③ ④
22. ① ② ③ ④	47. _____	72. _____	97. ① ② ③ ④
23. ① ② ③ ④	48. ① ② ③ ④	73. ① ② ③ ④	98. ① ② ③ ④
24. ① ② ③ ④ ⑤ ⑥	49. ① ② ③ ④	74. ① ② ③ ④	99. ① ② ③ ④
25. ① ② ③ ④	50. ① ② ③ ④	75. ① ② ③ ④	100. ① ② ③ ④

Answer Sheet

Practice Test 3

100 Questions – 150 minutes

Directions: This test matches the current NCSBN NCLEX-RN test plan. You may encounter the following types of questions:

1. **Multiple-choice** questions that will have only one correct answer.
2. **Multiple-answer** questions that will have more than one correct answer.
3. **Fill-in-the-blank** questions that will require math calculations.
4. **Hot spot** questions, where you will mark a very specific location on an image.

Each item will require you to perform critical thinking. It is important that you identify exactly what the question is asking before moving on to the answer choices. For multiple-choice and multiple-response questions, read all the answer choices, choose the best answer(s), and fill in the corresponding circle(s) on the answer sheet. Take care to not just pick the first answer that makes sense. For fill-in-the-blank questions, use the appropriate math calculation and fill in the correct answer in the blank provided. For hot spot questions, follow the directions provided in the question to indicate the correct answer. An answer key and explanations follow the practice test.

1. The nurse is reviewing the laboratory results of a client scheduled for a procedure requiring general anesthesia. Which finding is of **most** concern to the nurse?

   1. White blood cells—12,000
   2. Sodium—145 mEq/L
   3. Potassium—3.3 mEq/L
   4. Platelets—140,000

2. Which **initial** action will the nurse take before removing a nasogastric tube?

   1. Flush the tubing.
   2. Clamp the tubing.
   3. Stop the wall suction.
   4. Disconnect the tubing.

3. Which technique will the nurse include when obtaining a sterile culture from a wound?

   1. Insert the sterile swab into the exudate.
   2. Use only sterile water to cleanse the wound.
   3. Obtain the culture after cleansing the wound.
   4. Apply clean gloves before irrigating the wound.

4. The nurse is preparing a postoperative plan of care for an infant undergoing the repair of a cleft palate. Which **immediate** postoperative interventions should the nurse include in the care? **Select all that apply.**

   1. Upright seating
   2. Elbow immobilizers
   3. Feeding as tolerated
   4. Nonnutritive sucking
   5. Orthodontic appliances
   6. Administration of analgesia

5. The nurse has provided education for a client with a fracture who will require traction. Which statement made by the client indicates further teaching is needed?

   1. "The traction will help reduce pain."
   2. "The traction will prevent infection."
   3. "The traction will reduce muscle spasms."
   4. "The traction will help immobilize the injury."

6. Which statement made by a client with a new plaster cast should be of concern to the nurse?

   1. "I will allow the cast to air-dry."
   2. "I will keep my casted arm elevated."
   3. "I will keep the joint below my injury immobilized."
   4. "I will apply ice packs around the cast to reduce the pain."

7. The nurse has completed the education for a client with an ileostomy. Which statement made by the client indicates an understanding of the teaching?

   1. "I will decrease the amount of sports drinks when I lose fluids."
   2. "If I get constipated, I can irrigate my ostomy."
   3. "I will use only enteric-coated prescriptions."
   4. "I will decrease my intake of insoluble fiber."

8. The nurse is preparing to care for a child receiving moderate sedation. Which assessment finding should the nurse anticipate?

   1. Cognitive function may be impaired.
   2. The client responds to verbal commands.
   3. The ability to maintain the airway may be impaired.
   4. The client can be easily aroused with painful stimuli.

9. Which findings should the nurse be **most** concerned about for a client who is recovering from a coronary artery bypass graft (CABG)? **Select all that apply.**

   1. Decreasing somnolence
   2. Jugular venous distention
   3. Chest tube drainage of 50 mL/hr.
   4. Cessation of previously heavy mediastinal drainage
   5. Blood pressure of 20 mmHg or higher on inspiration than expiration
   6. A pulmonary arterial wedge pressure higher than the right atrial pressure

10. For which type of brain imaging should the nurse anticipate preparing for a client who is suspected of having a brain attack (stroke)?

    1. Ultrasound evaluation
    2. Positron emission tomography (PET)
    3. Magnetic resonance imaging (MRI) with contrast
    4. Computerized tomography (CT) without contrast

11. Which cerebral spinal fluid (CSF) assessment findings will the nurse anticipate for a client with bacterial meningitis? **Select all that apply.**

    1. Clear appearance
    2. Elevated glucose
    3. Increased sodium
    4. Decreased protein
    5. Elevated CSF pressure
    6. Increased white blood cells

12. Which **initial** position should the nurse assist the client into during preparation for a lumbar puncture?

    1. Prone
    2. Supine
    3. Semi-Fowler's
    4. Lateral recumbent

13. The nurse has completed the postprocedural teaching for a client scheduled for cerebral angiography. Which statement made by the client indicates further education is required?

   1. "I will need to increase my fluids."

   2. "I will have to lay flat for a while."

   3. "I will be sleepy after the procedure."

   4. "I will be able to put ice on the injection area."

14. The nurse notes the injection site of a client post cerebral angiography is slightly swollen. Which intervention should the nurse implement?

   1. Palpate the site.

   2. Apply ice to the site.

   3. Elevate the extremity.

   4. Apply a pressure dressing.

15. The nurse is monitoring the lab values for a client receiving oxygen therapy. Which finding indicates adequate gas exchange is occurring?

   1. pH 7.36 mmHg

   2. PaO_2 92 mmHg

   3. HCO_3 25 mEq/L

   4. $PaCO_2$ 34 mmHg

16. Which assessment finding will the nurse be **most** concerned about for the client post electroconvulsive therapy?

   1. Jaw pain

   2. Disorientation

   3. Muscle tremors

   4. Retrograde amnesia

17. Which should the nurse anticipate documenting for a client who is to receive a blood transfusion? **Select all that apply.**

   1. Client education

   2. Clinical indication

   3. Informed consent

   4. Blood compatibility

   5. Name of the component

   6. Donor identification number

18. The nurse has provided discharge teaching for a client with a halo fixation device. Which statement indicates further education is required?

   1. "I will not drive my vehicle."

   2. "I will avoid touching the pin sites."

   3. "I will use a straw when drinking fluids."

   4. "I can use a small pillow while sleeping."

19. Before administering a prescription, which should the nurse recognize as placing the client at a higher risk for adverse reactions? **Select all that apply.**

   1. Genetics

   2. Cognition

   3. Drug allergies

   4. Pathophysiology

   5. Capacity for self-care

   6. Lifespan considerations

20. Which factor alters the absorption of oral medication in a newborn infant?

   1. Increased gastric acidity

   2. Increased gastric emptying time

   3. Decreased absorption in the stomach

   4. Decreased drug absorption in the intestine

21. Which current medications should the nurse be concerned about for a client who states she has begun taking black cohosh? **Select all that apply.**

   1. Aspirin

   2. Labetalol

   3. Melatonin

   4. Metformin

   5. Evening primrose oil

   6. Estradiol/norgestimate

Practice Test 3

22. A client tells the nurse the prescription that is about to be administered is incorrect. Which action should the nurse take?
    1. Review the client's medical history.
    2. Consult with the health care provider.
    3. Review the health care provider's prescriptions.
    4. Educate the client about the purpose of the prescription.

23. The nurse who has been caring for a post-operative client on the unit is updating the charge nurse about the client's condition. Which statement should be of concern to the charge nurse?
    1. "I have raised the half-side rails at the head of the bed."
    2. "I have instructed the client to call for help before getting out of bed."
    3. "I have communicated to the health care team the client's risk for falling."
    4. "I have monitored the client's risk for falls based on the score of the fall risk assessment."

24. The educator is preparing to discuss intimate partner violence with the nursing staff. Which will the educator include when presenting the risk factors? **Select all that apply.**
    1. Chronic illness
    2. Unemployment
    3. Social isolation
    4. Low self-esteem
    5. Religious beliefs
    6. Unplanned pregnancy

25. The nurse notes that a client's IV pump has been programmed incorrectly by a nurse on the previous shift. After correcting the rate and assessing the client, which **initial** action should the nurse take?
    1. Disclose the incident to the client.
    2. Discuss the finding with the nurse.
    3. Report the incident to risk management.
    4. Document the occurrence in the client's record.

26. The nurse has provided education regarding exercise and health for an older female client. Which statement made by the client indicates further teaching is required?
    1. "Stretching will improve my range of motion."
    2. "Exercise will help increase my triglyceride levels."
    3. "I will use resistance training to prevent osteoporosis."
    4. "Aerobic exercise will improve the blood flow to my heart."

27. The health care provider has prescribed diazepam 6 mg IV push. The nurse has diazepam 5 mg/mL available. How many mL will the nurse administer? _____ mL

28. The nurse observes a health care provider who is not on a client's treatment team reading the client's records. Which action should the nurse take?
    1. Immediately notify risk management of the incident.
    2. Ask the health care provider why he is reading the client's records.
    3. Ask the client if the health care provider has been permitted to review the records.
    4. Review the client's records for written permission for the health care provider to access the information.

29. Which action should the nurse take when documenting additional information in a client's record several hours after the original documentation has been recorded?

    1. Document the information based on the time it occurred.

    2. Document the information by adding a late entry to the record.

    3. Provide a note as to why the information was not documented previously.

    4. Delete the original documentation and concisely redocument the information.

30. What is the BMI for a client who is 5 feet 6 inches tall, weighing 113 lbs.? **Round to the nearest tenth.** _____

31. The educator has reviewed the fundamental components of quality nursing documentation with the nurse. Which statement made by the nurse indicates further teaching is required?

    1. "I have documented the support I provided the client."

    2. "I have documented the client's response to the treatment."

    3. "I have documented a list of tasks that I have accomplished."

    4. "I will document the client's concerns about her treatment."

32. For which developmental change reported by the parent of an adolescent should the nurse be concerned?

    1. "My child has become difficult to wake up for school."

    2. "My child seeks out friends for advice instead of the family."

    3. "My child has become completely disrespectful of my rules."

    4. "My child does not want to spend much time with the family."

33. Which is the **most** appropriate referral for a family member who tells the nurse she is exhausted from caring for her parent with Alzheimer's disease?

    1. Respite care

    2. Counseling services

    3. Long-term care facility

    4. Community support group

34. The health care provider prescribes a 4 gram IV bolus of magnesium sulfate to be infused over 20 minutes. The nurse has available 4 grams of magnesium sulfate in 100 mL of D5W. What is the hourly rate for which the nurse will program the infusion pump? _____mL/hr.

35. After calculating the BMI of a client who is 5 feet 3 inches tall weighing 142 pounds, under which category will the nurse document the client's weight? **Round the calculation to the nearest tenth.**

    1. Underweight

    2. Normal weight

    3. Overweight

    4. Obese

36. A client asks the nurse how a 23-hour crisis stabilization can benefit him. Which information will the nurse provide to the client? **Select all that apply.**

    1. "The goal is to de-escalate the crisis quickly."

    2. "This service can prevent costly hospitalization."

    3. "This type of crisis service does not require payment."

    4. "You will be provided referrals for further treatment."

    5. "You will be stabilized and transferred to a residential program."

    6. "You will be provided support from others who have experienced psychiatric disorders."

Practice Test 3

37. Which is the **primary** goal during the initial interview of a client experiencing a crisis?

   1. Reduce symptoms of disorganization.

   2. Implement immediate problem solving.

   3. Stabilize the client's psychological condition.

   4. Determine what kind of crisis the client is experiencing.

38. Which of the following infectious diseases are mandated to be reported? **Select all that apply.**

   1. Tetanus

   2. Shingles

   3. Influenza

   4. Giardiasis

   5. Hepatitis A

   6. Cytomegalovirus

39. Which factors indicate a client can be safely transferred using a standing pivot method? **Select all that apply.**

   1. Poor posture

   2. Full weight-bearing

   3. Partial weight-bearing

   4. Able to follow directions

   5. Limited upper body strength

   6. Inability to follow instructions

40. A client newly diagnosed with human immunodeficiency virus expresses concern about her personal information being included in the mandated reporting. Which information should the nurse provide the client?

   1. "Your personal information is only reported to the state."

   2. "Your personal information is only reported to the CDC."

   3. "Your personal information is not shared with the state or the CDC."

   4. "Your personal information is kept confidential by the state and the CDC."

41. Which should the nurse incorporate into practice to prevent errors when receiving telephone orders from the health care provider? **Select all that apply.**

   1. Do not accept abbreviations.

   2. Read the order back to the prescriber.

   3. Request the indication for the prescription.

   4. Ensure required client identifiers have been verified.

   5. Transcribe the order directly into the client's record.

   6. Avoid taking telephone orders for high-risk medications.

42. Which ethical principles describe the client's right to know when an error has been made that requires additional treatment to correct? **Select all that apply.**

   1. Justice

   2. Veracity

   3. Autonomy

   4. Beneficence

   5. Nonmaleficence

   6. Right to self-determination

43. A health care provider prescribes 3 grams of magnesium sulfate per hour. The nurse has 40 grams of magnesium in 1,000 mL of D5W available. What setting will the nurse use when programming the infusion pump? _____ mL/hr.

44. Which assessment question will the nurse **initially** ask the client who has experienced intimate partner violence?

   1. "Do you have safe shelter?"

   2. "Do you feel like hurting yourself?"

   3. "Do you want me to call the police?"

   4. "Is there someone you would like me to call?"

45. Which intervention for comfort should the nurse anticipate for the client who had a transurethral resection of the prostate (TURP)?

  1. Toileting every two hours

  2. Intermittent catheterization

  3. Continuous bladder irrigation

  4. Intermittent bladder irrigation

46. Which statement made by a nurse caring for a client with an internal radiation implant indicates further education is required?

  1. "I will minimize the time in the client's room."

  2. "I have informed the client that she is radioactive."

  3. "I will make sure to wear a dosimeter film badge at all times."

  4. "I will keep all linens, trash, and food trays in the client's room."

47. At which location should the nurse place the bell of the stethoscope to auscultate the renal arteries? **Circle the correct location.**

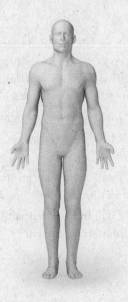

48. A client tells the nurse he is unsure if he wants to go through with the treatment plan. Which question will the nurse ask the client?

  1. "Can you tell me what you feel is best for you at this time?"

  2. "Can you tell me what you understand about your treatment plan?"

  3. "Can you tell me why you are so unsure about your treatment plan?"

  4. "Can you explain why you are considering refusal of the treatment plan?"

49. In which order will the nurse don PPE before entering a client's room?

  1. Mask, gown, gloves, goggles

  2. Gown, mask, goggles, gloves

  3. Mask, goggles, gown, gloves

  4. Gloves, gown, mask, goggles

50. The nurse has provided education for an older client receiving a pneumococcal vaccine. Which statement made by the client indicates an understanding of the information?

  1. "I will only need to get the pneumococcal vaccine once."

  2. "I will get my pneumococcal vaccine when I get my flu vaccine."

  3. "The pneumococcal vaccine will provide immunity against viruses."

  4. "The pneumococcal vaccine will help protect me against meningitis."

51. Which statement made by a new nurse about the family of a client who has died should be of concern to the educator?"

  1. "The family chose not to have the chaplain present."

  2. "I don't understand why the family does not seem upset."

  3. "I told a family member I just did not know what to say."

  4. "I shed a few quiet tears when I told the family I was sorry for their loss."

52. With which movement will the nurse intervene when observing a client using a cane?

   1. The client holds the cane on the strong side.

   2. The client looks down at his feet when walking with the cane.

   3. The client moves the cane and the affected leg together when taking a step.

   4. The client's bad leg assumes the first full weight-bearing step when descending the stairs.

53. Which statement made by a client regarding obtaining personal medical information indicates the client requires education?

   1. "I may have to pay to have my medical records copied."

   2. "I have to pay my medical bill before I can get my records."

   3. "I can access some of my medical information through a client portal."

   4. "I have the right to get my medical records within 30 days of my request."

54. The nurse has provided education about safe drinking water in the home for an immunocompromised client. Which statement made by the client indicates further teaching is required?

   1. "I will avoid drinking any fountain drinks."

   2. "I will drink commercially distilled water."

   3. "I will change the filter cartridge on my water filter."

   4. "I will avoid drinking water and ice from the refrigerator dispenser."

55. Which client will the postpartum nurse see **first**?

   1. A client six hours post vaginal delivery requesting pain medication for cramping

   2. A client three hours post vaginal delivery who needs assistance to the bathroom to void

   3. A client one day postoperative cesarean section requesting help with changing the newborn's diaper

   4. A client 24 hours postoperative cesarean delivery who is requesting to visit her baby in the neonatal intensive care unit

56. The health care provider has prescribed 60 mg of hydrocortisone. The nurse has available ampules of hydrocortisone containing 50 mg in 2 mL. Identify the volume of the drug to be drawn up. **Draw an arrow to the correct place.**

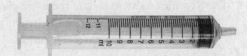

57. The nurse has provided education about the protection of skin integrity for a client in a wheelchair. Which statement made by the client indicates further teaching is needed?

   1. "I will report any weight gain."

   2. "I have obtained a foam seat cushion to sit on."

   3. "I will change my position in the chair every hour."

   4. "I will lift my body with my arms when transferring myself."

58. Which anatomical location should the nurse anticipate to assess the site of a pacemaker? **Circle the correct location.**

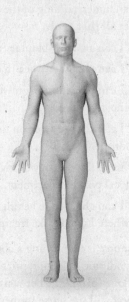

59. The nurse is providing education for a client and her spouse regarding the use of patient-controlled anesthesia (PCA) following surgery. Which information will the nurse include? **Select all that apply.**

   1. "The prescribed medication will eliminate your pain."
   2. "To receive a dose of medication, you just push the button."
   3. "You will be receiving a continuous low dose of pain medication."
   4. "There is a limit on the total dosage in a set time that you can receive."
   5. "The PCA will allow you and your spouse to control your pain effectively."
   6. "There is an automatic delay in the timing of the delivery of the medication."

60. A client who is hearing-impaired indicates she did not understand what the nurse has said. Which action will the nurse take?

   1. Repeat the sentence.
   2. Rephrase the sentence.
   3. Repeat the sentence raising the tone of voice.
   4. Repeat the sentence exaggerating the movements of the lips.

61. The nurse is evaluating the ECG tracing of a client with a pacemaker. Based on the evaluation of the tracing below, which part of the client's heart is paced?

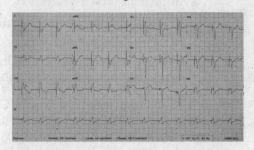

   1. Atria
   2. Ventricles
   3. Atria and ventricles
   4. Bundle of His

62. When making shift assignments on the telemetry unit, which client will the charge nurse assign to the new nurse?

   1. A client with atrial fibrillation receiving warfarin
   2. A client with angina scheduled for a cardiac catheterization
   3. A client with congestive heart failure receiving diuretics and digitalis
   4. A client who has returned to the unit after implantation of a pacemaker

Practice Test 3

63. Which intervention will the nurse implement for a client experiencing vomiting during a tube feeding?

1. Flush the tube.
2. Assess the residual.
3. Stop the tube feeding.
4. Decrease the rate of feeding.

64. After receiving the shift handoff, which client will the nurse see **first**?

1. A client with a deep vein thrombosis rating her pain a six out of ten
2. A client with hypothyroidism who is experiencing muscle weakness
3. A client with acute glomerulonephritis with a blood pressure of 170/98
4. A client with peripheral vascular disease experiencing intermittent claudication

65. A provider prescribes a client heparin 32 units per kg/hr. The client weighs 167 lbs. The heparin solution available is 20,000 units in 250 mL of 0.9% normal saline. For how many mL/hr. will the nurse program the pump? **Round to the nearest tenth.** _____ mL/hr.

66. Which will the nurse consider before choosing a topic for community health promotion?

1. Culture
2. Ethnicity
3. Spiritual practices
4. Socioeconomic status

67. The nurse is monitoring a client post pericardiocentesis. For which clinical finding will the nurse **immediately** notify the health care provider?

1. Fatigue
2. Tachycardia
3. Hypertension
4. Low-grade fever

68. The nurse has discussed the benefits of a psychiatric advanced directive with a client. Which statements made by the client indicate an understanding of the information? **Select all that apply.**

1. "I can avoid involuntary treatment."
2. "I can choose my health care providers."
3. "I can predetermine my treatment choices."
4. "I can choose a person to make decisions for me."
5. "I can leave a copy of my plan with the local police department."
6. "I can choose the health care facility where I would like treatment."

69. The nurse is monitoring a client treated for syndrome of inappropriate antidiuretic hormone (SIADH). For which assessment finding will the nurse **immediately** notify the health care provider?

1. Headache
2. Vomiting
3. Hypertension
4. Muscle weakness

70. Which **primary** intervention will the nurse initiate for a client with an electrical burn?

1. Initiate an IV.
2. Obtain an ECG.
3. Provide analgesics.
4. Maintain the temperature.

71. A nurse is preparing to provide education about the glucocorticoid prescribed for a client with gout. Which benefit of the treatment will the nurse discuss with the client?

1. Analgesic properties
2. Lowering uric acid levels
3. Anti-inflammatory effects
4. Facilitation of the excretion of uric acid

72. The nurse is discussing with a client where the tuning fork will be placed during the Weber test. Which location will the nurse identify? **Circle the correct location.**

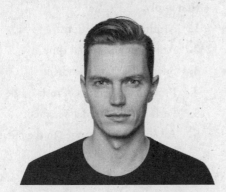

73. Which statement is appropriate to document in a client's record?
    1. The client appears to be sleeping.
    2. The client consumed all of his lunch.
    3. The client accidentally slipped on the floor.
    4. The client unintentionally pulled out the IV catheter.

74. The nurse has provided education for a client regarding acute pancreatitis. Which statement made by the client indicates an understanding of the information?
    1. "My urine may be darkened."
    2. "I will avoid drinking caffeine."
    3. "I plan on eating a low-sodium diet."
    4. "I may experience clay-colored stools."

75. Which position will the nurse use for the client with gastroesophageal reflux disease to decrease gastric acid reflux?
    1. Supine
    2. Left lateral
    3. Right lateral
    4. Semi-Fowler's

76. The nurse has provided a client education about the signs to expect before labor. Which statement made by a client indicates further education is needed?
    1. "My baby will become less active."
    2. "I may lose a few pounds before labor."
    3. "I will be able to breathe a little easier."
    4. "I may see blood-tinged vaginal mucous discharge."

77. A client discharged from the hospital with facial burns tells the nurse that even though she has been seeing a counselor, she is nervous about going out in public. Which intervention can a nurse suggest to help a client adapt to the changes?
    1. Reassure the client that the area is still healing.
    2. Suggest having friends visit at home for short periods.
    3. Inform the client she will eventually have plastic surgery.
    4. Encourage the client to discuss her feelings with the counselor.

78. Which assessment finding should the nurse be **most** concerned with for a client with acute diverticulitis?
    1. Melena
    2. Constipation
    3. Rigid abdomen
    4. Temperature of 101°F

79. The nurse is preparing to assess a client with a 10-year history of smoking 1.5 packs of cigarettes daily who has not had a cigarette in 48 hours. Which assessment finding should the nurse anticipate?
    1. Diarrhea
    2. Lethargy
    3. Insomnia
    4. Weight loss

Practice Test 3

80. Which will the nurse **not** include in the management of an arterial line?

1. Calibrating the monitor.
2. Performing square wave testing.
3. Ensuring the pressure bag is inflated to 100 mmHg.
4. Placing the transducer at the level of the left atrium.

81. The educator is discussing a client's plan of care with a nurse. Which statement made by the nurse indicates further education is required?

1. "I will evaluate the client's plan of care upon discharge."
2. "I will update the client's plan of care before the shift handoff."
3. "I have adjusted the client's interventions based on a change in condition."
4. "I have added another nursing diagnosis due to the change in the client's condition."

82. Which food will the nurse instruct the client prescribed oral calcium to limit in her diet?

1. Eggs
2. Yogurt
3. Spinach
4. Almonds

83. The nurse is reviewing the medical history of a 28-year-old client who is requesting oral contraceptives. For which finding should the nurse recognize that oral contraceptives are contraindicated?

1. Asthma
2. Dysmenorrhea
3. Raynaud's disease
4. Polycystic ovary syndrome

84. The nurse is preparing to conduct a routine physical assessment for an older client. Which interventions will the nurse plan to implement during the assessment? **Select all that apply.**

1. Minimize distractions.
2. Allow for additional time.
3. Speak clearly to the client.
4. Provide for periods of rest.
5. Perform a focused assessment.
6. Avoid sudden changes in the client's position.

85. Which interventions will the nurse implement to prevent contractures for a client with burns on his head, neck, and upper chest? **Select all that apply.**

1. Pillow
2. No pillow
3. Neck splint
4. Turn head side to side
5. A towel roll under the neck
6. Folded towel under the spine between the scapulae

86. When evaluating a client's arterial waveform, which will the nurse identify as the systolic and diastolic pressure? **Label both on the diagram below.**

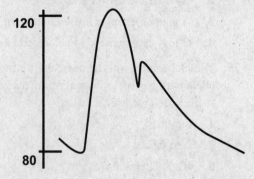

87. The nurse is assessing a client who had a chest tube inserted two hours prior. For which finding should the nurse **immediately** notify the health care provider?

   1. Oxygen saturation of 93%
   2. Chest tube stopped draining
   3. Erythema at the insertion site
   4. Fluctuation in the water seal chamber

88. The nurse has provided education for a client prophylactically prescribed nitrofurantoin. Which statement indicates further teaching is required?

   1. "My urine may turn brown."
   2. "I will take the prescription on an empty stomach."
   3. "The prescription is active against bacteria in the urine."
   4. "I will call my health care provider if I experience symptoms of a UTI."

89. The nurse is preparing to perform a cardiac assessment on a client with mitral valve prolapse. Which area of the client's chest should the nurse anticipate auscultating for a murmur?

   1. Fifth intercostal space (ICS), left mid-clavicular line
   2. Fourth left ICS, left sternal border
   3. Second left ICS, left sternal border
   4. Second right ICS, right sternal border

90. Which assessment finding should the nurse anticipate for a client with a tolerance to morphine?

   1. Epiphora
   2. Bradycardia
   3. Constipation
   4. Overnutrition

91. The nurse has received a dyspneic client suspected of having carbon monoxide poisoning. Which **initial** intervention will the nurse implement?

   1. Provide rescue breathing.
   2. Prepare the client for hyperbaric oxygen therapy.
   3. Administer 100% oxygen via a non-rebreather mask.
   4. Provide noninvasive continuous positive airway pressure.

92. The nurse is preparing to provide education for a client required to wear a pressure garment over the lower extremities as part of his burn rehabilitation. Which information will the nurse include in the teaching? **Select all that apply.**

   1. "The garment will reduce edema."
   2. "The garment will reduce scarring."
   3. "The garment promotes blood flow."
   4. "The garment is worn for 23 hours per day."
   5. "The garment may be worn for 12–24 months."
   6. "The garment will be applied after a skin graft procedure."

93. Based on the nurse's understanding of tissue injury, which reflects the fourth stage of wound healing?

   1. Thrombus has formed in the wound.
   2. Edema is present at the site of the injury.
   3. Reorganization of the collagen fiber occurs.
   4. Margins of the wound begin to pull together.

Practice Test 3

94. Which client condition may benefit from massage therapy?

1. Dermatitis

2. Osteoporosis

3. Rheumatoid arthritis

4. Congestive heart failure

95. At 1900 hours, a client's IV running at 75 mL/hr. has 600 mL remaining. What time should the nurse anticipate the infusion to be completed? _____

96. The nurse has provided information regarding the use of lemongrass oil for a client. Which statement made by the client indicates further education is required?

1. "I will discontinue the use of the oil if I suspect I am pregnant."

2. "I will avoid applying the oil directly to the mucous membranes."

3. "I will make sure the room I am using the oil in is well-ventilated."

4. "I will be sure to only apply a minimal amount directly to my skin."

97. Which type of immune response is a client exhibiting who has a poison ivy skin rash?

1. Cytotoxic reaction

2. Delayed hypersensitivity

3. Immune complex reaction

4. Immediate hypersensitivity reaction

98. At the end of the day, the nurse realizes a client's morning medication was overlooked when the pharmacy did not send it to the unit. Which option reflects the appropriate documentation in the client's records?

1. "0900 acetaminophen dose omitted, health care provider notified, no changes in the treatment plan, no changes in the client's condition."

2. "Health care provider notified of 0900 acetaminophen omission, no changes in client's condition, pharmacy notified of oversite."

3. "Health care provider and client informed of omission of the 0900 acetaminophen dose, occurrence report filed."

4. "Client did not receive the 0900 acetaminophen dose due to an oversight by the pharmacy, health care provider notified."

99. Which laboratory data will the nurse anticipate assessing before the initial administration of valproic acid?

1. Lipid levels

2. Liver function

3. Renal function

4. Platelet count

100. Which question should the nurse include in the **initial** assessment of an adolescent client with a major depressive disorder?

1. "How do you feel about your depression?"

2. "What do you do when you are feeling depressed?"

3. "When you feel depressed, what do you think about?"

4. "How has your depression affected your friendships?"

ANSWER KEY AND EXPLANATIONS

1. 3	**23.** 4	**45.** 3	**62.** 2	**82.** 3
2. 3	**24.** 2, 3, 4, 6	**46.** 2	**63.** 3	**83.** 3
3. 3	**25.** 3	**47.** LOCATION:	**64.** 2	**84.** 1, 2, 3, 4, 6
4. 1, 2, 3, 6	**26.** 2	to the right and	**65.** 30.4 mL/hr.	**85.** 2, 3, 4, 5, 6
5. 2	**27.** 1.2 mL	left sides of the	**66.** 2	**86.** POSITION:
6. 3	**28.** 2	abdomen, below	**67.** 1	arrows point to
7. 4	**29.** 2	the umbilicus	**68.** 2, 3, 4, 6	highest peak
8. 2	**30.** 18.2	**48.** 2	**69.** 3	and right end
9. 2, 4, 5	**31.** 3	**49.** 2	**70.** 2	of graph line
10. 4	**32.** 3	**50.** 4	**71.** 3	**87.** 2
11. 2, 5, 6	**33.** 1	**51.** 2	**72.** LOCATION:	**88.** 2
12. 4	**34.** 300 mL/hr.	**52.** 2	midline on the	**89.** 1
13. 3	**35.** 3	**53.** 2	client's head	**90.** 3
14. 1	**36.** 1, 2, 3, 4	**54.** 3	**73.** 2	**91.** 3
15. 2	**37.** 3	**55.** 2	**74.** 2	**92.** 1, 2, 3, 4, 5
16. 3	**38.** 1, 4, 5	**56.** 2.4 mL	**75.** 4	**93.** 3
17. 1, 5, 6	**39.** 1, 2, 3, 4, 5	**57.** 3	**76.** 1	**94.** 3
18. 2	**40.** 1	**58.** LOCATION:	**77.** 2	**95.** 0300
19. 1, 3, 4, 6	**41.** 1, 2, 3, 4, 5	under the col-	**78.** 3	**96.** 4
20. 2	**42.** 2, 3, 4, 5, 6	larbone on the	**79.** 3	**97.** 2
21. 1, 2, 4, 6	**43.** 75 mL/hr.	left side of the	**80.** 3	**98.** 1
22. 2	**44.** 2	chest wall	**81.** 1	**99.** 2
		59. 2, 3, 4, 6		**100.** 3
		60. 2		
		61. 1		

1. **The correct answer is 3.** Any potassium imbalance must be corrected before surgery. Hypokalemia places the client at risk for cardiac dysrhythmias and slows the recovery from anesthesia. An elevated white blood cell count (choice 1), a sodium level of 145 mEq/L (choice 2), or a platelet count of 140,000 (choice 4) are not the most concerning for the client who requires general anesthesia.

2. **The correct answer is 3.** Before removing a nasogastric tube, the wall suction is turned off. The tubing will then be disconnected (choice 4), flushed if needed (choice 1), and clamped (choice 2) so the secretions do not re-enter the tubing.

3. **The correct answer is 3.** Sterile normal saline should be used to irrigate the wound and remove the exudate before obtaining a culture. Use of sterile water instead of saline (choice 2) is not appropriate. The insertion

of a sterile swab into the exudate of a wound (choice 1) will contaminate the sterile specimen. The sterile swab should be used to obtain a culture from the wound after the exudate is removed. Sterile gloves (choice 4) are used when irrigating the wound.

4. **The correct answers are 1, 2, 3, and 6.** Immediate postoperative care includes upright seating to avoid aspiration of secretions and elbow immobilizers to prevent disruption of the suture line. The infant is fed as tolerated and analgesia is administered for pain. To prevent the disruption of the suture line, objects, such as a pacifier for nonnutritive sucking (choice 4), should not be inserted in the mouth. Orthodontic appliances (choice 5) may be used for long-term care to promote speech development, but are not part of the immediate postoperative interventions.

5. **The correct answer is 2.** If the client indicates that traction will prevent infection, then further teaching may be needed. Traction is used to help reduce pain (choice 1), reduce muscle spasms (choice 3), and immobilize the injury (choice 4), not reduce infection.

6. **The correct answer is 3.** To prevent complications, the client should not keep any joint either distal or proximal from the cast immobile. The cast should be allowed to air-dry (choice 1), the extremity should be elevated (choice 2), and ice packs can be used to help reduce the pain (choice 4).

7. **The correct answer is 4.** The client with an ileostomy is at risk for fluid and electrolyte imbalances. Decreasing the insoluble fiber intake will help to prevent obstruction. A client with an ileostomy should increase the amount of sports drinks consumed when there is a loss of fluids, not decrease as choice 1 indicates. An ileostomy should not be irrigated (choice 2) as it can increase the risk for dehydration. Enteric-coated or time-released prescriptions (choice 3) may not be adequately absorbed in clients with proximal ileostomies.

8. **The correct answer is 2.** The level of sedation the nurse should expect from a child receiving moderate sedation includes the ability to respond to verbal commands. The client's cognitive function will be impaired (choice 1), and the client's respiratory function (choice 3) will remain adequate. It is not necessary to use painful stimuli (choice 4) to arouse a client who has had moderate sedation.

9. **The correct answers are 2, 4, and 5.** The most concerning assessment findings for a client who has had a coronary artery bypass graft include jugular venous distention; cessation of previously heavy mediastinal drainage; and pulsus paradoxus, which is a blood pressure of 10 mmHg or higher on expiration than inspiration. Decreasing somnolence (choice 1) is an acceptable finding. Chest tube drainage of 50 mL/hr. (choice 3) following a CABG is insignificant, and the PAWP should be higher than the right atrial pressure (choice 6).

10. **The correct answer is 4.** A CT without contrast is used to diagnose a stroke. A CT scan is a quick, painless test that provides cross-sectional layers and detailed images of organs, tissues, bones, and tumors. Ultrasound evaluation (choice 1) is not used to diagnose a stroke. A PET scan (choice 2) requires the use of a radioactive tracer that is used to show images of bones and tissue, which is not helpful in the diagnosis of a stroke or identifying the type of stroke. Contrast medium (choice 3) is not used to diagnose a stroke because the stroke may have been hemorrhagic.

11. **The correct answers are 2, 5, and 6.** A client with bacterial meningitis will have elevated glucose and CSF pressure, as well as an increased WBC count. The appearance of the CSF will be cloudy rather than clear (choice 1), and the client will have an increased protein level (choice 4). The sodium (choice 3) in the CSF is not explicitly evaluated for a client suspected of having bacterial meningitis.

12. The correct answer is 4. The nurse will assist the client into a lateral recumbent position. Immediately before the procedure, the client will further be assisted into a fetal position. A lumbar puncture is not performed with a client in a prone (choice 1), supine (choice 2), or semi-Fowler's position (choice 3).

13. The correct answer is 3. The procedure does not require anesthesia; therefore, the client should not be sleepy after the procedure. The client should increase his fluids (choice 1) to help flush the iodinated contrast agent from the body and renal system. The client will keep his extremity flat and straight (choice 2) for a prescribed amount of time to decrease the risk of bleeding. Ice may be used on the injection site (choice 4) to help minimize discomfort and swelling.

14. The correct answer is 1. The client is at risk for a hematoma or bleeding at the injection site. The nurse will palpate the site for discomfort and assess for bleeding. Ice can be applied to the site (choice 2) after it is determined there are no abnormal assessment findings. The extremity should be kept straight and immobilized as prescribed by the health care provider, rather than being elevated (choice 3). The client will have a pressure dressing (choice 4) placed immediately after the procedure, so it is unnecessary to apply one at this point.

15. The correct answer is 2. The PaO_2 reflects the exchange of oxygen that passes through the alveoli into the arterial blood and is a primary measurement for effective respiratory gas exchange. A PaO_2 of 92 mmHg is within the normal range. The pH is the overall chemical balance in the body. A pH of 7.36 mmHg (choice 1) is on the low side. The HCO_3 is controlled by the kidneys and is the body's metabolic buffering system. An HCO_3 of 25 mEq/L (choice 3) is within the normal range. The $PaCO_2$ is a carbonic acid that is regulated by the respiratory system. A $PaCO_2$ of 34 (choice 4) is on the low side, which reflects a respiratory alkalotic state.

16. The correct answer is 3. A client who is post electroconvulsive therapy should not experience muscle tremors. The causative factor of the tremors should be identified, especially if the client is receiving other prescriptions included in her treatment. Jaw pain (choice 1), disorientation (choice 2), and retrograde amnesia (choice 4) may occur as a result of the procedure and are expected findings.

17. The correct answers are 1, 5, and 6. Anticipated documentation for a client who will receive blood products includes client education, name of the component, and the donor identification number. The clinical indication (choice 2), informed consent (choice 3), and blood compatibility (choice 4) should already be documented in the client's record and are included in the information that is verified.

18. The correct answer is 2. Further education may be required if the client indicates that she will avoid touching the pin sites. The client should be instructed to clean or have someone clean the pin sites as prescribed, in addition to inspecting the sites daily for drainage, redness, or any loosening. The client should not drive a car (choice 1), should use a straw when drinking (choice 3), and may use a small pillow while sleeping (choice 4).

19. The correct answers are 1, 3, 4, and 6. Genetics, drug allergies, pathophysiology, and lifespan are essential to consider before administering a prescription as they can be associated with the adverse effect of a prescription. Cognition (choice 2) does not specifically increase the client's risk of an adverse effect. The capacity for self-care (choice 5) is a consideration when the client will be required to manage his prescriptions, but is not a concern when being administered by the nurse.

20. The correct answer is 2. Gastric emptying time during the neonatal period is prolonged, which results in delayed absorption. Gastric acidity is decreased, rather than increased (choice 1). The absorption of drugs that are primarily absorbed in the intestine (choice 4) is delayed.

21. **The correct answers are 1, 2, 4, and 6.** Black cohosh may potentiate the effects of aspirin, labetalol, metformin, and estradiol/norgestimate. Melatonin (choice 3) and evening primrose (choice 5) are not contraindicated with the use of black cohosh.

22. **The correct answer is 2.** The nurse will discuss the client's concern with the health care provider. The client is regarded as an active participant in his care, and the nurse will listen to his concerns as the client may be aware of changes that may have been overlooked. Reviewing the client's medical history (choice 1), the health care provider's prescriptions (choice 3), and educating the client about the purpose of the prescriptions (choice 4) are inappropriate actions at this time.

23. **The correct answer is 4.** A fall risk scale is a tool used to identify clients at risk for falls; however, it is essential to consider other factors that place the client at risk for falls that may not be on the scale. Factors such as treatments, changes in physiological condition, or medications that may affect a client's reflexes or judgment all require the use of nursing judgment beyond the use of a scale. Full side rails (choice 1) require a health care provider's prescription. Communication (choice 3) and client education (choice 2) are essential for fall prevention.

24. **The correct answers are 2, 3, 4, and 6.** Risk factors for intimate partner violence include unemployment, social isolation, low self-esteem, and unplanned pregnancy. Chronic illness (choice 1) and religious beliefs (choice 5) are not directly associated with intimate partner violence.

25. **The correct answer is 3.** The nurse should report the medication error to the risk management department as well as the health care provider as soon as possible. After reporting, the nurse will collaborate with the risk management department and the health care provider as to how best to discuss the incident with the client (choice 1). While the nurse can discuss the finding with the nurse (choice 2), the initial priority is to report the occurrence as a medication error. Only pertinent clinical information should be documented in the client's record (choice 4).

26. **The correct answer is 2.** Further teaching may be required if the client indicates that exercise will help increase triglyceride levels. Exercise helps to *decrease* triglyceride levels and increase high-density lipoprotein. Stretching (choice 1) can improve the client's range of motion, weight-bearing exercise will help prevent osteoporosis (choice 3), and aerobic exercise (choice 4) improves blood flow to the heart.

27. **The correct answer is 1.2 mL.**

$$\frac{\text{Dose ordered}}{\text{Dose on hand}} \times \text{Quantity} =$$

$$\frac{6 \text{ mg}}{5 \text{ mg}} = 1.2 \text{ mL}$$

28. **The correct answer is 2.** The nurse must maintain the integrity of a client's records. Approaching the health care provider to ask why he is reading a client's records will provide information the nurse needs to have before implementing further action. It is premature to notify risk management (choice 1). Asking the client if the health care provider has permission to review his records (choice 3) can cause unnecessary alarm. Reviewing the client's records for written authorization for the health care provider to access the records (choice 4) delays intervening to protect the client's information.

29. **The correct answer is 2.** The nurse must maintain the integrity of the original documentation. A late entry can be added to the record to help supply additional information that was omitted from the original entry. The late entry should include the current date and time as well as the time of the occurrence. Additional entries should not be backdated or timed (choice 1), documentation as to why the information was initially

omitted (choice 3) is unnecessary, and deleting the initial documentation to "concisely" redocument the data (choice 4) is fraudulent.

30. **The correct answer is BMI = 18.2.**

Calculate the BMI using the formula:
$703 \times$ weight (lbs.) / [height (in)]^2

$$703 \times 113 = 79{,}439$$

Height is 66 inches, which is squared:

$$66 \times 66 = 4{,}356$$

$$\frac{79{,}439}{4{,}356} = 18.23 = 18.2$$

31. **The correct answer is 3.** Quality nursing documentation centers on the client, not a list of tasks. Documenting the support of a client (choice 1) reflects the nurse's work and time. Documentation of the client's response to treatments (choice 2) and concerns (choice 4) is appropriate and reflects quality nursing documentation.

32. **The correct answer is 3.** Adolescence is a time when independence is sought; however, complete disregard for the rules in the home is concerning behavior. A reluctance to get up early in the morning (choice 1) is a normal finding. Adolescents experience a delayed onset of sleep as a result of biological changes, but still require at least eight hours of sleep. Adolescents are seeking to assert independence, so it is normal to seek out peers (choice 2) and not want to spend as much time with the family (choice 4) as in the previous developmental stage.

33. **The correct answer is 1.** A caregiver who feels overburdened may benefit from a referral for respite care. Respite care can provide the caregiver a temporary break from the responsibility of caring for her family member. A referral for counseling services (choice 2) or to a long-term care facility (choice 3) is not appropriate. A community support group (choice 4) cannot provide the caregiver respite.

34. **The correct answer is 300 mL/hr.**

$$\frac{10 \text{ mL}}{20 \text{ min.}} \times 60 \text{ min.} = 300 \text{ mL/hr.}$$

35. **The correct answer is 3.**

Calculate the BMI using the formula:
$703 \times$ weight (lbs.) / [height (in)]^2

$$703 \times 142 \text{ lbs.} = 99{,}826$$

Height is 63 inches, which is squared:

$$63 \times 63 = 3{,}969$$

$$\frac{99{,}826}{3{,}969} = 25.15 = 25.2 \text{ (rounded)}$$

Based on the BMI index (shown below), a BMI of 25.2 indicates the client is overweight.

- Underweight BMI = less than 18.5
- Normal weight BMI = 18.5–24.9
- Overweight BMI = 25–29.9
- Obese BMI = 30 or more

36. **The correct answers are 1, 2, 3, and 4.** Goals of a 23-hour crisis stabilization include quick de-escalation of the crisis, prevention of costly hospitalization, and the provision of appropriate referrals for further treatment. As an additional advantage for the client, the 23-hour crisis stabilization does not require payment. The client who is stabilized (choice 5) is not necessarily transferred to a residential facility. Client support during a 23-hour crisis stabilization does not come from others who have experienced psychiatric disorders (choice 6); it is provided by health care professionals.

37. **The correct answer is 3.** During the initial interview, it is important to assist the client in feeling safe to help reduce anxiety, which will assist in stabilizing his psychological condition. Reduction of symptoms of disorganization (choice 1) and implementing problem solving (choice 2) will occur after the client has been psychologically stabilized. The type of crisis the client is

experiencing (choice 4) is determined when the client's thoughts are organized.

38. **The correct answers are 1, 4, and 5.** Tetanus, giardiasis, and hepatitis A are infectious diseases for which reporting is required. Shingles (choice 2), influenza (choice 3), and cytomegalovirus (choice 6) are not required to be reported.

39. **The correct answers are 1, 2, 3, 4, and 5.** A client who can be safely transferred using the standing pivot method can have poor posture and limited upper body strength, but must be able to bear weight (fully or partially) and follow directions. A client who cannot follow instructions (choice 6) cannot be safely transferred using the standing pivot method.

40. **The correct answer is 1.** The client's personal information is only reported to the state health department. The client's personal information is removed before sending the report to the CDC. The state maintains the confidentiality of the client's records; however, partner notification laws vary by state.

41. **The correct answers are 1, 2, 3, 4, and 5.** To prevent errors when taking a telephone order, the nurse should not accept abbreviations, will read the order back for verification, request the indication for the prescription, ensure the correct client has been identified, and transcribe the order directly into the client's record. Since there are emergent situations in which orders for high-risk medications are needed for a client, avoiding telephone orders (choice 6) is not a practical option.

42. **The correct answers are 2, 3, 4, 5, and 6.** The ethical principles associated with the client's right to know about an error which requires treatment include veracity, autonomy, beneficence, nonmaleficence, and the right to self-determination. Veracity requires that the client be provided comprehensive, objective information in a manner that helps her understand the information. Autonomy and the right to self-determination acknowledge the client's right to make

informed decisions regarding the additional treatment that is required. The principles of beneficence and nonmaleficence reflect the obligation to do what is best for the client and to avoid harm. Justice (choice 1) implies that all clients are treated fairly, which does not relate to this situation.

43. **The correct answer is 75 mL/hr.**

$$\frac{3 \text{ g}}{60 \text{ min.}} \times \frac{60 \text{ min.}}{1 \text{ hr.}} \times \frac{1,000 \text{ mL}}{40 \text{ g}} = \frac{180,000}{2,400}$$
$$= 75 \text{ mL/hr.}$$

44. **The correct answer is 2.** The safety of the client is always the nurse's first consideration, so the first step is to ensure the client does not intend to hurt herself. Establishing if the client has a safe shelter (choice 1), calling law enforcement (choice 3), or calling someone of the client's choice (choice 4) is not initial information to obtain.

45. **The correct answer is 3.** A client who has had a TURP will require an indwelling urinary catheter to provide continuous bladder irrigation. This is due to the client's decreased ability to void after the procedure, as well as the risk of blood clots forming and blocking the urine flow from the bladder. Continuous bladder irrigation is prescribed to maintain the client's comfort and ensure the urinary catheter is patent and draining.

46. **The correct answer is 2.** Further education would be required in the event that the nurse informed a client that she is radioactive. A client with an internal radiation implant is not radioactive; rather, the inserted implants are radioactive. No further education is required for the other answer choices. When caring for a client with an internal radiation implant, the nurse will minimize the time in the client's room (choice 1); wear a dosimeter at all times (choice 3); and keep all linens, trash, and food trays in the client's room (choice 4) while the client has the radiation implant in place. The health care facility's policy and procedures are followed for the restoration of the items to the client's

room after the client's radiation implants are removed.

47. The correct answer is shown below. The iliac arteries are located to the right and left sides of the abdomen, a couple of inches below the umbilicus.

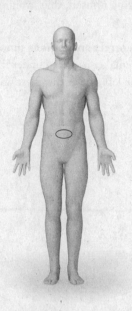

48. The correct answer is 2. The nurse should not assume a client understands a treatment plan and will seek clarification of the client's understanding. This action reflects advocacy for the client. If it is clear that the client understands the treatment, further discussion about what the client feels is best (choice 1) is pursued. Asking a client why he is unsure of his treatment plan (choice 3) is not helpful if he does not have a full understanding. Asking the client why he is considering refusal of the treatment plan (choice 4) does not foster therapeutic communication and also assumes that the client understands the plan of care.

49. The correct answer is 2. The order for donning PPE recommended by the CDC is the gown, mask, goggles, and gloves.

50. The correct answer is 4. The pneumococcal vaccine will help decrease the risk of meningitis. Choice 1 indicates that further clarification may need to be provided because

the CDC recommends two pneumococcal vaccines for adults over 65, so the client may receive the vaccine more than once. Choice 2 does not reflect an understanding of the information because pneumococcal vaccines should not be administered at the same time as a flu vaccine. Similarly, choice 3 does not reflect an understanding of the information as gram-positive bacteria may cause pneumococcal infections.

51. The correct answer is 2. Every family has their own manner of grieving. Making assumptions about a family's grief can interfere with the care that may be needed. The statement about the family's choice not to have the chaplain present (choice 1) conveys acknowledgment of the family's needs. Honesty with the family is essential, as it is not always easy to know what to say (choice 3). Nurse's may shed tears (choice 4), as long as it is not to the point where it is disruptive to the family's grieving.

52. The correct answer is 2. The nurse will intervene when the client looks down at his feet when walking with the cane. To avoid an accident, the client should look straight ahead. No intervention is needed if the cane is held on the strong client's strong side (choice 1) and is moved with the affected leg when taking a step (choice 3) on a flat surface. The nurse does not need to intervene if, when descending stairs, the client's bad leg assumes the first full weight-bearing step (choice 4).

53. The correct answer is 2. The client needs further education if she indicates that she will have to pay her medical bill before she can get her records. A client cannot be denied a copy of her medical records because the services have not been paid for. No further education is needed for the other answer options. There may be a reasonable cost-based fee associated with obtaining copies of medical records (choice 1). Client portals allow the client to view health care information (choice 3). HIPAA requires that copies of medical records be provided within 30 days of a request (choice 4).

54. The correct answer is 3. If an immunocompromised client indicates that he will change the water filter cartridge, then further teaching is required. The client should avoid touching the filter on the home water filtration system because the filters collect and may contain cryptosporidium and other infective bacteria or germs. Commercially distilled water (choice 2) is safe to drink. The client should avoid fountain drinks (choice 1), tap water, or using ice from the refrigerator dispenser (choice 4) because tap water may contain cryptosporidium.

55. The correct answer is 2. A client three hours post vaginal delivery who needs assistance to the bathroom to void should be seen first. A postpartum client with a full bladder can result in uterine atony, placing the client at risk for postpartum hemorrhage. The clients requesting a prescription for uterine cramping (choice 1), assistance with a diaper change (choice 3), and transport to the neonatal intensive care unit (choice 4) are not priorities.

56. The correct answer is 2.4 mL.

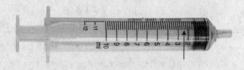

$$\frac{\text{Dose ordered}}{\text{Dosage on hand}} \times \text{Quantity} = \text{mL}$$

$$\frac{60 \text{ mg}}{50 \text{ mg}} \times 2 = 2.4 \text{ mL}$$

57. The correct answer is 3. If the client indicates that he will change his position in the chair every hour, then further teaching is needed. The client's weight should be shifted in the wheelchair every 15 minutes to help protect the integrity of the skin. No further teaching is needed if the client makes the statements listed in the other answer choices.

Any weight gain should be reported to the health care provider (choice 1) to evaluate the client's fit in the wheelchair. A foam seat cushion (choice 2) will help prevent skin breakdown. Lifting the body with the arms (choice 4) will prevent the client from dragging himself, thus avoiding injury to the skin.

58. The correct answer is as shown. Generally, a pacemaker is placed under the collarbone on the left side of the chest wall.

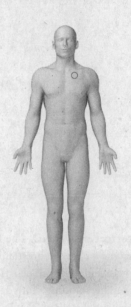

59. The correct answers are 2, 3, 4, and 6. The PCA pump allows a client to self-administer pain medication with a push of a button. The PCA pumps are programmed to deliver a prescribed amount of medication within a specific time frame and are also programmed to delay or lock out the further delivery of medication when the limit has been reached. A basal rate may be prescribed, which allows for continuous low dose delivery of the medication. The prescribed medication is not intended to eliminate the client's pain (choice 1). The client is the only person who should push the button (choice 5). A family member pressing the PCA button while the client is sleeping places the client at risk for respiratory depression and respiratory arrest.

60. **The correct answer is 2.** When a hearing-impaired client indicates she did not understand what the nurse has said, the nurse will rephrase the information. The sentence should not be repeated (choice 1) as it was stated the first time. Raising the tone of voice (choice 3) and exaggerating the movement of the lips (choice 4) will not improve the understanding or clarity of the information for the client who is hearing-impaired.

61. **The correct answer is 1.** Atrial pacemakers affect the sinoatrial node, which is reflected by a spike followed by the P wave and a normal QRS complex. When the ventricles are paced (choice 2), the spike follows a wider QRS complex. When both the atria and ventricles are sequentially paced (choice 3), the spike follows the atrial and ventricular complexes (P wave and QRS complex). The bundle of His (choice 4) is part of the electrical conduction system of the heart that transfers electrical impulses from the atrioventricular node to the ventricle of the heart and is responsible for electroconductivity through the ventricles (QRS complex).

62. **The correct answer is 2.** The client with angina scheduled for a routine procedure, such as a cardiac catheterization, is the most stable client and is an appropriate assignment for a new nurse. A client with atrial fibrillation receiving warfarin (choice 1) is at risk for pulmonary emboli, systemic emboli such as an embolic stroke, and bleeding from the treatment with warfarin. The client with congestive heart failure receiving diuretics and digitalis (choice 3) is at risk for fluid and electrolyte imbalances. A client who has had implantation of a pacemaker (choice 4) requires monitoring for hemorrhage as well as ECG monitoring to ensure the pacemaker is working correctly.

63. **The correct answer is 3.** The client who is vomiting during a tube feeding is at risk for aspiration. The nurse will stop the tube feeding. Neither flushing the tubing (choice 1) or decreasing the rate (choice 4) of the feeding will reduce the risk of client aspiration. Assessing the residual (choice 2) is not the first action to take.

64. **The correct answer is 2.** The nurse will see the client with hypothyroidism first. The client with hypothyroidism is at risk for a myxedema coma. Symptoms of a myxedema coma include hyponatremia, which is characterized by muscle weakness. Pain is expected to be associated with deep vein thrombosis (choice 1). Hypertension is a symptom of acute glomerulonephritis (choice 3). Intermittent claudication (choice 4) is an expected finding related to peripheral vascular disease.

65. **The correct answer is 30.4 mL/hr.**

$$\frac{167 \text{ lbs.}}{1} \times \frac{1 \text{ kg}}{2.2 \text{ lbs.}} \times \frac{32 \text{ units/hr.}}{1 \text{ kg}}$$
$$\times \frac{250 \text{ mL}}{20,000 \text{ units}} \times \frac{1,336,000}{44,000}$$
$$= 30.3636364 = 30.4 \text{ mL/hr.}$$

66. **The correct answer is 2.** The nurse will consider the ethnicity of the community when choosing a topic for health promotion. Some diseases are more prevalent in certain ethnicities, whereas the other choices are unlikely to relate to specific physiological disorders. Culture (choice 1) describes the values, beliefs, and behavior of groups of people. Spiritual practices (choice 3) are actions or activities undertaken that foster an individual's spiritual growth. Socioeconomic status (choice 4) can have a general effect on a community's health, but the educational topic chosen requires more specificity.

67. **The correct answer is 1.** The client who has had a pericardiocentesis is at risk for cardiac tamponade. Fatigue is one of the symptoms associated with cardiac tamponade. Other symptoms include bradycardia and hypotension, so tachycardia (choice 2) and hypertension (choice 3) would not need to be immediately reported to the health care provider. A low-grade fever (choice 4) does not warrant immediate reporting.

68. **The correct answers are 2, 3, 4, and 6.** A psychiatric advanced directive is used in a crisis and allows for the client to choose her preferred health care facility and health care provider, as well as allowing her to predetermine treatment choices and choose a person to make decisions for her. The document can *reduce* the risk of involuntary treatment (choice 1), but does not *prevent* involuntary treatment. A copy of the psychiatric advanced directive should be left in the client's home in a safe place with other important papers, where it can be easily located. A copy should be placed on file with the local hospital, rather than the police department (choice 5).

69. **The correct answer is 3.** When correcting SIADH, the client is at risk for hypernatremia, for which hypertension is a symptom. The nurse must immediately notify the health care provider if hypertension is present. A client with SIADH experiences dilutional hyponatremia characterized by expected symptoms of headache (choice 1), vomiting (choice 2), and muscle weakness (choice 4). As these choices are expected, they do not warrant immediate notification of the health care provider.

70. **The correct answer is 2.** The primary intervention in this case is to obtain an ECG. The client with an electrical burn requires ECG monitoring due to the risk of life-threatening cardiac arrhythmias. General management for clients with burn injuries includes the initiation of an IV (choice 1), analgesics for pain (choice 3), and maintenance of the body temperature (choice 4).

71. **The correct answer is 3.** Glucocorticoids reduce the inflammation resulting from gout. Glucocorticoids do not have analgesic properties (choice 1), nor do they lower uric acid levels (choice 2) or facilitate the excretion of uric acid (choice 4).

72. **The correct answer is shown below.** When conducting the Weber test, after gently striking the tuning fork, it is placed midline on the client's head to evaluate if the vibration is detected in both ears.

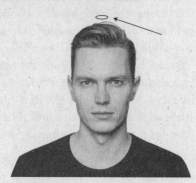

73. **The correct answer is 2.** Documentation of a client consuming all of his lunch is an objective statement and therefore suitable for inclusion in the client's record. Words such as *appears* (choice 1), *accidentally* (choice 3), and *unintentionally* (choice 4) are not objective and should be avoided when documenting assessment findings.

74. **The correct answer is 2.** Clients experiencing acute pancreatitis should avoid caffeine and alcohol. The client should notify the health care provider if he experiences darkened urine (choice 1) or clay-colored stools (choice 4). A low-fat diet, rather than a low-sodium diet (choice 3), is included in the treatment plan.

75. **The correct answer is 4.** The client with gastroesophageal reflux disease will be placed in a semi-Fowler's position to prevent reflux. Supine positioning (choice 1), left lateral (choice 2), and right lateral (choice 3) do not decrease acid reflux.

76. **The correct answer is 1.** Further education is needed if the client indicates that her baby will become less active. Fetal movement should not decrease before delivery. The client is instructed to monitor fetal movement using a method of kick counts and to contact the health care provider if decreased fetal movement is noted. A loss of 0.5 to 1.5 kg can occur in the later days preceding labor (choice 2). The presenting part of the fetus descends into the pelvis, making it easier for the client to breathe (choice 3), and the

client may notice a vaginal mucous discharge involving brownish or blood-tinged mucous (choice 4).

77. **The correct answer is 2.** Friends visiting the client at home for short periods offers the client the opportunity to socialize and may help the client begin to develop self-confidence as she continues through the recovery process. Reassuring the client that the burn areas are still healing (choice 1) or that she can have plastic surgery (choice 3) does not address her immediate feelings or concern, nor does referring her back to the counselor (choice 4).

78. **The correct answer is 3.** A client with diverticulitis is at risk for peritonitis, which is characterized by a rigid abdomen. Melena (choice 1), constipation (choice 2), and a temperature of 101°F (choice 4) are symptoms associated with acute diverticulitis and therefore should be expected.

79. **The correct answer is 3.** Symptoms of nicotine withdrawal, such as insomnia, begin about 24 hours after the last cigarette. Diarrhea (choice 1), lethargy (choice 2), and weight loss (choice 4) are not associated with nicotine withdrawal, although diarrhea is a symptom of nicotine toxicity. Other symptoms of nicotine withdrawal include irritability and increased appetite.

80. **The correct answer is 3.** The pressure bag should be inflated to 300 mmHg to prevent the retrograde flow of blood and to keep the arterial line patent with a heparinized normal saline solution. Square wave testing (choice 2) is performed to determine if the arterial wave is overdamped or underdamped. The monitor is calibrated (choice 1) and the transducer placed at the level of the left atrium (choice 4).

81. **The correct answer is 1.** The client's plan of care should be evaluated throughout the stay, not at the point of discharge. The plan of care can be updated before providing a shift handoff (choice 2). The client's interventions (choice 3) and nursing diagnosis (choice 4) are updated based on the client's condition.

82. **The correct answer is 3.** Foods that contain insoluble fiber and oxalic or phytic acid can suppress the absorption of calcium. Spinach contains oxalate, which inhibits the absorption of calcium. Eggs (choice 1), yogurt (choice 2), and almonds (choice 4) are all excellent sources of calcium that do not interfere with the absorption of prescribed oral calcium.

83. **The correct answer is 3.** Oral contraceptives can precipitate episodes of Raynaud's disease, which is characterized by painful arteriole and arterial spasms in the client's extremities. Oral contraceptives are not contraindicated with asthma (choice 1). Oral contraceptives can be used to treat dysmenorrhea (choice 2) and polycystic ovary syndrome (choice 4).

84. **The correct answers are 1, 2, 3, 4, and 6.** When assessing the older adult, the nurse will minimize distractions, allow for additional time, speak clearly to the client, provide for periods of rest, and avoid sudden changes in the client's positioning. A focused assessment (choice 5) is limited to a specific body system, current condition, or concern of the client and is not used for a routine assessment.

85. **The correct answers are 2, 3, 4, 5, and 6.** The goal when preventing contractures for a client with burns is to maintain neutral body alignment with minimal extension. A client with burns on his head, neck, and upper chest should not sleep on a pillow, but can use a neck splint or a towel rolled up and placed under the neck to prevent hyperextension. Turning the client's head side to side prevents a flexion contracture of the posterior neck. A folded towel under the client's spine placed between the scapula will help prevent shoulder retraction of the chest and upper chest area. The use of a pillow (choice 1) increases the client's risk of contractures resulting from the flexion of the neck.

86. **The correct answer is shown below.** The peak systolic pressure reflects the maximum left ventricular pressure or the systolic pressure on an arterial waveform. The diastolic value on the waveform reflects the amount of vasoconstriction in the arterial system.

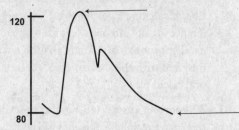

87. **The correct answer is 2.** The nurse should immediately notify the health care provider if the chest tube stopped draining. The drainage in the chest tube inserted two hours prior should not stop. Absent drainage may indicate displacement or clogging of the tube. The client's oxygen saturation (choice 1) will improve as the fluid from the pleural space drains. Erythema (choice 3) is present due to the trauma to the tissue during placement of the chest tube. A fluctuation in the water seal chamber (choice 4) is an expected finding.

88. **The correct answer is 2.** Further teaching is required if the client indicates that she will take the prescription on an empty stomach. The most common reaction to nitrofurantoin is gastrointestinal. The prescription should be taken with food or milk. The client's urine may turn brown (choice 1) and the prescription achieves antibacterial concentration in the urine (choice 3). The client should immediately notify the health care provider if she is experiencing symptoms of a UTI (choice 4).

89. **The correct answer is 1.** The mitral valve is auscultated in the fifth intercostal space (ICS), left mid-clavicular line. The tricuspid valve area is auscultated in the fourth left ICS, left sternal border (choice 2). The pulmonic valve is auscultated in the second left ICS, left sternal border (choice 3), and the aortic valve is auscultated in the second right ICS, right sternal border (choice 4).

90. **The correct answer is 3.** Constipation remains a chronic problem for a client with a tolerance to morphine. Epiphora, or excess tearing (choice 1), bradycardia (choice 2), or overnutrition (choice 4) are not specific findings associated with tolerance to morphine.

91. **The correct answer is 3.** The initial intervention for a client with carbon monoxide poisoning is to administer 100% oxygen via a non-rebreather mask. There is no indication that rescue breathing is indicated (choice 1), and preparing a client for hyperbaric oxygen therapy (choice 2) delays delivery of the oxygen. There is no indication the client requires noninvasive continuous positive airway pressure (choice 4).

92. **The correct answers are 1, 2, 3, 4, and 5.** A pressure garment is used as part of a burn rehabilitation to reduce edema and scarring, as well as to promote blood flow. For best results, the pressure garment should be worn 23 hours per day and may be worn for 12–24 months. The compression garment is applied after a skin graft procedure, but not until it has healed (choice 6).

93. **The correct answer is 3.** Reorganization of the collagen fibers occurs in the fourth stage of wound healing. During the first stage of wound healing a thrombus forms (choice 1). Edema (choice 2) is characteristic of the second stage of wound healing. During the third stage of healing, the margins of the wound begin to pull together (choice 4).

94. **The correct answer is 3.** Of the choices provided, massage is the only procedure that is not contraindicated for a client with rheumatoid arthritis. The client with dermatitis (choice 1) is at risk for skin impairment, and massaging a client with osteoporosis (choice 2) places the client at risk for a fracture. Massaging a client with congestive heart failure (choice 4) may increase the fluid load to the heart, further compromising the client by increasing the workload of the heart.

95. **The correct answer is 0300.** Add 8 hours to the initial time of 1900. The infusion will be completed at 0300 hours.

$$\frac{600 \text{ mL}}{75 \text{ mL/hr.}} = 8 \text{ hrs.}$$

96. **The correct answer is 4.** Further education is required if the client indicates that she will only apply a minimal amount of the lemongrass oil directly to the skin. The client should be instructed not to directly apply the lemongrass oil or any other oils to her skin without consulting the health care provider. The oil should be discontinued if the client suspects she is pregnant (choice 1). The client will be instructed to avoid applying the oil directly to the mucous membranes (choice 2) and to ensure the room is well-ventilated (choice 3) when using the oil.

97. **The correct answer is 2.** A poison ivy skin rash is an example of a delayed hypersensitivity reaction, also referred to as cell-mediated immunity. T cells, rather than antibodies, mediate the response. A cytotoxic reaction (choice 1) or type II reaction occurs when immunoglobulin G or immunoglobulin M antibodies bind to cell surface antigens, with subsequent complement fixation. A type III reaction or an immune complex reaction (choice 3) involves circulating antibody-antigen complexes. Immediate hypersensitivity (choice 4) or type I responses are associated with an immunoglobulin E mediated release of histamine and other mediators. The other mediators are released from mast cells and basophils.

98. **The correct answer is 1.** When an error has been made, factual information is documented in the client's records. For a missed dosage of medication, the nurse will document the omission, the notification of the provider, and the response. Failure to document the health care provider's response (choice 2) does not reflect accurate communication. The nurse should never document in a client's record that an occurrence report has been filed (choice 3), nor should the documentation reflect blame (choice 4) such as in the statement about an "oversight by the pharmacy."

99. **The correct answer is 2.** Liver function is assessed before the administration of valproic acid due to the risk of hepatoxicity. The client's lipid levels (choice 1), renal function (choice 3), or platelet count (choice 4) are not routinely evaluated before the administration of valproic acid.

100. **The correct answer is 3.** Clients with major depression can be preoccupied with death. Asking the client what he is thinking about when he is feeling depressed helps set the stage for the nurse to assess the risk of suicide. Exploring the client's feelings about his illness (choice 1), what he does when he is feeling depressed (choice 2), and how the depression has affected his friendships (choice 4) are essential to assess, but the client's safety is a priority.

PART V
APPENDICES

APPENDIX A   State Boards of Nursing
APPENDIX B   Nursing Organizations
APPENDIX C   Websites of Interest

State Boards of Nursing

Alabama*
Alabama Board of Nursing
RSA Plaza
770 Washington Avenue, Suite 250
Montgomery, AL 36104
Phone: 334-242-4060
Fax: 334-242-4360
Website: www.abn.state.al.us

Alaska
Alaska Board of Nursing
550 West 7th Avenue, Suite 1500
Anchorage, AK 99501-3567
Phone: 907-269-8160
Fax: 907-269-8195
Website: www.commerce.alaska.gov/web/cbpl/ProfessionalLicensing/BoardofNursing.aspx

Arizona*
Arizona State Board of Nursing
1740 W Adams Street, Suite 2000
Phoenix, AZ 85007
Phone: 602-771-7800
Website: www.azbn.gov

Arkansas*
Arkansas State Board of Nursing
University Tower Building
1123 South University Avenue, Suite 800
Little Rock, AR 72204-1619
Phone: 501-686-2700
Fax: 501-686-2714
Website: www.arsbn.org

California
California State Board of Registered Nursing
1747 N. Market Blvd., Suite 150
Sacramento, CA 95834-1924
Phone: 916-322-3350
Fax: 916-574-7699
Website: www.rn.ca.gov

*State participates in the Enhanced Nurse Licensure Compact (eNLC)

357

Colorado*

Colorado Board of Nursing
1560 Broadway, Suite 1350
Denver, CO 80202
Phone: 303-894-2430
Fax: 303-894-2821
Website: www.dora.state.co.us/nursing

Connecticut

Connecticut Board of Examiners for Nursing
Department of Public Health
410 Capitol Avenue, MS#13PHO
Hartford, CT 06134-0328
Phone: 860-509-7603
Fax: 860-509-8457
Website: https://portal.ct.gov/DPH/Public-Health-Hearing-Office/Board-of-Examiners-for-Nursing/
Board-of-Examiners-for-Nursing

Delaware*

Delaware Board of Nursing
Cannon Building
861 Silver Lake Blvd., Suite 203
Dover, DE 19904
Phone: 302-739-4500
Fax: 302-739-2711
Website: http://dpr.delaware.gov/boards/nursing

District of Columbia

District of Columbia Board of Nursing
Department of Health
Health Professional Licensing Administration
899 North Capitol Street, NE
Washington, DC 20002
Phone: 202-442-5955
Fax: 202-442-4795
Website: https://dchealth.dc.gov/bon

Florida*

Florida Board of Nursing
4052 Bald Cypress Way, Bin C-02
Tallahassee, FL 32399-3252
Phone: 850-245-4125
Website: www.doh.state.fl.us/mqa/nursing

*State participates in the Enhanced Nurse Licensure Compact (eNLC)

Georgia*

Georgia Board of Nursing
237 Coliseum Drive
Macon, GA 31217-3858
Phone: 844-753-7825
Fax: 877-371-5712
Website: http://sos.georgia.gov/plb/rn

Hawaii

Hawaii Board of Nursing
Professional and Vocational Licensing Division
Attn: Board of Nursing
P.O. Box 3469
Honolulu, HI 96801
Phone: 808-586-3000
Fax: 808-586-2689
Website: http://hawaii.gov/dcca/areas/pvi/boards/nursing

Idaho*

Idaho Board of Nursing
280 North 8th Street, Suite 210
Boise, ID 83720-0061
Phone: 208-334-3110
Fax: 208-334-3262
Website: http://cca.hawaii.gov/pvl/boards/nursing

Illinois

Illinois Board of Nursing
James R. Thompson Center
100 West Randolph, Suite 9-300
Chicago, IL 60601
Phone: 312-814-2715
Fax: 312-814-3145
Website: www.idfpr.com/profs/Nursing.asp

Indiana

Indiana Professional Licensing Agency
Attn: Indiana State Board of Nursing
402 West Washington Street, Room W072
Indianapolis, IN 46204
Phone: 317-234-2043
Fax: 317-233-4236
Website: www.in.gov/pla/nursing.htm

*State participates in the Enhanced Nurse Licensure Compact (eNLC)

Iowa*

Iowa Board of Nursing
400 S.W. 8th Street, Suite B
Des Moines, IA 50309-4685
Phone: 515-281-3255
Fax: 515-281-4825
Website: https://nursing.iowa.gov

Kansas*

Kansas State Board of Nursing
Landon State Office Building
900 SW Jackson Street, Suite 1051
Topeka, KS 66612-1230
Phone: 785-296-4929
Fax: 785-296-3929
Website: www.ksbn.org

Kentucky*

Kentucky Board of Nursing
312 Whittington Parkway, Suite 300
Louisville, KY 40222
Phone: 502-429-3300
Fax: 502-429-3311
Website: http://kbn.ky.gov

Louisiana*

Louisiana State Board of Nursing
17373 Perkins Road
Baton Rouge, LA 70810
Phone: 225-755-7500
Fax: 225-755-7584
Website: www.lsbn.state.la.us

Maine*

Maine State Board of Nursing
161 Capitol Street
158 State House Station
Augusta, ME 04333-0158
Phone: 207-287-1133
Fax: 207-287-1149
Website: www.maine.gov/boardofnursing

*State participates in the Enhanced Nurse Licensure Compact (eNLC)

Maryland*
Maryland Board of Nursing
4140 Patterson Avenue
Baltimore, MD 21215-2254
Phone: 410-585-1900
Fax: 410-358-3530
Website: www.mbon.org

Massachusetts
Massachusetts State Nursing Board
Commonwealth of Massachusetts
239 Causeway Street, Suite 500
Boston, MA 02114
Phone: 800-414-0168
Fax: 617-973-0984
Website: http://mass.gov/dph/boards/rn

Michigan
Office of Health Services
Michigan Department of Licensing and Regulatory Affairs
611 W. Ottawa
P.O. Box 30004
Lansing, MI 48909
Phone: 517-373-9102
Fax: 517-373-2179
Website: www.michigan.gov/lara

Minnesota
Minnesota Board of Nursing
2829 University Avenue SE, Suite 500
Minneapolis, MN 55414
Phone: 612-317-3000
Fax: 612-617-2190
Website: www.nursingboard.state.mn.us

Mississippi*
Mississippi Board of Nursing
713 Pear Orchard Road, Plaza II, Suite 300
Ridgeland, MS 39157
Phone: 601-957-6300
Fax: 601-957-6301
Website: www.msbn.state.ms.us

*State participates in the Enhanced Nurse Licensure Compact (eNLC)

Missouri*

Missouri State Board of Nursing
3605 Missouri Boulevard
P.O. Box 656
Jefferson City, MO 65102-0656
Phone: 573-751-0681
Fax: 573-751-0075
Website: http://pr.mo.gov/nursing.asp

Montana*

Montana State Board of Nursing
P.O. Box 200513
Helena, MT 59620-0513
Phone: 406-444-6880
Website: http://boards.bsd.dli.mt.gov/nur

Nebraska*

Office of Nursing and Nursing Support
DHHS, Division of Public Health
Licensure Unit 301
Centennial Mall South
Lincoln, NE 68509-4986
Phone: 402-471-4376
Fax: 402-742-2360
Website: http://dhhs.ne.gov/licensure/Pages/Nurse-Licensing.aspx

Nevada

Nevada State Board of Nursing
License Certification and Education
4220 S. Maryland Pkwy., Building B, Suite 300
Las Vegas, NV 89119-7533
Phone: 702-486-5803
Website: https://nevadanursingboard.org

New Hampshire*

New Hampshire Board of Nursing
121 South Fruit Street, Suite 102
Concord, NH 03301
Phone: 603-271-2323
Fax: 603-271-6605
Website: www.oplc.nh.gov/nursing

*State participates in the Enhanced Nurse Licensure Compact (eNLC)

New Jersey

New Jersey Board of Nursing
124 Halsey Street, 6th Floor
Newark, NJ 07102
Phone: 973-504-6430
Website: www.njconsumeraffairs.gov/nur/Pages/default.aspx

New Mexico*

New Mexico Board of Nursing
6301 Indian School Road NE, Suite 710
Albuquerque, NM 87110
Phone: 505-841-8340
Fax: 505-841-8347
Website: http://nmbon.sks.com

New York

New York State Board of Nursing
Education Building
89 Washington Avenue
2nd Floor West Wing
Albany, NY 12234
Phone: 518-474-3817, Ext. 120
Fax: 518-474-3706
Website: https://www.ncsbn.org/New%20York.htm

North Carolina*

North Carolina Board of Nursing
3724 National Drive, Suite 201
Raleigh, NC 27612
Phone: 919-782-3211
Fax: 919-781-9461
Website: www.ncbon.com

North Dakota*

North Dakota Board of Nursing
919 South 7th Street, Suite 504
Bismarck, ND 58504
Phone: 701-328-9777
Fax: 701-328-9785
Website: www.ndbon.org

*State participates in the Enhanced Nurse Licensure Compact (eNLC)

Ohio

Ohio Board of Nursing
17 South High Street, Suite 660
Columbus, OH 43215-3466
Phone: 614-466-3947
Fax: 614-466-0388
Website: www.nursing.ohio.gov

Oklahoma*

Oklahoma Board of Nursing
2915 North Classen Boulevard, Suite 524
Oklahoma City, OK 73106
Phone: 405-962-1800
Fax: 405-962-1821
Website: www.ok.gov

Oregon

Oregon State Board of Nursing
17938 SW Upper Boones Ferry Rd.
Portland, OR 97224
Phone: 971-673-0685
Website: www.osbn.state.or.us

Pennsylvania

Pennsylvania State Board of Nursing
Penn Center, 2601 N 3rd Street
Harrisburg, PA 17110
Phone: 717-787-8503
Fax: 717-783-0510
Website: www.dos.state.pa.us/bpoa/site/default.asp

Rhode Island

Rhode Island Board of Nurse Registration and Nursing Education
105 Cannon Building, Three Capitol Hill
Providence, RI 02908
Phone: 401-222-5700
Fax: 401-222-3352
Website: www.health.ri.gov/licenses/detail.php?id=231

South Carolina*

South Carolina State Board of Nursing
Synergy Business Park
Kingstree Building
110 Centerview Drive
Columbia, SC 29210
Phone: 803-896-4300
Website: www.llr.state.sc.us/pol/nursing

*State participates in the Enhanced Nurse Licensure Compact (eNLC)

South Dakota*

South Dakota Board of Nursing
4305 South Louise Avenue, Suite 201
Sioux Falls, SD 57106-3305
Phone: 605-362-2760
Fax: 605-362-2768
Website: http://doh.sd.gov/boards/nursing

Tennessee*

Tennessee Board of Nursing
665 Mainstream Drive, 2nd Floor
Nashville, TN 37243
Phone: 1-800-778-4123
Website: www.tn.gov/health/health-program-areas/health-professional-boards/nursing-board/nursing-board/about.html

Texas*

Texas Board of Nurse Examiners
333 Guadalupe, Suite 3-460
Austin, TX 78701-3944
Phone: 512-305-7400
Fax: 512-305-7401
Website: www.bne.state.tx.us

Utah*

Utah State Board of Nursing
Heber M. Wells Building, 4th Floor
160 East 300 South
Salt Lake City, UT 84111
Phone: 801-530-6628
Fax: 801-530-6511
Website: https://dopl.utah.gov/nurse/index.html

Vermont

Office of Professional Regulation
Board of Nursing
89 Main Street, Floor 3
Montpelier, VT 05620-3402
Phone: 802-828-2396
Fax: 802-828-2484
Website: www.sec.state.vt.us/professional-regulation/list-of-professions/nursing.aspx

*State participates in the Enhanced Nurse Licensure Compact (eNLC)

Virginia*

Virginia Board of Nursing
Dept of Health Professions
Perimeter Center
9960 Mayland Drive, Suite 300
Richmond, VA 23233-1463
Phone: 804-367-4515
Fax: 804-527-4455
Website: www.dhp.virginia.gov/Boards/Nursing/

Washington

Washington State Nursing Care Quality Assurance Commission
111 Israel Rd SE
Tumwater, WA 98501
Phone: 360-236-4703
Fax: 360-236-4738
Website: www.doh.wa.gov/LicensesPermitsandCertificates/NursingCommission

West Virginia*

West Virginia Board of Examiners for Registered Professional Nurses
90 MacCorkle Ave. SW, Suite 203
South Charleston, WV 25303
Phone: 304-744-0900
Fax: 304-744-0600
Website: www.wvrnboard.com

Wisconsin*

Wisconsin Department of Regulation and Licensing
4822 Madison Yards Way
Madison, WI 53705
Phone: 608-266-2112
Fax: 608-266-2264
Website: https://dsps.wi.gov/Pages/Professions/RN/Default.aspx

Wyoming*

Wyoming State Board of Nursing
130 Hobbs Ave, Ste B
Cheyenne, WY 82002
Phone: 307-777-7601
Fax: 307-777-3519
Website: http://nursing.state.wy.us

*State participates in the Enhanced Nurse Licensure Compact (eNLC)

Nursing Organizations

The following organizations have been formed to help promote continuing education, publish registered nursing journals, and to establish nursing standards. In addition, these organizations provide a means for RNs to communicate with each other.

American Nurses Association

1. One of the largest national associations, with connections at the state level as well.

2. Publishes *American Nurse Today*, a monthly, peer-reviewed professional publication.

3. Publishes the *Online Journal of Issues in Nursing*, as well as provides webinars and other online benefits to members.

4. Publishes *The Code of Ethics for Nurses with Interpretive Statements*, also referred to as "The Code."

5. Subsidiaries include the American Academy of Nursing, American Nurses Foundation, and the American Nurses Credentialing Center.

> American Nurses Association
> 8515 Georgia Avenue, Suite 400
> Silver Spring, MD 20910-3492
> *Phone:* 1-800-284-2378
> *Website:* www.nursingworld.org/ana

Hospice and Palliative Nurses Association

1. Publishes the bi-monthly *Journal of Hospice and Palliative Nursing* and the monthly *Journal of Palliative Medicine*, available online and in print.

2. Provides specialized types of membership levels, including one specifically for RNs.

3. Offers online e-learning courses that qualify for continuing nursing educational credits (CNEs).

> Hospice and Palliative Nurses Association
> One Penn Center West, Suite 425
> Pittsburgh, PA 15276
> *Phone:* 412-787-9301
> *Email:* hpna@hpna.org
> *Website:* https://advancingexpertcare.org

National League for Nursing (NLN)

1. Publishes a variety of journals, newsletters, and books (see www.nln.org/ publications).

2. Publishes professional directories.

3. Prepares and scores selection and achievement tests.

4. Accredits schools of practical and registered nursing.

5. Provides continuing education.

> NLN
> 61 Broadway, 33rd Floor
> New York, NY 10006
> *Phone:* 212-363-5555
> *Fax:* 212-812-0393
> *Email:* generalinfonln.org
> *Website:* www.nln.org

Emergency Nurses Association (ENA)

1. Provides a wide variety of emergency nursing education options that qualify for continuing education credit.

2. Supports regulatory and legislative interests in federal and state government related to emergency nursing.

3. Maintains a large collection of online resources, including practice guidelines and toolkits.

4. Provides a networking platform for over 42,000 emergency nursing professionals.

> Emergency Nurses Association
> 930 E. Woodfield Road
> Schaumburg, Illinois 60173
> *Phone:* 800-900-9659 ext. 4000
> *Email:* contact@ena.org
> *Website:* www.ena.org

American Association of Critical-Care Nurses (AACN)

1. World's largest specialty nursing organization, with 100,000 members internationally.

2. Offers critical care certification resources and continuing education opportunities.

3. Provides an online library of clinical resources.

4. Publishes *Critical Care Nurse, American Journal of Critical Care*, and *AACN Advanced Critical Care*, as well as *AACN Bold Voices*, a monthly membership publication.

> American Association of Critical-Care Nurses
> 101 Columbia
> Aliso Viejo, CA 92656-4109
> *Phone:* 800-809-2273
> *Website:* www.aacn.org

Websites of Interest

Nursing Community Websites

www.nln.org
This is the website for the National League for Nursing and includes site information on testing and nursing education for PNs, VNs, and RNs.

www.allnurses.com
This is an online network of nurses. It features health care and nursing news, a career center, clinical references, and continuing education.

www.clinicaltrials.gov
A US listing by the National Library of Medicine that lists all ongoing clinical trials in the US involving treatments for serious illnesses.

www.ec-online.net
An information database on rehabilitation providers, retirement communities, and long-term nursing care facilities. Useful for clients as well as hospitals and health care providers.

www.afscme.org
The website of the United Nurses of America, which is part of AFSCME, a union of health care employees. The United Nurses of America includes 76,000 RNs and PNs. The site includes clinical news, legal issues, and union activities. There is also a Spanish version.

www.nurse.com
This website offers online training and continuing education. It provides career information, study aids, and a national job search tool.

www.ama-assn.org
This is a website for physicians and clients. It lists almost every MD in the United States and also contains journal information, women's health, and other features.

RN Job Posting Websites

www.hospitaljobsonline.com
www.healthdirection.com
www.nursingjobs.com
www.hospitalsoup.com
www.onwardhealthcare.com
www.degreehunter.com/nursing_jobs.html
www.nurse.com/jobs
www.jobs.ana.org
www.jobs.registerednursing.org

> **TIP**
> Registered nurse positions are also consistently posted on more general employment sites, such as Indeed or Monster. com, as well as on websites for state and local health care facilities.